Emergency Medicine

Editors

JUSTINE A. LEE
LISA L. POWELL

VETERINARY CLINICS OF NORTH AMERICA: SMALL ANIMAL PRACTICE

www.vetsmall.theclinics.com

July 2013 • Volume 43 • Number 4

ELSEVIER

1600 John F. Kennedy Boulevard • Suite 1800 • Philadelphia, Pennsylvania, 19103-2899
http://www.vetsmall.theclinics.com

**VETERINARY CLINICS OF NORTH AMERICA: SMALL ANIMAL PRACTICE Volume 43, Number 4
July 2013 ISSN 0195-5616, ISBN-13: 978-0-323-18592-9**

Editor: John Vassallo; j.vassallo@elsevier.com
Developmental Editor: Teia Stone

Photocopying

Single photocopies of single articles may be made for personal use as allowed by national copyright laws. Permission of the Publisher and payment of a fee is required for all other photocopying, including multiple or systematic copying, copying for advertising or promotional purposes, resale, and all forms of document delivery. Special rates are available for educational institutions that wish to make photocopies for non-profit educational classroom use. For information on how to seek permission visit www.elsevier.com/permissions or call: (+44) 1865 843830 (UK)/(+1) 215 239 3804 (USA).

Derivative Works

Subscribers may reproduce tables of contents or prepare lists of articles including abstracts for internal circulation within their institutions. Permission of the Publisher is required for resale or distribution outside the institution. Permission of the Publisher is required for all other derivative works, including compilations and translations (please consult www.elsevier.com/permissions).

Electronic Storage or Usage

Permission of the Publisher is required to store or use electronically any material contained in this periodical, including any article or part of an article (please consult www.elsevier.com/permissions). Except as outlined above, no part of this publication may be reproduced, stored in a retrieval system or transmitted in any form or by any means, electronic, mechanical, photocopying, recording or otherwise, without prior written permission of the Publisher.

Notice

No responsibility is assumed by the Publisher for any injury and/or damage to persons or property as a matter of products liability, negligence or otherwise, or from any use or operation of any methods, products, instructions or ideas contained in the material herein. Because of rapid advances in the medical sciences, in particular, independent verification of diagnoses and drug dosages should be made.

Although all advertising material is expected to conform to ethical (medical) standards, inclusion in this publication does not constitute a guarantee or endorsement of the quality or value of such product or of the claims made of it by its manufacturer.

Veterinary Clinics of North America: Small Animal Practice (ISSN 0195-5616) is published bimonthly by Elsevier Inc., 360 Park Avenue South, New York, NY 10010-1710. Months of issue are January, March, May, July, September, and November. Business and Editorial Offices: 1600 John F. Kennedy Blvd., Ste. 1800, Philadelphia, PA 19103-2899. Customer Service Office: 3251 Riverport Lane, Maryland Heights, MO 63043. Periodicals postage paid at New York, NY and additional mailing offices. Subscription prices are $294.00 per year (domestic individuals), $473.00 per year (domestic institutions), $143.00 per year (domestic students/residents), $390.00 per year (Canadian individuals), $580.00 per year (Canadian institutions), $433.00 per year (international individuals), $580.00 per year (international institutions), and $208.00 per year (international and Canadian students/residents). To receive student/resident rate, orders must be accompained by name of affiliated institution, date of term, and the *signature* of program/residency coordinator on institution letterhead. Orders will be billed at individual rate until proof of status is received. Foreign air speed delivery is included in all *Clinics* subscription prices. All prices are subject to change without notice. **POSTMASTER:** Send address changes to *Veterinary Clinics of North America: Small Animal Practice*, Elsevier Health Sciences Division, Subscription Customer Service, 3251 Riverport Lane, Maryland Heights, MO 63043. Customer Service (orders, claims, online, change of address): Elsevier Periodicals Customer Service, Elsevier Health Sciences Division Subscription Customer Service 3251 Riverport Lane Maryland Heights, MO 63043. Tel: 1-800-654-2452 (U.S. and Canada); 314-447-8871 (outside U.S. and Canada). Fax: 314-447-8029. E-mail: journalscustomerservice-usa@elsevier.com (for print support); journalsonlinesupport-usa@elsevier.com (for online support).

Reprints. For copies of 100 or more of articles in this publication, please contact the Commercial Reprints Department, Elsevier Inc., 360 Park Avenue South, New York, NY 10010-1710. Tel.: 212-633-3812; Fax: 212-462-1935; E-mail: reprints@elsevier.com.

Veterinary Clinics of North America: Small Animal Practice is also published in Japanese by Inter Zoo Publishing Co., Ltd., Aoyama Crystal-Bldg 5F, 3-5-12 Kitaaoyama, Minato-ku, Tokyo 107-0061, Japan.

Veterinary Clinics of North America: Small Animal Practice is covered in *Current Contents/Agriculture, Biology and Environmental Sciences, Science Citation Index, ASCA, MEDLINE/PubMed (Index Medicus), Excerpta Medica,* and *BIOSIS.*

Printed and bound by CPI Group (UK) Ltd, Croydon, CR0 4YY

Contributors

EDITORS

JUSTINE A. LEE, DVM
Diplomate, American College of Veterinary Emergency and Critical Care; Diplomate, American Board of Toxicology; Associate Director of Veterinary Services, Pet Poison Helpline, a Division of SafetyCall International, Bloomington, Minnesota

LISA L. POWELL, DVM
Diplomate, American College of Veterinary Emergency and Critical Care; Full Clinical Professor, Small Animal Emergency and Critical Care, Veterinary Medical Center, University of Minnesota, St Paul, Minnesota

AUTHORS

ANUSHA BALAKRISHNAN, BVSc
Resident, Section of Emergency and Critical Care, Department of Clinical Studies-PHL, University of Pennsylvania School of Veterinary Medicine, Philadelphia, Pennsylvania

MANUEL BOLLER, Dr med vet, MTR
Diplomate, American College of Veterinary Emergency and Critical Care; Senior Lecturer Emergency and Critical Care, Faculty of Veterinary Science, The University of Melbourne, Werribee, Victoria, Australia

SØREN R. BOYSEN, DVM
Diplomate, American College of Veterinary Emergency and Critical Care; Associate Professor, Department of Veterinary Clinical and Diagnostic Sciences, Faculty of Veterinary Medicine, University of Calgary, Calgary, Alberta, Canada

BETH DAVIDOW, DVM
Diplomate, American College of Veterinary Emergency and Critical Care; Medical Director, Animal Critical Care and Emergency Services, Seattle, Washington; Adjunct Assistant Professor, Department of Clinical Sciences, College of Veterinary Medicine, Washington State University, Pullman, Washington

TERESA C. DEFRANCESCO, DVM
Diplomate, American College of Veterinary Internal Medicine (Cardiology); Diplomate, American College of Veterinary Emergency and Critical Care; Professor in Cardiology and Critical Care, Department of Clinical Sciences, College of Veterinary Medicine, North Carolina State University, Raleigh, North Carolina

JENNIFER J. DEVEY, DVM
Diplomate, American College of Veterinary Emergency and Critical Care; Saanichton, British Columbia, Canada

JILLIAN DIFAZIO, DVM
Resident, Section of Emergency and Critical Care, Cornell University Hospital for Animals, Ithaca, New York

KENNETH J. DROBATZ, DVM, MSCE
Diplomate, American College of Veterinary Internal Medicine; Diplomate, American College of Veterinary Emergency and Critical Care; Professor, Chief, Section of Emergency and Critical Care, Director of the Emergency Service, Department of Clinical Studies-PHL, University of Pennsylvania School of Veterinary Medicine, Philadelphia, Pennsylvania

DANIEL J. FLETCHER, PhD, DVM
Diplomate, American College of Veterinary Emergency and Critical Care; Assistant Professor of Emergency and Critical Care, Department of Clinical Sciences, College of Veterinary Medicine, Cornell University, Ithaca, New York

KATE HOPPER, BVSc, PhD
Diplomate, American College of Veterinary Emergency and Critical Care; Assistant Professor, Department of Veterinary Surgical and Radiological Sciences, University of California, Davis, California

AMIE KOENIG, DVM
Diplomate, American College of Veterinary Internal Medicine (Small Animal Internal Medicine); Diplomate, American College of Veterinary Emergency and Critical Care; Associate Professor, Department of Small Animal Medicine and Surgery, College of Veterinary Medicine, University of Georgia, Athens, Georgia

JUSTINE A. LEE, DVM
Diplomate, American College of Veterinary Emergency and Critical Care; Diplomate, American Board of Toxicology; Associate Director of Veterinary Services, Pet Poison Helpline, a division of SafetyCall International, Bloomington, Minnesota

GREGORY R. LISCIANDRO, DVM
Diplomate, American College of Veterinary Emergency and Critical Care; Hill Country Veterinary Specialists, Emergency Pet Center, Inc, San Antonio, Texas

ELISA MAZZAFERRO, DVM, MS, PhD
Diplomate, American College of Veterinary Emergency and Critical Care; Cornell University Veterinary Specialists, Stamford, Connecticut

GARRET PACHTINGER, VMD
Diplomate, American College of Veterinary Emergency and Critical Care; Veterinary Specialty and Emergency Center, Department of Emergency and Critical Care, Levittown, Pennsylvania

LISA L. POWELL, DVM
Diplomate, American College of Veterinary Emergency and Critical Care; Full Clinical Professor, Small Animal Emergency and Critical Care, Veterinary Medical Center, University of Minnesota, St Paul, Minnesota

JANE QUANDT, DVM, MS
Diplomate, American College of Veterinary Anesthesia and Analgesia; Diplomate, American College of Veterinary Emergency and Critical Care; Associate Professor in Comparative Anesthesia, Department of Small Animal Medicine and Surgery, College of Veterinary Medicine, University of Georgia, Athens, Georgia

ELIZABETH ROZANSKI, DVM
Diplomate, American College of Veterinary Emergency and Critical Care; Diplomate, American College of Veterinary Internal Medicine (Small Animal Internal Medicine); Associate Professor, Department of Clinical Sciences, Tufts University Cummings School of Veterinary Medicine, North Grafton, Massachusetts

CATHERINE SUMNER, DVM
Diplomate, American College of Veterinary Emergency and Critical Care; Emergency Clinician and Intensivist, Emergency and Critical Care Section, Tufts VETS, Walpole, Massachusetts

Contents

care of the poisoned patient includes the use of fluid therapy, gastrointestinal support (eg, antacids), central nervous system support (eg, muscle relaxants, anticonvulsants), sedatives/reversal agents (eg, phenothiazines, naloxone, flumazenil), hepatoprotectants, and miscellaneous antidotal therapy.

Internal injuries are common and often life-threatening conditions that can be challenging to detect based on physical examination, radiographs, and centesis. Recently, ultrasound has been introduced and evaluated in human and veterinary emergency medicine as a point-of-care test for a variety of emergent conditions. This article discusses the indications for point-of-care emergency ultrasound of dogs and cats in the emergency and critical care setting. Techniques for performing focused emergency evaluations are described and the current veterinary and human literature is contrasted, with emphasis on abdominal, pleural, pericardial, and pulmonary evaluation.

Management of respiratory distress involves careful consideration of the history, physical examination, and diagnostic testing. Supplemental oxygen is useful. Urgent procedures, such as intubation, thoracocentesis, or tracheostomy, may be required. The prognosis is dependent on the underlying disease, but is often favorable. This article reviews the approach, differential diagnoses, and the approach to management for dogs and cats with respiratory distress.

Cardiac emergencies are life-threatening conditions that must be diagnosed quickly to avoid delays in therapy. A timely and accurate diagnosis leads to early relief of symptoms and improved survival. This article provides both a comprehensive review and updated management recommendations for common cardiac emergencies in dogs and cats. Specifically, the article confers updates for the efficient clinical recognition of decompensated cardiac patients, including focused echocardiography, cardiac biomarkers, and electrocardiogram interpretation. This article also reviews the latest recommendations for the treatment of heart failure (including the use of pimobendan) and the management of arrhythmias, pericardial effusion, and aortic thromboembolism.

This article focuses on some of the most commonly seen urinary tract emergencies in dogs and cats, with emphasis on basic pathophysiology, diagnosis, and emergency management of these cases.

> Respiratory failure may occur due to hypoventilation or hypoxemia. Regardless of the cause, emergent anesthesia and intubation, accompanied by positive pressure ventilation, may be necessary and life saving. Long-term mechanical ventilation requires some specialized equipment and knowledge; however, short-term ventilation can be accomplished without the use of an intensive care unit ventilator, and can provide oxygen supplementation and carbon dioxide removal in critical patients.

> For dogs and cats that experience cardiopulmonary arrest, rates of survival to discharge are 6% to 7%, as compared with survival rates of 20% for people. The introduction of standardized cardiopulmonary resuscitation guidelines and training in human medicine has led to substantial improvements in outcome. The Reassessment Campaign on Veterinary Resuscitation initiative recently completed an exhaustive literature review and generated a set of evidence-based, consensus cardiopulmonary resuscitation guidelines in 5 domains: preparedness and prevention, basic life support, advanced life support, monitoring, and postcardiac arrest care. This article reviews some of the most important of these new guidelines.

VETERINARY CLINICS OF NORTH AMERICA: SMALL ANIMAL PRACTICE

THE CLINICS ARE NOW AVAILABLE ONLINE!
Access your subscription at:
www.theclinics.com

Preface

Emergency Medicine

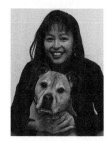 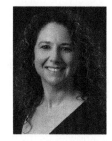

Justine A. Lee, DVM, DACVECC, DABT   Lisa L. Powell, DVM, DACVECC

Editors

It has been 8 years since *Veterinary Clinics of North America: Small Animal Practice* covered emergency medicine. It has been an honor to follow in the footsteps of Ken Drobatz, DVM, DACVIM, DACVECC, MSCE, in providing the most updated edition.

Our goals as editors were to provide unique viewpoints through different passions: Dr Lee's for emergency medicine and toxicology, and Dr Powell's for the critically ill patient.

The aim of this volume is to provide practical, cutting-edge updates in small animal emergency medicine. This volume is designed to be a thorough—but practical—approach for veterinary emergency practitioners. This edition is a general review of new, clinically relevant "hot topics" of emergency and critical care.

Topics include a global and organ-based approach to the emergent patient, including monitoring of the emergent patient and management of respiratory, cardiac, urinary tract, endocrine, and neurologic emergencies. As emergency clinicians are commonly presented with poisoning cases, one article is dedicated to emergency management and treatment of the poisoned patient. Key diagnostic updates in emergency medicine, including the use of the FAST and TFAST ultrasound, are reviewed. Images and photographs were included to help the practitioner feel comfortable with this rapid, inexpensive, diagnostic tool.

Included in this latest version are focuses on treatment, including fluid therapy, transfusion medicine, surgical considerations, and analgesia and anesthesia of the emergent patient. Although less commonly performed in the emergency room (as compared to the ICU), the approach to basics of mechanical ventilation was also discussed. Last, the RECOVER project was reviewed in the CPR article and reiterated the importance of a "team approach" to veterinary medicine.

We would like to thank John Vassallo and Elsevier for their support in this project. The editors are also exceedingly grateful to all their colleagues, friends, coworkers, and authors who contributed to make this a useful, state-of-the art publication. These

Vet Clin Small Anim 43 (2013) xiii–xiv
http://dx.doi.org/10.1016/j.cvsm.2013.03.015
0195-5616/13/$ – see front matter © 2013 Published by Elsevier Inc.

vetsmall.theclinics.com

experts— ranging from academia to busy private specialty clinics—do this every day to help save lives and improve the quality of care in veterinary medicine.

By knowing the updates in emergency and critical care and treating each patient as if they were our own pet, we provide a life-saving service to two-legged and four-legged alike. Thank you to everyone out there who "treats and streets" and saves lives.

ACKNOWLEDGMENTS

To all the unnamed colleagues (including front desk staff, veterinary technicians, intern mates, resident mates, veterinary students, nursing staff, clinicians, colleagues, faculty, and veterinary specialists) who taught me—and continue to teach me—how to be a jack of all trades in the exciting, challenging field of ER. — Justine Lee

Thanks to my many wonderful friends and colleagues that have made this edition possible. I'd also like to acknowledge my great friend Dr Justine Lee, who is the major force behind this issue, and whose friendship I couldn't live without. Finally, to Carter, Jalen, Claire, and Morgan, you are my life and my love. — Lisa Powell

Justine A. Lee, DVM, DACVECC, DABT
Pet Poison Helpline, a division of SafetyCall International
3600 American Boulevard West, Suite 725
Bloomington, MN 55431, USA

Lisa L. Powell, DVM, DACVECC
Small Animal Emergency and Critical Care
University of Minnesota Veterinary Medical Center
1365 Boyd Avenue
St. Paul, MN 55108, USA

E-mail addresses:
jlee@petpoisonhelpline.com (J.A. Lee)
powel029@umn.edu (L.L. Powell)

Monitoring of the Emergent Small Animal Patient

Garret Pachtinger, VMD

KEYWORDS

- Emergency • Monitoring • Triage • Diagnostics • Small animals

KEY POINTS

- Careful monitoring of the emergent patient is crucial in assessment and treatment of potentially life-threatening conditions.
- Monitoring equipment does not replace the clinical evaluation of the patient. Hands-on serial patient assessment can recognize patient changes before clinical deterioration.
- Major body systems assessed include the respiratory system (eg, airway, breathing), cardiovascular system (eg, circulation), and neurologic system (eg, dysfunction).
- Assessment of the cardiovascular system begins with hands-on patient assessment, followed by timely serial assessments, and is supplemented with diagnostics including electrocardiography and monitoring of blood pressure.
- Assessment of the respiratory system begins with observation of the patient from afar, followed by hands-on assessment. It can then be supplemented with diagnostics including radiographs, pulse oximetry, and arterial blood gases.

Monitoring of the emergent patient is a challenging aspect in both the emergency room and intensive care unit (ICU). When people think of "monitoring," the immediate reaction is monitoring with equipment. Monitoring equipment does not replace the clinical evaluation of the patient. Hands-on monitoring is an important aspect of patient evaluation and patient care, and allows one to better focus the diagnostics and treatment plan. While useful, there are limitations of monitoring systems that are important to be cognizant of, as invasive monitoring may have potential negative consequences in a critically ill patient.

The condition of an emergent patient can dramatically change on a minute-to-minute basis, not only making the initial assessment valuable, but emphasizing the importance of serial assessment as part of thorough patient management. Although diagnostics can be performed to supplement the physical examination, diagnostics do not replace a thorough examination. Moreover, with the increasing costs of veterinary medicine, clients may have significant limitations, preventing advanced diagnostics.

Disclosures: None.
Department of Emergency and Critical Care, 301 Veterans Highway, Levittown, PA 19056, USA
E-mail address: gpachtinger@vsecvet.com

Vet Clin Small Anim 43 (2013) 705–720
http://dx.doi.org/10.1016/j.cvsm.2013.03.014
0195-5616/13/$ – see front matter © 2013 Elsevier Inc. All rights reserved.

As a result, the use of physical examination findings to help fine-tune appropriate diagnostics will allow for overall better patient care.

In the patient that presents on emergency, the initial focus is on triage and the primary survey. Triage is the art of giving priority to patients and their problems on presentation to the hospital. Triage involves a concise history, including the patient signalment, primary complaint, and time of onset. The signalment (eg, age, breed, sex) helps provide a differential diagnosis list, as younger patients may have a different differential list (eg, trauma, poisoning) in comparison with older patients (eg, neoplasia, metabolic disease), and intact dogs (eg, pyometra, prostatic abscess) may have a differential list different to that of spayed or neutered patients. A triage examination to assess the major body systems is then completed. In veterinary medicine, emergent findings which warrant immediate care may include trauma, toxin exposure, urethral obstruction, seizures, bleeding, heat prostration, shock, wounds, anemia, or reproductive emergencies.[1]

Following the triage examination, a primary survey is performed. This survey is designed to rapidly identify abnormalities associated with life-threatening conditions. Major body systems assessed include the respiratory system (eg, airway, breathing), cardiovascular system (eg, circulation), and neurologic system (eg, dysfunction). Failure to recognize an abnormality in any of these systems can result in immediate life-threatening deterioration of the patient. There are several pneumonics used to aid in primary survey evaluation, including ABC-LOC (airway, breathing, circulation, level of consciousness) and ABCD (airway, breathing, circulation, drug use/exposure/dysfunction).

RESPIRATORY (AIRWAY AND BREATHING)

Assessment of the respiratory system begins with simple observation of the patient from afar, followed by hands-on assessment. Visual assessment of the respiratory system includes making sure the patient has a patent airway and is ventilating adequately. Because the patient may be most comfortable with the owner, the respiratory visual examination is often performed while taking a triage history from the owner to obtain a sense of the respiratory status before handling, as stress, pain, or anxiety may alter the respiratory pattern and make the respiratory assessment difficult.

During the normal respiratory cycle, the primary work of breathing is through contraction and relaxation of the diaphragm. During inspiration, contraction of the diaphragm results in the chest wall and abdomen moving outward in a coordinated manner. During expiration the diaphragm relaxes, and the chest and abdominal walls move inward.[2] In patients with respiratory distress, clinical signs of increased work of breathing, tachypnea, cyanosis, orthopnea, open-mouth breathing, restlessness, or an inability to lie down may be seen. Other abnormalities may include short and shallow breathing with absent chest wall motion or flaring of the nares. With severe respiratory distress, paradoxic respiration may be seen (eg, when the chest wall and abdominal wall move in opposite directions). Paradoxic abdominal movement is seen in conditions preventing adequate lung inflation, including upper respiratory tract obstruction, diaphragmatic injury, decreased lung compliance, and pleural effusion.

Posture is another visual cue when assessing the respiratory system. A patient in respiratory distress may display orthopnea, most commonly seen as head and neck extension and abducted elbows. Elevation of the head and extension of the neck allows straightening the trachea while abduction of the elbows minimizes compression of the chest wall. Clinical signs of orthopnea are often associated with advanced, severe respiratory fatigue and potentially imminent respiratory arrest or failure.

Anatomic localization of the origin of the respiratory disease may be determined based on respiratory patterns. There are 5 breathing patterns commonly seen in patients that present for respiratory distress.

1. An increased respiratory rate (eg, tachypnea) does not always indicate pathologic pulmonary disease (eg, panting, healthy canine patient). When presented with a tachypneic patient, work of breathing, auscultation, and ancillary testing (eg, pulse oximetry) should be assessed; if normal, other causes of tachypnea such as "non-respiratory lookalikes" (eg, anemia, pain, anxiety, fever, metabolic acidosis) should be considered.
2. Pleural space disease is visually characterized by shallow, rapid respirations. Auscultation may reveal the presence of dull lung sounds and muffled heart sounds. Differentials for pleural space disease include pneumothorax, pleural effusion (eg, hemothorax, pyothorax, chylothorax), and diaphragmatic hernia.
3. Upper airway obstruction is characterized by inspiratory stridor or stertor. With upper airway obstruction the respiratory rate may be normal; however, respiratory effort may be dramatic owing to ventilation through a narrowed airway. Differentials include laryngeal paralysis, tracheal collapse, nasopharyngeal polyp, neoplasia, granulomatous disease, coagulopathy (resulting in bleeding into the upper airway), and brachycephalic airway syndrome.
4. Lower airway disease is typically characterized by tachypnea with a prolonged expiration and an expiratory push. Expiratory wheezing may also be found on auscultation. Common differentials include feline allergic airway disease, pulmonary fibrosis, and chronic bronchitis.
5. Pulmonary parenchymal disease is characterized by both labored inspiration and expiration. On auscultation, common findings may include harsh lung sounds, pulmonary crackles, and wheezes. Common differentials include infectious pneumonia (eg, bacterial, fungal, viral, protozoal, parasitic), aspiration pneumonia (eg, infectious and chemical pneumonitis), interstitial lung diseases, pulmonary edema (cardiogenic and noncardiogenic), coagulopathies (eg, long-acting anticoagulants), and neoplasia.

Following visual examination and hands-on examination (eg, auscultation), diagnostic tools may be used to supplement the examination of the respiratory system. In general, diagnostics such as thoracic radiographs are not considered a first line of defense when assessing the respiratory system, as this poses a stressful threat to a compromised patient. Once stabilized, however, advanced diagnostics can be performed. Such methods include pulse oximetry, arterial blood gas (ABG) or venous blood gas (VBG) analysis, thoracic radiography, and Thoracic Focused Assessment with Sonography for Trauma (TFAST). Please see the article "The Use of Ultrasound for Dogs and Cats in the Emergency Room (AFAST and TFAST)" elsewhere in this issue for more information.

Pulse oximetry (Spo_2) is a noninvasive, readily available diagnostic monitoring tool that can be used to evaluate oxygenation, and is often considered the first objective method for assessing severity of hypoxemia in a patient. Pulse oximetry works by spectrophotometry and measures 2 forms of hemoglobin that circulate in arterial blood: oxyhemoglobin (saturated hemoglobin) and deoxyhemoglobin (unsaturated hemoglobin).[3] A combination of light reflectance and absorption is used to measure the concentrations of oxyhemoglobin and hemoglobin present within red blood cells (RBC). The measurements are placed in a formula to calculate the percentage of saturation ($Sao_2 = [Hbo_2/Hbo_2 + Hb] \times 100$). Pulse oximetry allows clinicians to measure Spo_2 and therefore extrapolate the partial pressure of oxygen (Pao_2) based on the oxyhemoglobin dissociation curve (**Fig. 1**). Although pulse oximeters estimate

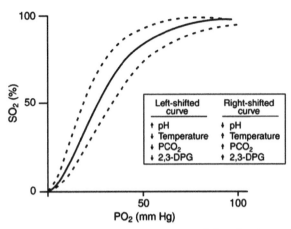

Fig. 1. Oxyhemoglobin dissociation curve. 2,3-DPG, 2,3-diphosphoglycerate. (*From* Odom-Forren J. Postanesthesia recovery. In: Nagelhout JJ and Plaus K, editors. Nurse Anesthesia, 4th edition. St Louis: Mosby;2010; with permission.)

hemoglobin saturation, they do not assess oxygen delivery or tissue perfusion. The pulse oximeter can be used for intermittent monitoring of oxygen saturation, or alternatively to provide a continuous real-time assessment, which is particularly useful for monitoring general anesthesia or sedation.

Common testing sites for using the pulse oximeter include the mucous membranes (eg, tongue, buccal membrane) or thin, nonpigmented skin found on the pinnae, back of the hock, prepuce, vaginal fold, or interdigital hairless areas of the paw. In healthy patients, the Spo_2 when breathing room air (fraction of inspired oxygen [Fio_2] 21%) is expected to be at least 96%. Spo_2 measurements of less than 93% to 94% require further evaluation, and typically require oxygen supplementation. An Spo_2 of 90% indicates severe hypoxemia, and is consistent with a Pao_2 of 60 mm Hg (normal 80–100 mm Hg, at sea level).

One must keep in mind, however, that the pulse oximeter cannot differentiate between oxyhemoglobin, carboxyhemoglobin (eg, from carbon monoxide toxicosis), methemoglobin (eg, from acetaminophen toxicosis), or cyanide toxicity. Of note, cyanide poisoning may result in a falsely elevated Spo_2 because it reduces the oxygen extraction from the arterial blood.[4,5] As a result, this tool has limited use for patients with carbon monoxide poisoning or methemoglobinemia. Severe anemia, hypotension, or vasoconstriction may also result in a falsely low Spo_2. Dark skin pigmentation will result in light interference and be difficult to interpret. On the pulse oximeter the signal strength, detected heart rate, and waveform oscillation should always be assessed (eg, matching) when evaluating the reading to ensure accurate results.

ABG analysis is the gold standard for direct assessment of pulmonary function (eg, oxygenation and ventilation) and provides information about the metabolic acid-base status of the body.[6] The most commonly evaluated parameters include pH, Pao_2, partial pressure of carbon dioxide ($Paco_2$), and bicarbonate (HCO_3). Normal Pao_2 is expected to be 80 to 100 mm Hg (Fio_2 21%).[7] Normal $Paco_2$ is 35 to 45 mm Hg. Advanced blood gas machines may also assess electrolytes, blood urea nitrogen (BUN), creatinine, and blood lactate concentrations.

Common locations for ABG sampling include the dorsal pedal artery, the auricular artery, or the femoral artery. Owing to physical restraint, an ABG analysis may not be possible because of the added stress of a patient already in respiratory distress (eg, feline patient). Rather, a VBG analysis may be a substitute when evaluating the pH, P_{CO_2}, electrolytes, and blood lactate. As $P_{venous}CO_2$ is typically within 5 mm Hg of $P_{arterial}CO_2$ when perfusion is adequate, ventilation—not oxygenation—can be adequately assessed on VBG analysis.[8] Increases in P_{CO_2} indicate compromised ventilatory function and may result in increasing acidosis, mental depression, and vasodilation. Decreases in P_{CO_2} may be seen in hyperventilating patients or may be related to poor gas exchange. Oxygenation cannot be adequately assessed on VBG analysis, and should only be assessed with ABG. However, the combined use of a VBG analysis and pulse oximetry reading can be used to provide information similar to that obtained with ABG, based on extrapolation from an oxygen hemoglobin dissociation curve (see **Fig. 1**).

When assessing an ABG with oxygen supplementation, the P_{aO_2} should be 5 times the inspired oxygen concentration with normal pulmonary function. For example, when breathing room air (F_{iO_2} 21%), the P_{aO_2} should be 100 mm Hg (21 × 5 = 105 mm Hg). Under anesthesia (F_{iO_2} 100%), the P_{aO_2} should be 500 mm Hg (100 × 5 = 500 mm Hg). Another way of assessing oxygenation is by calculating the alveolar-arterial (A-a) gradient $(P_{A}O_2 = [(P_B - P_{H2O}) \times F_{iO_2}] - P_{aCO_2} (1/RQ))$ (where RQ is respiratory quotient), or $P_{aO_2}{:}F_{iO_2}$ ratio. These formulations provide a more objective assessment of respiratory function. Patients with an A-a gradient greater than 10 to 15 mm Hg[9,10] or a $P_{aO_2}{:}F_{iO_2}$ ratio less than 300 mm Hg have respiratory compromise, and may require further intervention ranging from supplementation oxygen administration to mechanical ventilation. These latter 2 formulations should only be assessed based on an ABG analysis.

CARDIOVASCULAR SYSTEM (CIRCULATION)

Assessment of the cardiovascular system also begins with hands-on patient assessment, followed by timely serial assessments. Patient assessment should include heart rate and rhythm, pulse quality, mucous membrane color, and capillary refill time. Ancillary monitoring devices for the emergent patient include electrocardiography (ECG) and blood pressure monitoring.

ECG records the electrical activity generated by the heart from electrodes attached to the skin of the patient. It allows one to assess if the electrical activity is normal, thus providing information on the expected contraction of the heart. The ECG assesses heart rate and rhythm, but does not measure or assess cardiac output or tissue perfusion.[11]

Monitoring of the critically ill patient with initial, intermittent, or even continuous ECG evaluation is important, particularly in patients with underlying cardiac disease, metabolic disease, neoplasia, or at risk for development of arrhythmias. Arrhythmias result from abnormalities of impulse generation that alter the heart rate, heart rhythm, origin of excitation, or atrial and ventricular depolarization owing to interference with electrical conduction. If the electrical current is abnormal, the clinician must determine if the abnormality is a result of primary cardiac abnormalities resulting in abnormal impulse generation and conduction (eg, dilated cardiomyopathy), a systemic illness (eg, ventricular premature contractions [VPCs] seen following splenectomy), or other underlying conditions such as electrolyte abnormalities, hypoxia, trauma, or those secondary to medications.[11,12]

The ECG should be used to look for the presence of dysrhythmias, bradycardia, or tachycardia. Both tachyarrhythmias and bradyarrhythmias may result in decreased cardiac output (because of poor ventricular delivery or poor ventricular filling), potentially resulting in congestive heart failure, secondary end-organ failure (eg, acute renal failure, "shock gut") and sudden death. **Table 1** lists examples of tachyarrhythmias and bradyarrhythmias. The overall prognosis for a malignant arrhythmia depends on the underlying cause or disease and response to treatment. In general, the following parameters should warrant immediate intervention if detected on ECG:

- Dog: heart rate (HR) less than 50 beats/min or greater than 180 beats/min
- Cat: HR less than 120 beats/min or greater than 240 beats/min
- Presence of severe VPCs including R-on-T phenomenon (often predisposing to serious ventricular arrhythmias such as ventricular fibrillation)
- Ventricular tachycardia greater than 180 beats/min
- Pulse deficits
- Hypotension
- Clinical symptoms of poor perfusion (eg, prolonged capillary refill time, dull mentation)

When evaluating an arrhythmia, common questions that must be answered to determine if the arrhythmia requires therapy include:

1. Is the arrhythmia hemodynamically significant (eg, causing HR changes, absent pulses, weakness, collapse, blood pressure changes, and resulting overall in clinical signs associated with poor perfusion)?
2. Is the arrhythmia one that can lead to further morbidity and mortality (eg, R-on-T phenomenon, sustained ventricular tachycardiac, HR >180 beats/min)?
3. Can you identify an underlying cause for the arrhythmia (eg, T waves may be large relative to the R waves during hyperkalemia)?
4. What are the risks of beginning therapy? Do the benefits outweigh the risks (keeping in mind that antiarrhythmic therapies have the potential to be proarrhythmogenic)?

The readers are referred to a cardiology resource for additional information of treatment of cardiac arrhythmias. Emergency cardiac drug dosing can be found in Table 9 of the article elsewhere in this issue on emergency management and treatment of the poisoned small animal patient.

BLOOD PRESSURE MONITORING

Blood pressure monitoring in the emergent or critically ill patient is an important monitoring tool in the diagnosis of hypotension or hypertension. Hypotension is more commonly seen in the emergency room or ICU setting following hypovolemia,

Table 1 Types of cardiac arrhythmia	
Tachyarrhythmias	Atrial tachycardia
	Atrioventricular (AV) nodal tachycardia
	Ventricular tachycardia
	Ventricular fibrillation
	Atrial fibrillation
Bradyarrhythmias	Sick sinus syndrome
	Severe second-degree AV block
	Third-degree AV block
	Atrial standstill
	Asystole

hemorrhage, sepsis, and so forth, and must be treated aggressively and rapidly to ensure adequate tissue perfusion. However, when assessing blood pressure, it is important that it is not directly correlated with perfusion; rather, it is an assessment of overall global tissue perfusion. The assumption is that if the patient is hypotensive, blood flow in tissue will be inadequate, leading to decreased tissue perfusion.[13,14]

The primary treatment for hypotension should be directed at the underlying cause, as there are many variables that affect blood pressure (**Fig. 2**). Hypotension as a result of hypovolemia is treated with intravenous fluid therapy. Isotonic crystalloid boluses of 10 to 30 mL/kg or colloid boluses with hydroxyethyl starch (eg, Hetastarch) of 5 to 10 mL/kg over 15 to 30 minutes can increase the circulating fluid volume and improve the blood pressure. Patients with underlying cardiac disease (eg, chronic valvular heart disease, dilated or hypertrophic cardiomyopathy) that require fluid resuscitation warrant the use of judicious fluid therapy (eg, smaller volumes such as 5–10 mL/kg of an isotonic crystalloid or 2–5 mL/kg of a colloid over 30–60 minutes) followed by careful reassessment to determine if additional fluid boluses are warranted. Large volume resuscitation is not appropriate for every hypovolemic patient with normal cardiac function.

Hypotensive resuscitation is a form of fluid resuscitation for stabilization of the presurgical patient with uncontrolled hemorrhage. The most commonly practiced form of limited-volume resuscitation in veterinary medicine is permissive hypotension. This form of fluid resuscitation consists of administration of conservative volumes of intravenous fluids before definitive control of hemorrhage, with the target of a systolic blood pressure of 60 to 80 mm Hg. The goal is to provide adequate perfusion to the vital organs (eg, brain, kidneys, heart) without an increased risk of further massive hemorrhage.[15,16] Conversely, hypotension is not always a product of hypovolemia, and when hypotension exists despite an adequate circulating fluid volume, other therapies may be necessary. Inotrope therapy with blood pressure medications such as dopamine (5–20 µg/kg/min), dobutamine (2–20 µg/kg/min), or norepinephrine (0.05–0.4 µg/kg/min) may be needed.

In hypertensive patients (mean arterial pressure [MAP] >160 mm Hg or systolic pressure >200 mm Hg), several factors must be addressed, including toxicant ingestion (eg, selective serotonin reuptake inhibitor [SSRI] antidepressants, amphetamines), agitation, pain, underlying metabolic disease (eg, heart disease, renal disease, hyperadrenocorticism, immune-mediated hemolytic anemia), and neoplasia (eg, pheochromocytoma), among others. The use of judicious sedation/analgesia, anxiolytics, vasodilators, or angiotensin-converting enzyme inhibitors may be necessary. If the hypertension is toxicant related and concurrent agitation is simultaneously observed, the repeated use of sedatives may be required in cardiovascularly stable patients

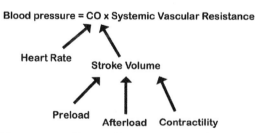

Fig. 2. Summary of factors controlling cardiac output: Central determinants of blood pressure are stroke volume and heart rate, both of which influence cardiac output. Changes in either will affect cardiac output.

(eg, phenothiazines). In patients failing to respond to sedative/anxiolytic therapy, the use of antihypertensives or other cardiac medications may be indicated to prevent vascular injury or secondary complications (eg, retinal detachment).

There are several methods for measuring blood pressure, including measurement of direct arterial blood pressure (DABP), Doppler blood pressure, and oscillometric blood pressure; these are listed in order of accuracy.

Monitoring of Direct Arterial Blood Pressure

Monitoring of direct arterial blood pressure is considered the gold standard for blood pressure measurement in both veterinary and human patients, and allows the clinician to assess trends in pressure changes. It requires placement of an arterial catheter, typically in the dorsal pedal artery. Other sites for arterial catheter placement include the femoral artery and the auricular artery.[17,18] Placement of an arterial catheter allows for rapid blood sampling and ABG analysis in the critically ill patient.

To monitor DABP, a catheter must be connected to a pressure transducer and monitor; this transducer then converts the pressure wave to an electrical impulse, which is transmitted to the monitor for display. This process allows for continuous monitoring of systolic pressure, diastolic pressure, and MAP. One must keep in mind that false results may be seen with compliant tubing, clot formation within the catheter, air bubbles in the tubing, or malfunction of catheter or tubing. Additional complications seen with arterial catheter placement include catastrophic hemorrhage (eg, from accidental disconnection of the arterial line), hematoma formation at the site of arterial puncture, thrombosis of the artery (more common in cats), necrosis of the tissues distal to the catheter (notably in cats that have an indwelling catheter for more than 6–12 hours), and infection.[19] Despite many advantages, DABP monitoring is often limited to critically ill patients or those patients under anesthesia (eg, intraoperative or receiving mechanical ventilation), where there is little movement and the benefits outweigh the risks of arterial catheter placement.

Monitoring of Noninvasive Blood Pressure

Monitoring of noninvasive blood pressure is based on inflation of a cuff to levels greater than systolic pressure to occlude arterial flow, followed by measurement of the pressure at which flow returns; this is typically measured by Doppler or oscillometric measurement. Doppler blood pressure measures systolic pressure, and is preferred because of its accuracy in smaller animals such as cats and small dogs. The Doppler unit consists of a probe, amplifier, speaker, and rechargeable battery. The probe consists of two piezoelectric crystals, one transmitting a continuous ultrasonic wave at a set frequency while the other crystal acts as a receiver. The Doppler method is preferred in patients with hypotension or in those with arrhythmias or tachycardia, which make the oscillometric results inaccurate. An appropriately sized cuff (measuring about 40%–60% of the limb or tail circumference) is placed proximal to the Doppler probe. This cuff is inflated to a pressure greater than the expected systolic pressure, resulting in absence of the sound signal. Once the signal is lost, the pressure in the cuff is slowly reduced. When the flow in the artery returns, the return of the audible pulse signal indicates the systolic arterial pressure.[20]

Oscillometric blood pressure devices measure oscillations within a cuff bladder using a microprocessor. Examples of oscillometric devices used in veterinary medicine include brands such as the Dinamap (ie, Device for Indirect Noninvasive Automatic Mean Arterial Pressure) and Cardell. Common locations for blood pressure measurement and cuff placement include just below the elbow, above the hock, below the hock, or on the tail base. Following cuff placement, the cuff is pressurized. The pressure is held constant while the microprocessor samples pressure oscillations and is incrementally deflated. During cuff deflation the microprocessor measures the pressure, averaging the amplitude of pressure oscillations.[21,22] The peak amplitude of oscillations equals the MAP. Systolic pressure equals the pressure at which oscillations are first detected, and diastolic pressure equals the pressure at which oscillations decrease rapidly. The HR calculated by the blood pressure machine should be compared with the patient's pulse rate on examination or heart rate on auscultation to ensure accuracy; one that does not match is generally considered inaccurate.[21] Many factors can adversely affect oscillometric blood pressure measurement. Common causes for erroneous readings include movement of the patient, arrhythmias, tachycardia, and inappropriate cuff width. A cuff that is too wide will result in an artifactual lower reading, and a cuff that is not wide enough will result in a falsely elevated reading.

NEUROLOGIC ASSESSMENT (DYSFUNCTION)

Primary neurologic evaluation should include both an extracranial and intracranial assessment. Extracranial assessment for life-threatening injuries includes hemorrhage, respiratory distress, and trauma. Triage of the ABCDs should initially be cursory to allow rapid identification and stabilization of a problem; therefore, although a full neurologic examination is not immediately performed, dysfunction is still considered a priority in initial monitoring of the emergency patient. Patients in severe hypovolemic shock may have decreased mentation, and should be frequently assessed during volume resuscitation to evaluate if the neurologic dysfunction improves. Likewise, patients should be assessed for appropriate neurologic dysfunction before the administration of analgesics, which may skew further assessment. Although the initial examination is important, serial patient assessment will allow for detection of changes in mental status. If detected, this should prompt a more in-depth patient evaluation and investigation of underlying causes. Once life-threatening issues are assessed, intracranial priorities include maintaining cerebral perfusion pressure (CPP) and ensuring oxygen delivery to the brain.[23] CPP, which is the difference between intracranial pressure (ICP) and MAP, can be enhanced by decreasing ICP (eg, mannitol, 15°–30° head elevation) and maintaining MAP (eg, fluid therapy, oxygen therapy).

When assessing the emergent patient neurologically, the Modified Glasgow Coma Scale (GCS) may be used. The modified GCS is a quantitative assessment of neurologic function assessing level of consciousness, brainstem reflexes, and motor activity and posture. Each category has a scale ranging from 1 to 6, with 6 being normal and 1 being recumbent, nonresponsive, and areflexic with dilated, unresponsive pupils and an absent oculocephalic reflex. Once the assessment is complete, the scores for each of the 3 systems are cumulated. The total score provides a 48-hour survival prognosis, with 3 to 8 being grave, 9 to 14 being guarded, and 15 to 18 yielding a good prognosis. One must exercise caution when prognosticating a neurologically impaired patient based on an initial assessment, as the trend over time is more valuable when predicting the final outcome.[24,25] The reader is referred to the article elsewhere in this issue on updates in the management of the neurologic trauma small animal patient for further information.

In the veterinary patient, common variables assessed in the neurologic examination/dysfunction include:

- Mentation:
  - Alert
  - Obtunded (dull, but can be aroused by nonnoxious stimuli)

- o Stuporous (semiconscious/somnolent, rousable with a noxious stimulus)
- o Comatose (unconscious, cannot be roused by a noxious stimulus)
- o Brain dead (no cerebrocortical electrical activity, no brainstem reflex function)
- Pupils: size, symmetry, pupillary light reflexes
- Presence and direction of nystagmus
- Menace response
- Facial asymmetry
- Posture
- Pain sensation, conscious proprioception, and withdrawal reflexes in limbs

In patients suspected of having increased ICP, careful and frequent monitoring of HR and systemic blood pressure are imperative to rule out the rapid onset of the Cushing reflex. The Cushing reflex (also referred to as the vasopressor response) is a physiologic nervous system response to increased ICP, and is clinically detected based on an acute onset of bradycardia and severe hypertension. Physiologically an increased ICP results in an increase in the cerebrospinal fluid pressure. When the ICP exceeds the MAP, the arterioles in the cerebrum become compressed. Compression results in diminished blood supply to the brain, leading to cerebral ischemia. Cerebral ischemia activates the parasympathetic and sympathetic nervous systems; activation of the sympathetic nervous system results in arterial vasoconstriction, increasing the total resistance of blood flow and elevating the systemic blood pressure. Systemic hypertension is produced in an attempt to restore blood flow to the ischemic cerebral arterioles. Baroreceptors in the carotid arteries detect the hypertensive compensation and trigger a parasympathetic response via the vagus nerve, resulting in bradycardia.[26,27] When clinical signs of Cushing reflex are seen, imminent herniation may occur; therefore, the patient should be treated aggressively and immediately (eg, with mannitol).

TEMPERATURE

Monitoring a patient's body temperature provides valuable information and does not require expensive equipment, and is most commonly performed rectally or via placement of the probe in the axilla. If using a rectal thermometer in the axilla, it is recommended to add 1 Fahrenheit degree for an equivalent approximate rectal temperature, as this modality is generally not considered to be as accurate.[28]

When an elevated rectal temperature is detected, it is important for the clinician to differentiate hyperthermia from a true fever. Heat balance occurs through the actions of heat-gaining and heat-dissipating mechanisms. Heat gain is seen with hypermetabolism, exercise, increased muscle activity (eg, tremors, seizures), and elevated ambient temperature (eg, heat stroke, when locked in a car). Heat-dissipating methods include behavioral changes such as finding a cool location, panting, and peripheral vasodilation. When heat gain exceeds the ability of the body to dissipate heat, hyperthermia occurs. Risk factors for developing hyperthermia include upper airway obstruction, laryngeal paralysis, brachiocephalic airway syndrome, high ambient humidity, and collapsing trachea.[29,30] With fever, differentials such as underlying infectious, inflammatory, or neoplastic processes should be considered. As fever is an endogenous source of heat, patients presenting with fever should not be cooled, in contrast to exogenous sources of heat (eg, hyperthermia), which should be cooled.

When hyperthermia is present, rapid cooling measures should be instituted when body temperatures exceed 104° to 105°F/40° to 40.5°C in the dog or 106°F/41.1°C in the cat.[29-31] Hyperthermia may result in decreased perfusion to the mesentery and thermal injury to the gastrointestinal tract, hematemesis, hematochezia, bacterial translocation, hypoglycemia, disseminated intravascular coagulation (DIC),[32] neuronal damage, cerebral edema, hemorrhage, and seizures.

Convection is the most effective cooling method,[31,33,34] which can be accomplished by wetting the patient with cool (not cold) water and using a fan to disperse the heat. Applying ice or cold water is discouraged, as this may cause peripheral vasoconstriction and delay heat loss. To prevent rebound hypothermia, cooling measures should be discontinued when body temperature reaches 103°F/39.4°C.

Although hyperthermia is more common in emergent patients, hypothermia is equally concerning. Again, rule-outs include an exogenous versus endogenous cause for hypothermia. An exogenous source (eg, a fall through ice, heat loss by anesthesia) warrants active warming, in contrast to an endogenous source (eg, severe dehydration or hypovolemia resulting in poor blood flow to the rectal area, resulting in hypothermia). With endogenous sources of hypothermia, warming should only be performed with resolution of the cause of the hypothermia; in other words, the concurrent use of intravenous fluid therapy to help perfuse the patient while simultaneously warming the patient is warranted.

Mild hypothermia is defined as a body temperature anywhere from 96° to 98°F/35.6° to 36.7°C, whereas moderate hypothermia is 94° to 96°F/34.4° to 35.6°C and severe hypothermia is 90° to 94°F/32.2° to 34.4°C. A temperature lower than 90°F/32.2°C must be addressed rapidly, as this is considered life-threatening hypothermia. Severe hypothermia can lead to cardiac abnormalities, vasodilation, and decreased blood flow. Heat support is provided with gloves or bottles filled with warm water, or blankets with circulating warm water. To prevent rebound hyperthermia, warming measures should be discontinued when body temperature reaches 99° to 100°F/37.2° to 37.8°C.[35]

BODY WEIGHT

Hospitalized patients should be weighed at least once a day (ideally on the same scale). Recording body weight in the metric scale is advantageous, as 1 kg = 1000 mL. Azotemic, oliguric, or anuric patients should be weighed at least 3 to 6 times per day. This simple monitoring tool can be used to assess changes in hydration status based on weight gain or weight loss. Acute changes in body weight are caused by changes in fluid balance rather than body mass. Once hydrated, an acute gain in body weight would be a concern for excess fluid accumulation (eg, edema). Conversely, acute weight loss may indicate ongoing fluid losses or continued dehydration. For example, a 30-kg dog that is 10% dehydrated requires 3 L to replace dehydration. As 1 L equates to 1 kg, this patient is expected to gain approximately 3 kg with appropriate fluid resuscitation. A 0.1-kg change in body weight translates to 100 mL of fluid gained or lost.[36]

URINE OUTPUT

Urine output (UOP) is often an underused tool in the critically ill patient or even in the patient with urethral obstruction. Along with body weight, UOP can be an important tool in assessing hydration status. Normal UOP ranges from 1 to 2 mL/kg/h. A decreased UOP despite adequate hydration and perfusion, reported as less than 0.5 mL/kg/h, is referred to as oliguria. Total lack of UOP is referred to as anuria.[37,38] Fluid intake ("ins") measurement is often easy, quantified by the digital fluid pump. By contrast, urine output ("outs") can be monitored grossly (eg, quantified either during walks or measurement of absorbent pads within the cage) or via measurement with a closed-system urinary catheter collection. A closed urinary collection system allows continuous urine collection and measurement to compare with fluid intake (ins), to ultimately assess fluid balance within the body, as ins should match the outs to ensure adequate hydration.[37,38]

The placement of a urinary catheter and a closed urinary collection system is not without risk. Nosocomial and ascending bacterial urinary tract infections, along with sedation risks and possible urethral injury, can occur, albeit rarely. Urinary catheter placement should be performed using a strict aseptic technique, and removed as soon as clinically possible to help prevent secondary infection.[39]

Aside from volume measurement, the urine-specific gravity (USG) can provide information regarding hydration. First, the USG should ideally be assessed before any administration of fluid; this will allow adequate evaluation of underlying renal function. Once a patient has been treated with intravenous fluids USG can be evaluated, as patients with ongoing fluid deficits will concentrate their urine, resulting in a hypersthenuria (cat >1.040, dog >1.025). Ideally, patients on intravenous fluids should be isosthenuric (eg, USG 1.015–1.018), as this indicates appropriate hydration.

Measurement of ins and outs, UOP, urine volume, and USG should all be assessed together to evaluate the clinical picture of the patient. An increased USG with a lower UOP (eg, USG 1.038, UOP 0.5 mL/kg/h) often indicates dehydration, and warrants an increase in fluid therapy. Conversely, a decreased UOP with concurrent isosthenuria or hyposthenuria (eg, USG 1.015, UOP 0.5 mL/kg/h) in an adequately hydrated and euvolemic azotemic patient may warrant diuretics such as furosemide or vasopressor support (to increase renal blood flow), if appropriate. Patients should be adequately hydrated based on additional assessment measures (eg, physical examination, evidence of hemodilution, weight gain, central venous pressure [CVP]) before instituting medications to increase UOP (eg, furosemide, mannitol); otherwise these drugs may result in increased UOP at the expense of dehydrating the patient.

MINIMUM DATABASE MONITORING

A basic emergency minimum database should include packed cell volume (PCV), total solids (TS), BUN, blood glucose (BG), and a blood smear. Depending on the capabilities of the clinic and the stability of the patient, further diagnostics may include electrolytes, creatinine, lactate, VBG, pulse oximetry, ECG, and blood pressure. Patients on intravenous fluids should have a daily minimum database (eg, PCV/TS/BG/BUN) and electrolytes (eg, Na^+, K^+) performed. Additional types of point-of-care machines are becoming more common in private practice settings, offering rapid assessment of variables that once took 24 hours to obtain.

LACTATE

Hand-held lactate machines can be used as an inexpensive monitoring point-of-care test in the emergency room or ICU. Hyperlactatemia occurs commonly in emergent and critically ill patients, likely secondary to a lactic acidosis following poor perfusion. Hyperlactatemia may result from hypoperfusion, liver failure, sepsis, lactate-containing fluid therapy, toxins, and drug therapy.[40] Hyperlactatemia is defined as a plasma lactate level above normal, commonly greater than 2.5 mmol/L.[41] In the 1990s an elevation in initial lactate was used to prognosticate for certain conditions[42]; since then, a recent push has been made to use serial lactate measurements to assess response to therapy instead.[43]

COAGULATION TESTING

Coagulopathies are common in emergency patients. Diagnostics to evaluate the coagulation system include activated clotting time, prothrombin time, activated partial thromboplastin time, platelet count, and d-dimers. Evaluation of red cell morphology as part of the complete blood count and blood smear may reveal the presence of red cell fragments, schistocytes, anisocytosis, and polychromasia. The in-house use of coagulation testing is readily available in veterinary medicine, and is beneficial in the diagnostic workup (eg, long-acting anticoagulant toxicosis, evidence of DIC, response of heparin therapy) in the critically ill patient.

CENTRAL VENOUS PRESSURE

CVP, also known as right atrial pressure (RAP), describes the pressure of blood in the thoracic vena cava. The CVP reflects the amount of blood returning to the heart and the ability of the heart to pump the blood into the arterial system (ie, preload). The most common access point for a central venous catheter is the external jugular vein. A peripherally inserted central line (PICC) may also be used for CVP measurement; this can be done by placing the PICC into the medial (cat) or lateral (dog) saphenous vein. Note, however, that this can only be performed when severe intra-abdominal hypertension is not present. Moreover, accurate CVP measurements can only be evaluated when the PICC line is placed to the level of the abdomen, as close as possible to the heart, for an accurate approximation of RAP.

The use of CVP is an important, simple diagnostic monitoring tool to help guide and monitor fluid therapy. It is of particular benefit in a potentially volume overloaded, azotemic, anuric patient with cardiac disease. CVP is influenced by blood volume, venous tone and compliance, cardiac function, and intrathoracic pressure (eg, CVP measurements are inaccurate when the patient is receiving continuous positive pressure ventilation). CVP can be measured using an electronic pressure transducer or extension tubing and manometer. The normal CVP ranges between 0 and 5 cm H_2O or 0 to 10 mm Hg.

A significantly elevated CVP (eg, >15 cm H_2O) is suggestive of cardiac tamponade, right-sided heart failure, or potentially abnormal catheter placement. In general, caution should be used when evaluating a single CVP measurement, which does not provide as much useful information as serial measurements. Repeated measurements of CVP are valuable for establishing trends when monitoring fluid therapy,[44] as it provides important information about the cardiovascular status. As intravenous fluids are administered the intravascular volume expands, thus both venous return and CVP will increase. When a fluid challenge is given to the patient, a euvolemic patient with normal cardiac function may demonstrate a small transient increase in CVP (2–4 mm Hg), which returns to baseline within 15 minutes. If there is an increase of less than 2 to 4 mm Hg or no increase at all in CVP, this would indicate a reduced vascular volume (potentially warranting more aggressive fluid therapy). If a fluid challenge is given and there is a large increase in CVP (eg, >4 mm Hg), the concern would be for either reduced cardiac compliance or increased venous blood volume (or both).

CAPNOGRAPHY

Capnography measures end-tidal carbon dioxide ($ETco_2$) concentration in exhaled gases, estimating alveolar carbon dioxide concentration. Capnometers use the absorption of infrared light at a specific wavelength projected through the gas mixture to determine the amount of carbon dioxide present. Carbon dioxide readily diffuses across the capillary membrane and quickly equilibrates with alveolar gas, thus $ETco_2$ closely approximates arterial carbon dioxide and, therefore, ventilation. However, with increased dead-space ventilation (eg, significant ventilation-perfusion mismatch from pulmonary atelectasis or lung consolidation), $ETco_2$ will be measured as erroneously low. Capnometry may also be used to assess the effectiveness of cardiopulmonary resuscitation and return of spontaneous circulation.[45,46] Unfortunately, the limitations of capnography are typically to intubated (eg, heavily sedated) patients. Nevertheless, the use of $ETco_2$ is of particular use in an intubated, sedated seizure patient to ensure adequate ventilation (eg, a dog excessively sedated secondary to being loaded on anticonvulsant therapy).

COLLOID OSMOTIC PRESSURE

Colloid osmotic pressure (COP), otherwise known as oncotic pressure, can be measured and used to guide fluid therapy. The COP is a force created by large plasma proteins within the vascular space that do not move freely across capillaries. Normal COP values are often documented to be 18 to 25 mm Hg.[47] A colloid osmometer is used to measure COP. When testing, the patient's plasma is forced across a membrane on the osmometer. The molecules exert a pressure in the sample chamber, sensed by the transducer, which is then converted to electrical energy and displayed in mm Hg. A low COP is consistent with a hypo-oncotic states (eg, protein-losing nephropathy, protein-losing enteropathy, sepsis, liver failure), and warrants supplementation with synthetic colloids (eg, hydroxyethyl starch) or albumin. See the article "Fluid Therapy for the Emergent Small Animal Patient: Crystalloids, Colloids, and Albumin Products" elsewhere in this issue for additional information.

SUMMARY

Management of the emergent or critically ill patient requires early recognition of life-threatening disturbances (eg, ABCDs) followed by serial patient assessment and monitoring. The clinician should be ready to intervene when life-threatening changes are documented, to prevent patient compromise. Emphasis on serial patient examination and assessment, accompanied by appropriate ancillary testing, is the best way to improve outcomes in emergent patients.

REFERENCES

1. Aldrich J. Global assessment of the emergency patient. Vet Clin North Am Small Anim Pract 2005;35:281–305.
2. Lumb AB. Nunn's applied respiratory physiology. 5th edition. Boston: Butterworth-Heinemann; 2000.
3. West JB. Respiratory physiology, the essentials. 6th edition. Baltimore (MD): Lippincott Williams & Wilkins; 2000.
4. Bozeman WP, Myers RA, Barish RA. Confirmation of pulse oximetry gap in carbon monoxide poisoning. Ann Emerg Med 1997;30:608–11.
5. Rausch-Madison S, Mohsenifar Z. Methodologic problems encountered with co-oximetry in methemoglobinemia. Am J Med Sci 1997;314:203–6.
6. Sorrell-Raschi L. Blood gas and oximetry monitoring. In: Silverstein DC, Hopper K, editors. Small animal critical care medicine. St Louis (MO): Saunders; 2009. p. 878–82.

7. De Morais, DiBartola. Acid-Base Disorders. In: Kirk RW, editor. Current veterinary therapy XIV. Philadelphia: WB Saunders; 2009. p. 54–60.
8. Ilkiw JE, Rose RJ, Martin IC. A comparison of simultaneously collected arterial, mixed venous, jugular venous, and cephalic venous blood samples in the assessment of blood gas and acid–base status in dogs. J Vet Intern Med 1991;5:294–8.
9. Muggenburg BA, Mauderly JL. Cardiopulmonary function of awake, sedated, and anesthetized beagle dogs. J Appl Phys 1974;37:152–7.
10. Mauderly JL, Pickrell JA, Hobbs CH, et al. The effect of inhaled 90Y fused clay aerosol on pulmonary function and related parameters of the beagle dog. Radiat Res 1973;56:83–96.
11. Tilley LP. Essentials of canine and feline electrocardiography. 3rd edition. Philadelphia: Lea & Febiger; 1992.
12. Edwards NJ. Bolton's handbook of canine and feline electrocardiography. Philadelphia: WB Saunders Co; 1987.
13. Moens Y, Coppens P. Patient monitoring and monitoring equipment. In: Seymour C, Duke-Novakovski T, editors. BSAVA manual of canine and feline anaesthesia and analgesia. 2nd edition. Gloucester: British Small Animal Veterinary Association; 2007. p. 62–79.
14. Stepien RL. Blood pressure measurement in dogs and cats. In Pract 2000;22: 136–45.
15. Bickell WH, Wall MJ, Pepe PE, et al. Immediate versus delayed fluid resuscitation for hypotensive patients with penetrating torso injuries. N Engl J Med 1994;331: 1105–9.
16. Dutton RP, Mackenzie CF, Scalea TM. Hypotensive resuscitation during active hemorrhage: impact on in-hospital mortality. J Trauma 2002;52:1141–6.
17. Waddell L. Blood pressure monitoring for the critically ill. In: Proceedings of the Western Veterinary Conference. Las Vegas (NV): 2004.
18. Haskins. Monitoring critical patients. In: Macintire DK, Drobatz KJ, Haskins SC, editors. Manual of small animal emergency & critical care medicine. Philadelphia: Lippincott Williams & Wilkins; 2005. p. 71–88.
19. Scheer BV, Perel A, Pfeiffer UJ. Clinical review: complications and risk factors of peripheral arterial catheters used for haemodynamic monitoring in anaesthesia and intensive care medicine. Crit Care 2002;6(3):199–204.
20. Macintire DK. Hypotension. In: Ettinger SJ, Feldman EC, editors. Textbook of veterinary internal medicine. 5th edition. Philadelphia: WB Saunders; 2000. p. 183–6.
21. Binns SH, Sisson DD, Buoscio DA, et al. Doppler ultrasonographic, oscillometric sphygmomanometric, and photoplethysmographic techniques for noninvasive blood pressure measurement in anesthetized cats. J Vet Intern Med 1995;9(6): 405–14.
22. Grady DL, Dunlop CI, Hodgson DS, et al. Evaluation of the Doppler ultrasonic method of measuring systolic arterial blood pressure in cats. Am J Vet Res 1992;53:1166.
23. Syring RS. Assessment and treatment of central nervous system abnormalities in the emergency patient. Vet Clin North Am Small Anim Pract 2005;35: 343–58.
24. Platt SR, Radaelli ST, McDonnell JJ. The prognostic value of the modified Glasgow Coma Scale in head trauma in dogs. J Vet Intern Med 2001;15(6):581–4.
25. Dewey C, Budsberg S, Oliver J. Principles of head trauma management in dogs and cats—Part II. Comp Cont Edu Pract Vet 1993;15(2):177–92.

26. Sande A, West C. Traumatic brain injury: a review of pathophysiology and management. J Vet Emerg Crit Care (San Antonio) 2010;20(2):177–90.
27. Fletcher D, Syring R. Traumatic brain injury. In: Silverstein D, Hopper K, editors. Small animal critical care medicine. St Louis (MO): Saunders; 2009. p. 658–62.
28. Morley CJ, Hewson PH, Thornton AJ, et al. Axillary and rectal temperature measurements in infants. Arch Dis Child 1992;67(1):122–5.
29. Johnson SI, McMichael M, White G. Heatstroke in small animal medicine: a clinical practice review. J Vet Emerg Crit Care (San Antonio) 2006;16(2):112–9.
30. Bruchim Y, Klement E, Saragusty J, et al. Heat stroke in dogs: a retrospective study of 54 cases (1994–2004) and analysis of risk factors for death. J Vet Intern Med 2006;20:38–46.
31. Drobatz KJ, Macintire DK. Heat-induced illness in dogs: 42 cases (1976-1993). J Am Vet Med Assoc 1996;209(11):1894–9.
32. Aroch I, Segev G, Loeb E, et al. Peripheral nucleated red blood cells as a prognostic indicator in heatstroke in dogs. J Vet Intern Med 2009;23:544–51.
33. Flournoy WS, Wohl JS, Macintire DK. Heatstroke in dogs: pathophysiology and predisposing factors. Comp Cont Cont Edu Pract Vet 2003;25:410–8.
34. Flournoy WS, Wohl JS, Macintire DK. Heatstroke in dogs: clinical signs, treatment, prognosis and prevention. Comp Cont Cont Edu Pract Vet 2003;25:422–31.
35. Oncken AK, Kirby R, Rudloff E. Hypothermia in critically ill dogs and cats. Comp Cont Edu Pract Vet 2001;23(6):506–20.
36. DiBartola S, editor. Fluid therapy in small animal practice. 2nd edition. Philadelphia: W.B. Saunders; 2000.
37. Lees GE. Early diagnosis of renal disease and renal failure. Vet Clin North Am Small Anim Pract 2004;34(4):867–86.
38. Labato MA. Strategies for management of acute renal failure. Vet Clin North Am Small Anim Pract 2001;31(6):1265–87.
39. Smarick S. Urinary catheterization. In: Hopper K, Silverstein D, editors. Small animal critical care medicine. St Louis (MO): Saunders Elsevier; 2008. p. 603–7.
40. Hughes Dez. Lactate measurement: diagnostic, therapeutic and prognostic implications. In: Bonagura, editor. Kirks' current veterinary therapy XIII. Philadelphia: WB Saunders Co; 2000. p. 112–6.
41. Karagiannis MH, Reniker AN, Kerl ME, et al. Lactate measurement as an indicator of perfusion. Compendium 2006;28:287–98.
42. de Papp E, Drobatz KJ, Hughes D. Plasma lactate concentration as a predictor of gastric necrosis and survival among dogs with gastric dilatation-volvulus: 102 cases (1995-1998). J Am Vet Med Assoc 1999;215:49.
43. Stevenson CK, Kidney BA, Duke T, et al. Serial blood lactate concentrations in systemically ill dogs. Vet Clin Pathol 2007;36(3):234–9.
44. Hansen BD. Technical aspects of fluid therapy. In: DiBartola SP, editor. Fluid, electrolyte, and acid-base disorders in small animal practice. 3rd edition. St Louis (MO): Saunders Elsevier; 2006. p. 344–76.
45. Plunkett SJ, McMichael M. Cardiopulmonary resuscitation in small animal medicine: an update. J Vet Intern Med 2008;22:9–25.
46. ECC Committee, Subcommittees and Task Forces of the American Heart Association. 2005 American Heart Association Guidelines for cardiopulmonary resuscitation and emergency care. Circulation 2005;112(Suppl IV):IV-1–6.
47. Chan DL, Rozanski EA, Freeman LM, et al. Colloid osmotic pressure in health and disease. Comp Cont Edu Pract Vet 2001;23(10):896–90.

Fluid Therapy for the Emergent Small Animal Patient
Crystalloids, Colloids, and Albumin Products

Elisa Mazzaferro, DVM, MS, PhD[a], Lisa L. Powell, DVM[b],*

KEYWORDS

- Intravenous fluids • Crystalloids • Colloids • Albumin • Volume resuscitation
- Dehydration

KEY POINTS

- Fluid therapy is essential in the treatment of emergent veterinary patients and includes crystalloid solutions, blood component therapy, concentrated albumin solutions, and synthetic colloids.
- Bolus intravenous (IV) fluid therapy can restore perfusion and stabilize critically ill and injured patients for further diagnostics and treatment.
- Synthetic colloids help maintain colloid osmotic pressure (COP) and improve blood pressure but should be used with caution in coagulopathic patients or those with cardiac disease.
- Concentrated albumin solutions may have a role in the treatment of critically ill veterinary patients with severe hypoalbuminemia (eg, septic peritonitis); further prospective, comparative studies are needed to fully elucidate the role of albumin solutions in dogs and cats.
- The pros and cons of the use of human serum albumin (HSA) and canine serum albumin (CSA) will be reviewed.

Water is essential for life. Without adequate fluid intake, normal body functioning becomes impaired and ultimately can lead to death. A fluid therapy plan should be considered for any small animal patient that has either inadequate fluid intake, excessive fluid loss, or both. A simplified approach to fluid therapy begins with an understanding of the composition of fluid and its distribution within the body. Next, consideration of electrolyte loss, acid-base disturbances, perfusion impairment, and loss of protein also becomes important when replenishing deficits by using various fluids that are commercially available to small animal practitioners.

---

[a] Cornell University Veterinary Specialists, 880 Canal Street, Stamford, CT 06902, USA;
[b] Veterinary Medical Center, Department of Veterinary Clinical Sciences, University of Minnesota College of Veterinary Medicine, 1365 Boyd Avenue, #D335, St Paul, MN 55108, USA
* Corresponding author.
E-mail address: powel029@umn.edu

Vet Clin Small Anim 43 (2013) 721–734
http://dx.doi.org/10.1016/j.cvsm.2013.03.003   **vetsmall.theclinics.com**
0195-5616/13/$ – see front matter © 2013 Elsevier Inc. All rights reserved.

TOTAL BODY WATER AND FLUID COMPARTMENTS WITHIN THE BODY

A discussion of IV fluid administration is incomplete without an understanding of total body water (TBW) and fluid balance between the various compartments within the body. Approximately 60% of a healthy animal's total body weight is water. This value can change slightly depending on age, lean body mass, degree of leanness or obesity, and gender. Total body water has been estimated as approximately 534 mL/kg to 660 mL/kg in healthy dogs and cats.[1]

Conceptually, the body can be divided into the intracellular and extracellular compartments. Fluid located within cells is known as intracellular fluid (ICF) and contributes approximately two-thirds (66%) to TBW. Extracellular fluid (ECF) is that located outside of cells and contributes approximately one-third (33%) to TBW; the ECF can be further subdivided into the intravascular and interstitial compartments. Fluid contained within blood vessels is intravascular fluid. The intravascular fluid contains plasma water, cellular components, proteins, and electrolytes. The interstitial extravascular compartment is the space located outside of the blood vessels. Intravascular fluid contributes only 8% to 10% of TBW, and interstitial fluid contributes 24% of TBW. A small amount of fluid is known as transcellular fluid and is located within the gastrointestinal tract, joints, cartilage, and cerebrospinal space.[1] Total intravascular fluid volume has been estimated as 80 mL/kg to 90 mL/kg in dogs and cats. Of that, the fluid component, or intravascular plasma water volume, has been estimated as approximately 45 mL/kg to 50 mL/kg.[1]

GOALS OF FLUID THERAPY

Administration of IV fluids requires an understanding of the type of fluid lost, the presence of underlying disease processes, an animal's hydration and intravascular volume status, acid-base and electrolyte derangements, an animal's ability to retain fluid within the intravascular space, and determinants of resuscitation endpoints when treating dehydration or various forms of hypovolemia. An understanding of electrolyte and protein composition within the body is also essential to help maintain homeostasis and to use the variety of crystalloid fluids that are available to treat specific abnormalities. Thus, the goals of fluid therapy are to replenish interstitial, intracellular, and intravascular fluid deficits; to correct and maintain electrolyte and acid-base derangements; and to maintain normal TBW in the face of excessive loss or lack of adequate intake.

CRYSTALLOID FLUIDS

A crystalloid fluid contains water and various forms of electrolytes (including salt) or sugar crystals (**Table 1**).[1,2] Some crystalloid fluids also contain buffers (eg, acetate, gluconate, and lactate) that are metabolized to bicarbonate to increase serum pH. Crystalloid fluids are categorized according to their osmolality relative to that of plasma. An isotonic crystalloid fluid has an osmolality similar to or equal to that of plasma and the extracellular compartment (eg, approximately 300 mOsm/L). Fluids with tonicity lower than that of the extracellular space are called hypotonic fluids (eg, 0.45% dextrose and 5% dextrose in water [D5W]) and can cause fluid influx into red blood cells (RBCs) and hemolysis.[1,2] Fluids with tonicity greater than that of the ECF compartment (eg, >300 mOsm/L) are called hypertonic solutions (eg, 7.2% and 23.4% hypertonic saline) and can be used to expand intravascular fluid volume in a hypovolemic animal by pulling water from the interstitial into the intravascular space. It has been estimated that approximately 80% of an isotonic crystalloid fluid

Table 1
Various crystalloid fluids and their components

Fluid	Osmolarity	Buffer	Sodium	Chloride	Potassium	Calcium	Magnesium	Glucose
Normosol-R	296	Acetate 27 Gluconate 23	140	98	5	0	3	0
PlasmaLyte-A	294	Acetate 27	140	98	5	0	3	0
0.9% Saline	308	0	154	154	0	0	0	0
LRS	272	Lactate 28	130	109	4	3	0	0
D5W	252	0	0	0	0	0	0	50 g/L
0.45% NaCl + 2.5% dextrose	280	0	77	77	0	0	0	25 g/L
Normosol-M + 5% dextrose	364	Acetate 16	40	40	13	0	3	50 g/L
PlasmaLyte-M	363	Acetate 16	40	40	13	0	3	110
PlasmaLyte-56	110	Acetate 16	40	40	13	0	3	0
3% NaCl	1026	0	513	513	0	0	0	0
7% NaCl	2567	0	1283	1283	0	0	0	0

administered IV leaves the intravascular compartment and move to the interstitial compartment within 1 hour of infusion.[3]

Isotonic fluids have sodium concentrations similar to that of plasma and the ECF compartment.[1,2,4] Water and sodium are intimately associated within the body's fluid compartments. Wherever sodium goes, water must follow. For this reason, the concentration of sodium in a crystalloid fluid becomes important when selecting a particular fluid to treat a specific disease state. Other important components of isotonic crystalloid fluids to consider include the presence or absence of buffers or various electrolytes (calcium, magnesium, potassium, chloride, and so forth).

Fluids used to replace intravascular and interstitial volume deficit should contain 130 mEq/L to 154 mEq/L of sodium. Several solutions are used for replacement of fluid volume, electrolyte abnormalities, and correction of acid-base abnormalities, including Normosol-R, PlasmaLyte-A, normal (0.9%) saline, and lactated Ringer solution (LRS) (also called Hartmann solution).

Maintenance crystalloid solutions contain lower concentrations of sodium and other compounds compared with the extracellular space[1,2,4] and are used primarily to replace sensible fluid losses that can be measured and insensible fluid losses that can be estimated.[3] An example of a maintenance isotonic crystalloid fluid is 0.45% sodium with 2.5% dextrose, PlasmaLyte-M, and PlasmaLyte 56. If such fluids are used as replacement solutions, a patient's serum sodium can decrease and lead to a state of hyponatremia.

HYPERTONIC SALINE

Hypertonic sodium (eg, 7.2 and 23.4% NaCl) contains the highest concentration of sodium (eg, 1283 mEq/L of sodium and approximately 4000 mEq/L). Infusion of hypertonic saline should only be considered in a hypovolemic patient with normal interstitial and intracellular hydration (ie, only lacking fluid within the intravascular space). Infusion of hypertonic saline increases intravascular sodium concentration, and the intravascular space has a higher osmolality compared with the interstitial and intracellular space. To maintain fluid equilibrium, water diffuses down a concentration gradient by osmosis, from an area of higher water concentration (lower osmolality). After infusion of hypertonic saline, water moves from the intracellular and interstitial space into the intravascular space and causes intravascular volume expansion at the expense of the interstitium. The effect is short-lived for 20 to 30 minutes unless the hypertonic saline is administered concurrently with a colloid to retain the fluid within the intravascular space.[5,6] Hypertonic saline (23.4%) can be diluted with a synthetic colloid at a ratio of 1 part hypertonic saline with 2.5 parts colloid, which creates a 7.5% solution.[7] Hypertonic saline in combination with a synthetic colloid (dogs: 5–10 mL/kg of the combination; cats: 2 mL/kg of the combination; total dose in either species should not exceed 1 mL/kg/min as a bolus)[7] can also be used to initially treat hypovolemic shock, provided a patient is not clinically dehydrated.

After correction of intravascular hypovolemia, replacement crystalloid fluids must be administered after administration of hypertonic saline (with or without colloids) to replenish that fluid borrowed from the interstitial and intracellular compartments to rehydrate them. Potential complications of hypertonic saline administration include rapid respiratory rate, hypotension, bradycardia, and hypernatremia.[1,7]

SODIUM

Sodium is the major extracellular cation (ie, positive charged molecule) in the body. Normal sodium concentrations are 140 mEq/L 150 mEq/L for dogs and 150 mEq/L to 160 mEq/L for cats.[8] The sodium content of most isotonic crystalloid fluids ranges from 130 mEq/L to 140 mEq/L. Normal (0.9%) saline is the isotonic crystalloid fluid with the highest sodium concentration (154 mEq/L) and is used as a replacement fluid. Fluids used to replace intravascular and interstitial volume deficit should contain 130 mEq/L to 154 mEq/L of sodium. In the realm of isotonic crystalloid fluids, LRS contains the lowest concentration of sodium (130 mEq/L) relative to plasma. Conditions that promote hyperaldosteronemia and sodium retention, such as congestive heart failure and hepatic failure, may benefit from infusion of lower concentrations of sodium.

Maintenance fluids can be used to replace daily ongoing sodium losses. Fluids, such as Plasmalyte-M and Plasmalyte 56, contain approximately 40 mEq/L sodium. If such fluids were used as replacement solutions, a patient's serum sodium could be decreased and lead to a state of hyponatremia.

Rapid changes in serum sodium concentration can be detrimental, depending on the how quickly an animal's sodium balance and serum sodium concentration become deranged. Diarrhea, heat-induced illness, hyperthermia, and lack of access to water can cause varying degrees of hypernatremia. Hypernatremia largely is characterized by a free water deficit, a deficit of fluid in excess of electrolytes. Ideally, serum sodium concentration should not be lowered by more than 15 mEq in a 24-hour period. Similarly, syndromes, such as hypoadrenocorticism, can cause decreases in serum sodium concentration. Overzealous administration of sodium-containing fluids, such as normal (0.9%) saline, can result in cerebral edema and central pontine myelinolysis.[9]

CHLORIDE

Chloride is a major extracellular anion (ie, negative charged molecule). Chloride can be lost in vomitus caused by an upper gastrointestinal obstruction, from administration of diuretics (eg, furosemide) or from loss in diarrheic feces. The presence of a hypochloremic metabolic alkalosis is typically less common in veterinary medicine and is often characteristic of the causes discussed previously. Normal (0.9%) saline contains supraphysiologic concentrations of chloride (154 mEq/L) and is used as a chloride replacement fluid in cases of hypochloremia. Other isotonic crystalloid fluids contain varying concentrations of chloride (55–103 mEq/L). Although chloride is important, consideration of sodium and other electrolyte concentrations is more important when selecting a replacement fluid for a specific disease state.

POTASSIUM

Potassium is the major intracellular cation. Serum potassium can become elevated due to severe dehydration, hypoadrenocorticism, metabolic acidosis, diabetic ketoacidosis (DKA), renal failure, or obstructive uropathies. Most replacement and maintenance crystalloid fluids contain minimal supplementation of potassium (eg, 4 mEq/L of potassium in LRS) and typically need to be supplemented in the form of potassium chloride. In animals with hyperkalemia, it is ideal to avoid the administration of a potassium-containing fluid whenever possible; however, studies have shown that as long as the underlying disease mechanism is promptly treated, the small amount of potassium with replacement or maintenance fluids is rarely consequential.[10] Administration of IV fluids alone dilutes serum potassium as intravascular fluid volume is replenished, even if the fluid contains small amounts of potassium. In animals with hypokalemia, potassium supplementation is commensurate with the degree of hypokalemia.[5,8] It is advisable to not exceed administration of more than 0.5 mEq/kg/h of potassium IV.

MAGNESIUM

Magnesium is required for regulation and normal functioning of the sodium-potassium-ATPase pump. Some maintenance fluids (eg, PlasmaLyte and Normosol) contain trace amounts of magnesium. In general, most healthy patients do not require additional supplementation of magnesium. In animals with refractory hypokalemia (eg, DKA), animals with endocrine diseases predisposing them toward significant electrolyte changes (eg, DKA), or in critically ill patients, magnesium should be supplemented (eg, 0.75 mEq/kg/d or 0.375 mmol/kg/d) in addition to potassium, because both electrolytes follow similar physiologic paths within the body. Total body magnesium is a function of absorption and loss as well as redistribution throughout body compartments. Any physiologic condition that can cause a lack of intake and absorption, increased loss in diarrheic feces, renal tubular loss, or redistribution can cause hypomagnesemia. For example, in animals with DKA and whole-body magnesium depletion secondary to glucose/osmotic diuresis, administration of insulin and dextrose for treatment causes magnesium to rapidly shift to the intracellular space and result in a serum ionized hypomagnesemia. Although the crystalloid fluids contain small quantities of magnesium, the amount is insufficient to replenish a whole-body magnesium deficit in some populations of critically ill patients.

CALCIUM

Calcium is an important cation that is necessary for normal muscle conduction and coagulation. Calcium is present in small amounts in LRS (3 mEq/L) and typically does not need to be supplemented in healthy patients above this amount. In cases of puerperal tetany (eg, eclampsia), however, LRS may be the preferred fluid as adjunct therapy to those that do not contain calcium and to those that promote calcium excretion (0.9% NaCl). Additionally, the preemptive use of a calcium-containing fluid, such as LRS, may be beneficial in helping to prevent hypocalcemia during the postoperative period after surgical removal of the parathyroid gland.

Hypercalcemia can be seen due to a variety of causes. Administration of a calcium-containing fluid is contraindicated in hypercalcemic patients if other crystalloid fluids are available. Normal (0.9%) saline is the treatment of choice in cases of hypercalcemia not only because the fluid does not contain calcium but also because the higher sodium content (eg, 154 mEq/L) promotes calciuresis at the Na_2Ca exchanger.[11]

BUFFERS

A buffer is a compound that is converted or metabolized in the body to bicarbonate to help maintain normal physiologic blood pH. The most common buffers found in IV fluids include lactate, acetate, and gluconate. Medical conditions that cause metabolic acidosis (lactic acidosis secondary to poor perfusion, DKA, uremia, ethylene glycol toxicosis, salicylate toxicosis, and so forth) should ideally be treated with a crystalloid fluid that contains a buffer. Certain medical conditions, however, may warrant the judicious use or the more appropriate use of certain buffers. In cases of hepatic dysfunction, the liver's ability to convert lactate to bicarbonate may be diminished; therefore, LRS is contraindicated. Acetate and gluconate, commonly found in Normosol-R or PlasmaLyte, are buffers that are metabolized to bicarbonate in the liver and muscle tissue. Therefore, in patients with LSA or whose liver function is suboptimal, crystalloid fluids that contain acetate and gluconate may be preferable to lactate-containing solutions. Acetate, which has been reported to potential hypotension with large, massive infusions (eg, dialysis),[12] should ideally be avoided in patients requiring large, rapid boluses (eg, anesthetic-induced hypotension).

Normal (0.9%) saline contains no buffers and is known as an acidifying crystalloid fluid because it promotes excretion of bicarbonate by the renal tubules.[5] In cases of a hypochloremic metabolic alkalosis, an acidifying solution, such as 0.9% saline without additional buffers, is preferred, to avoid administration of additional sources of bicarbonate and to replenish chloride ions lost in the vomitus.

DEXTROSE

Dextrose-containing fluids, such as D5W and 0.45% sodium chloride with 2.5% dextrose, are not common fluid choices in the dehydrated patients, and their use is typically limited to patients with severe hypernatremia, patients that cannot tolerate a large amount of sodium (eg, heart failure), or during treatment of conditions that cause hyperaldosteronism (hepatic failure, cardiac disease, and so forth). Dextrose-containing fluids are largely hypotonic compared with plasma; D5W is analogous to infusing a free water solution, once the dextrose is rapidly metabolized by the body. The remaining fluid redistributes within the intravascular, interstitial, and intracellular fluid compartments. Because free water alone is severely hypotonic (eg, 0 Osm/L) relative to plasma (eg, 300 Osm/L), infusion of free water causes rapid and severe hemolysis; hence, sterile water is not used. The addition of 5% dextrose (50 mg of dextrose/mL) makes the fluid isoosmolar and brings the tonicity of the fluid up to a safe acceptable range. The dextrose in these fluids is quickly metabolized but is insufficient to meet an animal's daily metabolic caloric requirements.

MAINTENANCE FLUID REQUIREMENTS

Many estimates of the maintenance fluid requirements for healthy dogs and cats have been recommended. In general, the estimates have been extrapolated from those recommended for humans or have been suggested based on experiments performed on healthy dogs and cats. The most recent swing of the fluid pendulum has been based on data obtained from calorimetry analysis in which fluid requirements are extrapolated from an animal's resting energy expenditure (REE) and lean body mass.[13,14] An animal's metabolic water requirements are equivalent to the number of basal calories required. During metabolism of 1 kcal of energy, 1 mL of water is consumed. By calculating the REE, or daily caloric requirements, a patient's daily fluid requirements for metabolic purposes can be calculated by the following linear formula: REE = mL H_2O^* = [(30 × body weight [kg]) + 70], where * denotes requirement for a 24-hour period.

This formula is accurate for animals greater than 2 kg and less than 100 kg. One caveat is that the REE is applicable to a healthy animal that is euvolemic, resting, and in a postprandial state. This formula denotes a starting point for dehydrated or hypovolemic animals or those with excessive fluid losses. Because some patients may become dehydrated when this formula is used, frequent evaluation of hydration status (body weight, evidence of hemodilution, urine specific gravity, and so forth) is essential during hospitalization. As a rule of thumb, 1 mL of water is equivalent to 1 g of body weight. Therefore, loss of 1 kg is equivalent to a loss of l L of water. Careful weighing of the animal on a regular basis allows clinicians to determine whether additional ongoing losses are occurring, allowing for accurate correction of interstitial and intracellular dehydration.

DEHYDRATION

Dehydration refers to the fluid deficit within the interstitial and intracellular fluid compartments. The extent of dehydration can be estimated based on subjective guidelines of skin turgor, mucous membrane dryness, and sunken appearance of the eyes within the orbit (**Table 2**). Once degree of dehydration is determined, the volume of fluid that must be administered to replace the fluid deficit can be calculated by the following formula:

Dehydration (%) × body weight in kg × 1000 = milliliters fluid deficit

The fluid deficit then should be added to the animal's maintenance fluid requirements and replaced over a 6-hour to 24-hour period, depending on a patient's stability and ability to handle the volume administered. There is no absolute correct method of replacing an animal's fluid deficit, as long as the deficit is considered in the calculation of the total amount of fluids that need to be administered to a dehydrated patient. Frequent weighing and calculation of urine, vomit, and diarrhea fluid output (again, knowing that 1 mL of fluid weighs 1 g) allow a clinician to determine whether a patient's fluid deficit and maintenance needs are met or whether IV crystalloid dose needs to be adjusted.

HYPOVOLEMIA

Hypovolemia denotes loss of fluid from the intravascular space and is semantically different than dehydration. This fluid loss may be relative or absolute, meaning that in conditions of vasodilation (eg, sepsis or an anesthetized patient), there is a relative intravascular fluid deficit. Absolute intravascular fluid deficits occur as a result of fluid loss, such as that associated with hemorrhage or excessive ongoing losses (vomiting, diarrhea, renal loss, and so forth), where fluid efflux from the interstitial space to compensate for intravascular fluid loss has been depleted. Likewise, if an isoosmolar fluid is lost (eg, blood), there is no osmotic gradient drive to pull fluid from the interstitial space into the intravascular space. Clinical signs of hypovolemia are manifested as abnormalities of perfusion and include tachycardia, peripheral vasoconstriction with cool

Table 2 Subjective parameters used to estimate the degree of dehydration	
Estimated Degree of Dehydration	**Clinical Signs**
<5%	History of vomiting or diarrhea or other fluid loss, normal mucous membranes, unable to detect <5% on physical examination
5%	History of vomiting or diarrhea or other fluid loss, tachy or dry mucous membranes
7%	History of vomiting or diarrhea or other fluid loss, dry mucous membranes, increased skin tenting, tachycardia, normal pulse quality and arterial blood pressure
10%	History of vomiting or diarrhea or other fluid loss, dry mucous membranes, increased skin tenting, tachycardia, weak pulses, hypotension
12%	History of vomiting or diarrhea or other fluid loss, dry mucous membranes, sunken eyes, increased skin tenting, tachycardia or bradycardia, weak to absent pulses, hypotension, cold extremities, hypothermia

extremities, hypothermia, prolonged capillary refill time, hypotension, pallor, and mental dullness. When an animal presents in hypovolemic shock, the location of the fluid deficit, the presence of electrolyte abnormalities, and whether interstitial or intracellular dehydration is a component of a fluid deficit or if the deficit is associated with the intravascular space alone must be considered. With hypovolemia, rapid fluid replacement is imperative to improve perfusion parameters. Previously, recommendations for the treatment of hypovolemic shock (eg, shock volume) in dogs and cats have been reported as 90 mL/kg and 44 mL/kg, respectively,[4,8,13,14] which represents the blood volume of a patient. Because administration of large volume of crystalloids can dilute coagulation factors, platelets, and RBCs, more recently, the use of smaller aliquots are recommended rather than replacing the whole blood volume at once **Table 3**.

Ideally, it is preferred to administer a one-fourth of the shock volume (eg, 20–30 mL/kg over 20 minutes) and reassess a patient's perfusion parameters. If normalizing, then moving to maintenance fluid rates and performing diagnostics can be considered to assess and treat the primary cause of the problem. If a patient fails to respond (eg, perfusion parameters have still not normalized), additional aliquots (eg, one-fourth shock bolus) of crystalloid fluids should be readministered once or twice more; additional therapy may warrant the use of a colloid thereafter. Once stabilized, a continuous rate of infusion of fluids should be maintained, because 80% of a crystalloid fluid volume

Table 3
Relative indications and relative contraindication for use of various isotonic, hypotonic, and hypertonic crystalloid fluids

Fluid	Indications	Relative Contraindications
Normosol-R	Replacement, metabolic acidosis, anorexia, vomiting, hypovolemic shock, diarrhea, renal failure	Hyperkalemia, metabolic alkalosis
PlasmaLyte-A	Replacement, metabolic acidosis, anorexia, vomiting, hypovolemic shock, diarrhea, renal failure	Hyperkalemia, metabolic alkalosis
0.9% NaCl	Replacement, hypovolemic shock, anorexia, vomiting, diarrhea, metabolic alkalosis, hyperkalemia, hypercalcemia acute hyponatremia, chronic hypernatremia, renal failure	Cardiac disease, liver disease, metabolic acidosis
LRS	Replacement, hypovolemic shock, vomiting, diarrhea, hypocalcemia, metabolic acidosis, renal failure	Hypercalcemia, hyperkalemia, lymphosarcoma, liver failure
D5W	Drug carrier, correction of hypernatremia and free water deficit, congestive heart failure	Does not provide sufficient calories to be used as a form of parenteral nutrition
0.45% NaCl + 2.5 dextrose	Maintenance, replacement of insensible losses, correction of free water deficit	Not to be used as a replacement fluid
Normosol-M	Replacement of insensible losses	Hyponatremia, not to be used as a replacement fluid
PlasmaLyte-M	Replacement of insensible losses	Hyponatremia, not to be used as a replacement fluid
3% NaCl	Intravascular volume expansion, hypovolemic shock	Interstitial dehydration, hypernatremia
7% NaCl	Intravascular volume expansion, hypovolemic shock	Interstitial dehydration, hypernatremia

infused leaved the intravascular space within 1 hour of infusion, if not administered along with a colloid.[3]

COLLOID OSMOTIC PRESSURE

COP is the pressure exerted on membranes primarily due to the presence of albumin. Normal plasma COP in dogs and cats has been reported as 16.7 mm Hg to 28.9 mm Hg and 21 mm Hg to 34 mm Hg, respectively.[15–17] Normal whole blood COP in dogs and cats has been reported as 17.9 mm Hg to 27.1 mm Hg and 21 mm Hg to 34 mm Hg, respectively.[15,16] Starling's law governs the movement of fluid between the intracellular and extracellular (intravascular and interstitial) space:

$$J_v = K_f[(P_c - P_i) - \sigma(\pi_c - \pi_i)]$$

where J_v is net fluid movement between compartments, K_f is filtration coefficient, P_c is capillary hydrostatic pressure, P_i is interstitial hydrostatic pressure, σ is reflection coefficient, π_c is COP, and π_i is interstitial osmotic pressure.

The filtration coefficient (K_f) is a measure of how well a tissue allows fluid to efflux and is a product of the surface area of the tissue and how permeable the capillary wall is to water (also referred to as hydraulic conductivity). The reflection coefficient (σ) is a measure of protein permeability in the membrane. If a membrane is completely impermeable to protein, then the osmotic forces are able to exert their full effect, making the reflection coefficient equal to 1.0. For example, the cerebrospinal fluid and the glomerular filtrate are impermeable to protein, and, therefore, the reflection coefficient for protein in these capillaries is close to 1. Proteins cross the walls of the hepatic sinusoids easily, so the reflection coefficient for protein in the sinusoids is low. The reflection coefficient in the pulmonary capillaries is approximately 0.5. Hydrostatic pressure (P) tends to force fluid out of the capillary, and the osmotic pressure (π) acts to pull inward, keeping fluid within the intravascular space.

COLLOID SOLUTIONS

Colloid solutions contain high molecular weight (MW) particles thereby increasing plasma COP and more efficiently holding fluid within the intravascular space. Colloids can be further classified as natural or synthetic. Natural colloid solutions include blood products (eg, plasma and whole blood) and concentrated albumin. Synthetic colloids include dextrans and hydroxyethyl starches (HESs).

NATURAL COLLOIDS

Blood products include whole blood, component therapy (eg, plasma), and concentrated albumin solutions. Packed RBCs (pRBCs) have a lower COP (eg, 5 mm Hg) and are not considered a true colloid compared with whole blood (eg, because the plasma proteins have been separated out of the solution). If an anemic patient is euvolemic (eg, due to hemolysis of RBCs), pRBC transfusion is most appropriate, because the risk of hypervolemia can be avoided.

Plasma transfusions, with a COP of 20 mm Hg, are most appropriate in patients with coagulation abnormalities rather than hypoproteinemic patients. Although the COP of fresh frozen plasma or frozen plasma is comparable to normal plasma, the volume of plasma needed to significantly increase albumin by 1 mg/dL is large (eg, 45 mL/kg, IV) compared with the volume necessary to correct a coagulopathy (eg, 6–20 mL/kg, IV). This is usually cost prohibitive and increases the risk of fluid overload and triggering for future transfusion reactions.

Whole blood transfusions are indicated when both plasma and RBCs are required for transfusion. Whole blood also contains platelets; however, the number of platelets is not sufficient to support patients with severe thrombocytopenia. Also, platelet function within a unit of whole blood is negated once the unit has been refrigerated (Please see the article "Transfusion Medicine in Small Animals" elsewhere in this issue for more information). In patients with severe thrombocytopenia hemorrhaging into life-threatening tissue (eg, brain or lung), a whole blood transfusion or the use of lyophilized platelets may be indicated to attempt hemostasis.

Concentrated albumin solutions, including 25% HSA and CSA, have been used in critically ill canine and feline patients to help support blood pressure and to aid in the treatment of significant hypoalbuminemia. Studies have been published assessing the utility of HSA in the treatment of critically ill, hypoalbuminemic dogs and cats.[18–20] These studies are descriptive and retrospective; at the time of this publication, there is no published prospective, comparative study on the use of HSA in veterinary medicine. Studies assessing the use of HSA in healthy dogs have been published, however, and have unmasked the occurrence of hypersensitivity reactions in some dogs, including immediate anaphylactoid reactions and delayed events, including urticaria, vasculitis, lethargy, and edema 1 week postinfusion.[21,22] In addition, a study evaluating dogs that had received HSA revealed the presence of HSA autoantibodies in all dogs, increasing the risk for type III hypersensitivity reactions.[21,23] In critically ill dogs and cats receiving HSA, there were few reported hypersensitivity reactions, which may be due to their immunoparalyzed state. In these studies, dogs and cats with higher serum albumin levels were more likely to survive compared with those with lower serum albumins.[19,20] It is unknown if transfusing concentrated albumin solutions actually improves survival or if albumin is simply a marker of improved clinical outcome.

More recently, CSA has been produced and available through a national veterinary blood bank (Animal Blood Resources International, Dixon, California, and Stockbridge, Michigan; abrint.net). This may be a better, safer option with less risk for hypersensitivity reaction than with the human product. CSA is a lyophilized product and is currently sold in 5-g bottles at an estimated $125 per bottle. The published dose, based on company safety studies in healthy beagles, is 800 mg/kg to 844 mg/kg over 6 hours. (Animal Blood Resources International, package insert, lyophilized canine albumin; abrint.net) The use of CSA has been evaluated in a prospective, blinded, comparative study in dogs with septic peritonitis.[24] This study showed that CSA was safe in this population of dogs and caused an initial increase in serum albumin that was significantly different than the untreated dogs. At the time of discharge or death, however, there was no significant difference in serum albumin levels between the 2 groups. Some limitations to the study included a small population (n = 14 total dogs) and dogs receiving CSA were only administered 1 dose (eg, after surgical intervention for septic peritonitis). It is unknown if multiple dosing, if indicated, would improve albumin levels for a longer period of time, providing a prolonged duration of effect. In addition, the study was not powered to assess outcome, so it is still not known if there is a survival benefit or decreased hospitalization when dogs with septic peritonitis are administered CSA.

Based on these studies, the use of HSA should be reserved for critically ill veterinary patients with a life-threateningly low albumin (eg, septic peritonitis). It should not be routinely used for patients with a low COP; rather, a safer synthetic colloid, such as an HES, can be used. If considering use of an albumin source (rather than a synthetic colloid), the alternative use of CSA over HSA seems a safer option for use in dogs; however, it is unclear if the use of concentrated albumin products decrease hospitalization time or improve survival compared with dogs with similar disease that do not receive albumin products. A comparative, prospective veterinary study is required to more fully answer these questions.

SYNTHETIC COLLOIDS

Synthetic colloids, such as dextrans and HESs, are fluids that can be used to increase blood pressure and support COP. The HESs (eg, hetastarch, tetrastarch, and pentastarch) are most commonly used, because dextrans were found to induce renal disease in humans. In veterinary medicine, the use of synthetic colloids in the form of HES are most common, because they are readily available, inexpensive, and carry fewer potential side-effects compared with albumin.

HESs are esterified amylopectin-containing starches that remain in the intravascular space after administration due to its high MW. The differences between hetastarch, pentastarch, and tetrastarch are the average MW of the particles and the degree of substitution of glucose units on the starch particle with a hydroxyethyl group. Hetastarch (450 kDa) has the highest average MW, with pentastarch (260 kDa) and tetrastarch (130 kDa) having lower MWs. The MW of the product and the degree of substitution (hetastarch 0.5, pentastarch 0.45, and tetrastarch 0.4) determine the exerted COP of the fluid and the degradation time. The higher the substitution with hydroxyethyl groups, the longer the fluid persists in the intravascular space. Therefore, hetastarch lasts approximately 24 hours after administration, whereas pentastarch and tetrastarch lasts approximately 12 hours. Serum α-amylase degrades the HESs, and elimination occurs through the kidneys. When describing HES solutions, 3 numbers are used: the concentration of the HES solution, the MW, and the degree of substitution of hydroxyethyl groups/glucose unit.

Some key factors describing HES solutions include the following:

1. The concentration of HES solutions, commonly 6%, is iso-osmolar.
2. The higher the average MW of the HES solution, the longer the solution lasts, because larger molecules are more slowly degraded.
3. The degree of substitution of hydroxyethyl groups per glucose molecule is reported as a decimal percent. For example, hetastarch has a degree of substitution between 0.6 and 0.75, meaning that 60% to 75% of the glucose molecules contain a hydroxyethyl group at either the carbon-2 or carbon-6 position. The higher the degree of substitution, the longer the colloidal effects last, because the molecules are metabolized more slowly.

Side effects can also be seen with synthetic colloids and include influencing in vitro coagulation and increasing the potential for volume overload due to the efficacy of expanding intravascular volume. Coagulation abnormalities are more likely with the higher MW HES and at doses of greater than 20 mL/kg/d and include decreased circulating factor VIII and von Willebrand factor, platelet dysfunction, and decreased fibrin clot stabilization.[25] Clinical manifestation of coagulation abnormalities secondary to the use of high MW HES has not been reported in the veterinary literature. Synthetic colloid administration may be safer and more effective than using concentrated albumin solutions for the treatment of low COP due to lower risk of immune reactions and increased effectiveness as a colloid due to its variation in size (eg, molecules larger than albumin may not leak through vessels).

SUMMARY

Fluid therapy is essential in the treatment of emergent veterinary patients and includes crystalloid solutions, blood component therapy, concentrated albumin solutions, and synthetic colloids. Bolus IV fluid therapy can restore perfusion and stabilize critically ill and injured patients for further diagnostics and treatment. Synthetic colloids help to maintain COP and improve blood pressure but should be used with caution in coagulopathic patients or those with cardiac disease. Concentrated albumin solutions may have a role in the treatment of critically ill veterinary patients with severe hypoalbuminemia (eg, septic peritonitis); further prospective, comparative studies are needed to fully elucidate the role of albumin solutions in dogs and cats.

REFERENCES

1. Wellman ML, DiBartola SP, Kohn CW. Applied physiology of body fluids in dogs and cats. In: DiBartola SP, editor. Fluid, electrolyte and acid-base disorders in small animal practice. 3rd edition. St Louis (MO): Saunders- Elsevier; 2006. p. 3–26.
2. Rudloff E, Kirby R. Fluid therapy: crystalloids and colloids. Vet Clin North Am Small Anim Pract 1998;28(2):297–328.
3. Griffel MI, Kaufman BS. Pharmacology of colloids and crystalloids. Crit Care Clin 1992;8(2):235–53.
4. DiBartola SP, Bateman S. Introduction to fluid therapy. In: DiBartola SP, editor. Fluid, electrolyte, and acid-base disorders. 3rd edition. St Louis (MO): Saunders-Elsevier; 2006. p. 325–44.
5. Mathews KA. The various types of parenteral fluids and their indications. Vet Clin North Am Small Anim Pract 1998;28(3):483–513.
6. Silverstein DC, Aldrich J, Haskins SC, et al. Assessment of changes in blood volume in response to resuscitative fluid administration in dogs. J Vet Emerg Crit Care 2005;15(3):185–92.
7. Rozanski E, Rondeau M. Choosing fluids in traumatic hypovolemic shock: the role of crystalloids, colloids and hypertonic saline. J Am Anim Hosp Assoc 2002; 38(6):499–501.
8. Wingfield WE. Chapter 13 fluid and electrolyte therapy. In: Wingfield WE, Raffe MR, editors. The veterinary ICU Book. Jackson Hole (WY): Teton Newmedia; 2002. p. 170.
9. MacMillan KL. Neurological complications following treatment of canine hypoadrenocorticism. Can Vet J 2003;44(6):490–2.
10. Drobatz KJ, Cole SG. The influence of crystalloid fluid type on acid-base and electrolyte status of cats with urethral obstruction. J Vet Emerg Crit Care 2008; 18(4):355–61.
11. Rose BD. Ch 3: the proximal tubule. In: Clinical physiology of acid-base and electrolyte disorders. 4th edition. New York: Mc-Graw-Hill, Inc; 1994. p. 87.
12. Graefe U, Milutinovich J, Follette WC, et al. Less dialysis-induced morbidity and vascular instability with bicarbonate in dialysate. Ann Intern Med 1978;88: 332–6.
13. Walton RS, Wingfield WE, Ogilvie GK, et al. Energy expenditure in 104 Postoperative and traumatically injured dogs with indirect calorimetry. Vet Emerg Crit Care 1996;6(2):71–9.
14. O'Toole E, Miller CW, Wilson BA, et al. Comparison of the standard predictive equation for calculation of resting energy expenditure with indirect calorimetry in hospitalized and healthy dogs. J Am Vet Med Assoc 2004;225(1):58–64.
15. Culp AM, Clay ME, Baylor IA, et al. Colloid osmotic pressure and total solids measurements in normal dogs and cats. Abstract in: Proceedings of the 4th International Veterinary Emergency and Critical Care Symposium. San Antonio, Texas: Veterinary Emergency and Critical Care Society; 1994. p. 705.

16. Odunayo A, Kerl ME. Comparison of whole blood and plasma colloid osmotic pressure in healthy dogs. J Am Vet Emerg Crit Care 2011;21(3):236–41.
17. Brown SA, Dusza K, Boehmer J. Comparison of measured and calculated values for colloid osmotic pressure in hospitalized animals. Am J Vet Res 1994;55(7): 910–4.
18. Mathews K, Barry M. The use of 25% human serum albumin: outcome and efficacy in raising serum albumin and systemic blood pressure in critically ill dogs and cats. J Vet Emerg Crit Care 2005;15:110–8.
19. Trow A, Rozanski E, de Laforcade A, et al. Evaluation of the use of human albumin in critically ill dogs: 73 cases (2003-2006). J Vet Intern Med 2008;233:607–12.
20. Vigano F, Perissinotto L, Bosco V. Administration of 5% human serum albumin in critically ill small animal patients with hypoalbuminemia: 418 dogs and 170 cats (1994-2008). J Vet Emerg Crit Care 2010;20:237–43.
21. Martin L, Luther T, Alperin D, et al. Serum antibodies against human albumin in critically ill and healthy dogs. J Am Vet Med Assoc 2008;232:1004–9.
22. Cohn L, Kerl M, Lenox C, et al. Response of healthy dogs to infusions of human serum albumin. Am J Vet Res 2007;68:657–63.
23. Francis AH, Martin L, Haldorson G, et al. Adverse reactions suggestive of type III hypersensitivity in six healthy dogs given human albumin. J Am Vet Med Assoc 2007;320:873–9.
24. Craft EM, Powell LL. The use of canine-specific albumin in dogs with septic peritonitis. J Vet Emerg Crit Care 2012;22(6):631–9.
25. Chan DL. Colloids: current recommendations. Vet Clin North Am Small Anim Pract 2008;38(3):587–93.

Transfusion Medicine in Small Animals

Beth Davidow, DVM, DACVECC[a,b,*]

KEYWORDS

- Transfusion medicine • Red blood cells • Plasma • Platelets • Albumin • TRALI
- TACO • Transfusion reaction

KEY POINTS

- Transfusion medicine can be life saving and can be performed in veterinary clinics.
- Blood donors should be appropriately screened to minimize disease transmission.
- Blood typing is strongly recommended before transfusion in both dogs and cats.
- Crossmatching can be performed using gel technology.
- Red blood cell transfusions are the treatment of choice for anemia. Use of plasma is indicated for the treatment of active bleeding caused by coagulopathy. Other uses of plasma are controversial.
- Platelet transfusions can be used in small animal patients with active bleeding secondary to thrombocytopenia or thrombocytopathia.
- The use of human serum albumin is associated with a high risk of reactions.
- Reactions, both non–immune mediated and immune mediated, are a risk of transfusions.

Transfusions have been used as a life-saving modality for hundreds of years. The first documented transfusion in any species occurred in 1665 when Richard Lower withdrew blood from one dog and replaced it with blood from another dog. However, it was not until the 1950s that the use of transfusion medicine became more prominent in veterinary medicine because of the availability of equipment and techniques.[1] In the past 60 years, veterinary transfusion medicine has made remarkable advances. However, as knowledge has grown and the availability of different blood products has increased, transfusion therapy has become more complex. Availability of expanded donor screening, typing modalities, and crossmatching techniques make choosing the right donor unit for each patient potentially more complicated. Increased

Disclosures: The author has no funding sources or conflicts of interest to disclose.
[a] Animal Critical Care and Emergency Services, 11536 Lake City Way Northeast, Seattle, WA 98125, USA; [b] Department of Clinical Sciences, College of Veterinary Medicine, Washington State University, 100 Grimes Way ADBF 1020, Pullman, WA 99164-6610, USA
* Animal Critical Care and Emergency Services, 11536 Lake City Way Northeast, Seattle, WA 98125.
E-mail address: bdavidow@criticalcarevets.com

availability of different blood components gives the clinician more options to tailor therapy more appropriately while avoiding transfusion-related reactions. This article summarizes recent advances in veterinary transfusion medicine and provides the clinician with evidence to guide transfusion decision making.

BLOOD DONOR SCREENING

In human medicine, individual blood units are screened for infectious diseases. A limited number of diseases are screened because of test availability and cost. Careful interview of donors is used to minimize risk of other diseases. In the veterinary field, it is usually cost prohibitive to test individual units. Therefore, a combination of careful interview and blood screening of the donor is used to minimize the risk of infectious disease transmission.

In 2005, the American College of Veterinary Internal Medicine (ACVIM) Consensus Statement on infectious disease testing for blood donors was published.[2] Since publication, polymerase chain reaction (PCR) assays have become more readily available for many diseases of concern.[3] When positive, PCR assays indicate that the organism has been identified in the blood stream and active infection is present. False-negatives are possible if the organism is present only in small amounts, because only a small sample of blood is examined. Several veterinary diagnostic laboratories offer donor-screening PCR panels, which typically include at least *Ehrlichia* spp, *Babesia* spp, *Anaplasma* spp, and *Mycoplasma hemocanis* or *Mycoplasma haemofelis*. When assessing which screening tests to perform, it is important to evaluate whether the diseases included are transmitted in blood, are present in asymptomatic donors, are geographically appropriate, and whether the test specificity and sensitivity for pertinent infectious diseases is acceptable. **Table 1** gives general recommendations of clinicopathologic screening for dogs and cats.

ADVANCES IN BLOOD TYPING
Dogs

Different blood antigens have been known to exist in dogs since 1910 and antigen groups have been described since the 1940s.[4] Although approximately 20 antigen specificities in 13 groups were originally identified by researchers, only 6 of these

Table 1	
Recommended testing for canine and feline blood donors	
Canine Donors	**Feline Donors**
Blood type	Blood type
Complete blood count	Complete blood count
Chemistry panel	Chemistry panel
Fecal analysis	Fecal analysis
Heartworm antigen	FeLV
Babesia spp	FIV
Ehrlichia spp	*M haemofelis*
Neorickettsia spp	*Bartonella* spp
Bartonella spp	—
M hemocanis	*Ehrlichia, Anaplasma, Neorickettsia* spp (geographic)
Leishmania spp (geographic)	*Cytauxzoon felis* (geographic)
Trypanosoma cruzi (geographic)	
Brucella canis (breeding animals)	

Abbreviations: FeLV, feline leukemia; FIV, feline immunodeficiency virus.

antigens, dog erythrocyte antigen (DEA) 1.1, DEA 1.2, DEA 3, DEA 4, DEA 5, and DEA 7, can be routinely identified by typing.[5–7] A newer antigen, Dal, exists at high frequency in most dogs but is missing in some Dalmatians.[8] Antibodies against Dal in vitro seem to induce a strong agglutination reaction and could cause a severe transfusion reaction. Dal has been shown to be independent from known DEA antigens.[9] Dogs do not have natural antibodies to the DEA 1 system. It has been shown that natural antibodies are present in some dogs for DEA 3, DEA 5, and DEA 7, and in occasional dogs for less common antigens.[7,9,10] At present, a universal donor in dogs is considered to be negative for DEA 1.1, DEA 1.2, DEA 3, DEA 5, and DEA 7, and positive for DEA 4.

The DEA 1 system, with its allelic subtypes (DEA 1.1, DEA 1.2, and possibly DEA 1.3), is most important because of its high degree of antigenicity. Dogs that are DEA 1.1 negative do not react to DEA 1.1–positive blood on initial transfusion because of lack of natural antibodies to this allele. However, the second time a DEA 1.1–negative dog is given DEA 1.1–positive blood, it may develop a severe hemolytic reaction.[11] Likewise, natural antibodies to DEA 3, DEA 5, and DEA 7 can result in transfusion reactions that are usually mild or delayed; also, a significantly shorter survival time of the transfused red blood cells (RBCs) may be seen.[12]

In order to identify dogs that are true universal donors, typing must be done through a commercial laboratory (Animal Blood Resources International) rather than through point-of-care blood typing tests. Specific blood typing is done with polyclonal antibodies using a tube agglutination method. A gel column test using a monoclonal antibody against DEA 1.1 was developed; however, this is no longer commercially available. Research is ongoing to develop gel methodology for other DEA antigens. Availability of testing for DEA 3 and DEA 5 has been variable in recent years.

In-house typing kits are available; however, these only test for the most antigenic type system, DEA 1.1. Although this is typically beneficial for the emergent patient, it should not be used as a sole method for blood screening prospective donors. The most common in-house typing kits are the DMS card test (CARD; DMS Laboratories, NJ) and the Quick test DEA 1.1 (CHROM; Alvedia, France), both of which use different monoclonal anti–DEA 1.1 antibodies. The benefits of the CHROM testing system is that it is not affected by the presence of autoagglutination (ie, the agglutinates do not move across the test strip and therefore do not interfere with typing).[13] With the tube agglutination method or the CARD, autoagglutination can prevent accurate typing.

A recent study compared the gel column test, CARD, and CHROM tests in both healthy dogs and those who were sick, and found identical results in 69 of 88 samples (78%). In 6 cases, the CHROM result was DEA 1.1 negative, whereas the gel and CARD both were positive. In 18 cases, the CARD result was different from both the gel and CHROM, reading positive in 15 and negative in 3. Because of the disparity of results in these systems, it is strongly recommended that blood typing for donors be confirmed by an outside laboratory.[13] For recipients, it is better to use a test that has false-negative results, because this leads to a true DEA 1.1–positive dog receiving a negative blood unit, which is safe, rather than a test with a high false-positive rate, which could lead to true DEA 1.1–negative dog receiving a positive transfusion (after which a transfusion reaction is more apt to occur).

Cats

Cats are either type A, type B, or type AB. Recently, the MiK antigen has also been identified.[14] Note that there is no universal blood type in cats, and all cats must be tested before receiving any type of transfusion. Blood type is determined by 3 alleles, with A being dominant over the rare ab, which is dominant over b. Cats with a genotype A/A, A/ab, or A/b are type A, whereas only cats with b/b are type B. Rare AB cats are genotypically ab/ab or ab/b.

The distribution of these blood types varies geographically, with the highest incidence of B reported in Australia (36% in Sydney).[15] It was originally reported that 97% of cats in the United States were type A and that only 0.3% of cats in the northeast part of the United States were type B.[16] However, a 2005 study from the Animal Medical Center of New York City revealed a 6% incidence of the B blood type.[17] The B blood type is more common in certain exotic cat breeds, including Devon rex (41%), British shorthair (36%), Cornish rex (31%), exotic shorthair (27%), and Scottish fold (19%), but is also seen in domestic breed cats.[18] Type AB has been reported to occur in less than 1% of the general cat population. However, this incidence may be higher because new methodologies seem better at identifying these cats.[19]

Type A cats may have weak anti-B alloantibodies that can cause shortened RBC survival if a B donor is used. However, type B cats have strong anti-A antibodies and can have a fatal reaction from as little as 1 mL of transfused type A blood.[20] Type AB cats have no alloantibodies against either type A or B blood in their sera; they should receive either AB or A blood products if they need a transfusion because of the strong anti-A antibodies present in B serum. Most cats have MiK antigen but, in cats that do not, naturally occurring antibodies can lead to a hemolytic transfusion reaction with a first-time transfusion.

Original typing for cats was done using serum from type B cats with strong anti-A antibodies to identify type A cats. Anti-B antibodies are weaker in A serum but lectin from *Triticum vulgaris* reacts strongly with type B antigen.[21] At present, there are 2 commercially available in-house typing kits for cats (Rapid®-VetH Feline, DMS Laboratories, Flemington, NJ [CARD] and Quick test A+B, Alvedia, France [CHROM]). Both kits use monoclonal antibodies against type A and type B. In a recent study comparing typing methodologies in cats, the gold standard tube agglutination test, CARD, and CHROM gave identical results in 52 of 58 cats (89.7%). Overall, the CARD had 91.4% accuracy and CHROM had an overall accuracy of 94.8%. In 2 of the 6 cats with discordant resultants, feline leukemia (FeLV) infection was present.[22] It is recommended that B and AB cats be confirmed by a second method or through an outside laboratory.[19,22] At present, there is no in-house typing system available for the MiK antigen.

Blood typing is recommended before all transfusions in both dogs and cats. In an emergent situation in which time for blood typing is precluded, DEA 1.1–negative blood can be given to a dog of unknown type safely. However, typing and use of DEA 1.1–specific blood is recommended whenever possible to maximize the efficient use of canine blood donors that can be used. In cats, there are no universal donors and cats must always be blood typed before transfusion to prevent a life-threatening reaction.

CROSSMATCHING

In-house crossmatching can be used when blood typing is not available. It can also be used in conjunction with blood typing results. In dogs, crossmatching is recommended if transfusion history is unknown, if a hemolytic reaction is noted during a first transfusion, if more than 7 days has lapsed between administration of transfusions, or if the donor DEA 7 type is unknown.[7,23] In the past, crossmatching was recommended in dogs that had previously been pregnant. However, a recent study showed that pregnancy does not seem to sensitize dogs to antigens on RBCs.[8] In cats, both typing and crossmatching should be strongly considered before an initial transfusion, because of the identification of antigens such as MiK with naturally occurring antibodies and the potential for a potential fatal transfusion reaction (eg, when type A blood is given to a type B cat). In addition, because in-house typing methodologies are not perfect, both typing and crossmatching on the first transfusion helps to identify any missed type incompatibilities in cats.[7]

Crossmatching has historically been done using a manual procedure that includes both a wash and an incubation step. **Box 1** gives a description of the crossmatching technique.[24] The procedure is time consuming and interpretation has been shown to be operator dependent. Gel crossmatch technology has recently been developed. One benefit is that the gels can be saved to show to others for verification (vs blood typing cards, which dry up). Gel technology also requires less blood than a standard crossmatch (0.5 mL vs 2–3 mL). In addition, the gel crossmatch can be used even if the patient is autoagglutinating.[25] The gel allows agglutinates to be trapped in a matrix but free cells to sink to the bottom, allowing easier interpretation of compatibility. A gel system for companion animals is available for both major and minor crossmatches (RapidVet®-H, DMS Laboratories Inc., NJ) **Fig. 1**.[9]

TRANSFUSION COLLECTION AND ADMINISTRATION

Whole blood can be collected for transfusion in many hospitals when proper bags and preservatives are available. Dogs and cats should be appropriately screened and a full physical examination should be performed before to each donation to ensure general health and lack of ectoparasites. If sedatives are necessary (typically required for cats), acepromazine should be avoided because of potential effects on platelet function. Blood is usually drawn from the jugular vein once the area has been aseptically prepped (to avoid contamination of the blood product). Dogs can safely donate 15 to 20 mL/kg, whereas cats can donate 10 to 15 mL/kg (lean body weight).

Blood should ideally be collected with the use of an anticoagulant preservative (eg, citrate-phosphate-dextrose-adenine [CPDA-1], Adsol) at a ratio of 1 mL of anticoagulant per 9 mL of blood.[24] Note that blood cannot be stored in syringes long-term,

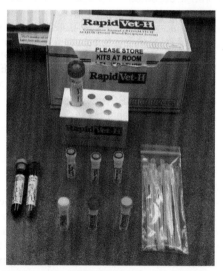

Fig. 1. Gel crossmatch kit for use in both dogs and cats. (*Courtesy of* RapidVet®-H Feline/ DMS Laboratories, Inc., Flemington, NJ; with permission.)

Box 1
Crossmatching technique

1. Obtain blood in both ethylenediamine tetraacetic acid (EDTA) tube (purple top) and in a nonadditive tube (red top) from both donor and recipient. If using a stored RBC unit, use one of the provided tags and empty the sample into a red-top tube to spin.

2. Centrifuge and separate plasma and serum from the RBCs. Save the removed serum in a separate tube. Discard the plasma from the EDTA tube.

3. Wash the RBCs from the EDTA tube (purple top).

   a. Place the RBC in a second tube 12 × 75 mm and fill three-quarters full with saline.

   b. Centrifuge for 1 minute, decant the saline, and repeat 3 times, removing the supernatant the last time.

4. Resuspend the cells to make a 2% to 4% solution (0.2 mL of blood in 4.8 mL of saline gives a 4% solution).

5. Label tubes to make the following mixtures:

   a. Major crossmatch: 2 drops patient serum with 1 drop donor RBC suspension

   b. Minor crossmatch: 1 drop patient RBC suspension with 2 drops donor serum

   c. Control: 1 drop patient RBC suspension with 1 drop patient serum

6. Incubate for 15 to 30 minutes at 37°C.

7. Centrifuge for 15 seconds.

8. Interpretation of results:

   a. If either hemolysis or hemagglutination is seen macroscopically, or if agglutination is seen microscopically, the donor is not a good match

Modified from Lanevschi A, Wardrop KJ. Principles of transfusion medicine in small animals. Can Vet J 2001;42:447–54.

---

and should only be stored if collected aseptically into sealed, gas-diffusible blood bags.

The process of transfusion administration can potentially affect the survival of the RBCs, and technique, use of delivery system, and filter use must be correct when transfusing a patient. All blood products should be warmed to body temperature before administration. Plasma should be thawed by double bagging the product and placing in a warm water bath. Microwaves should not be used to thaw or warm blood products because of potential RBC or protein damage. RBCs should ideally be administered through a large-bore peripheral catheter (ideally >22 gauge). Initial administration of transfusions should be done slowly (eg, 0.5–1 mL/kg/h for the first 15 minutes) to monitor for an acute reaction, time permitting. Vital signs should be monitored every 15 minutes during the first hour and every 30 to 60 minutes thereafter. All transfusions should be administered within 4 hours, to prevent increased risk of bacterial contamination of the unit.[7]

In 2011, a study showed a significant decrease in the short-term probability of RBC survival in those canine blood transfusions administered with either a volumetric or syringe pump.[26] However, a similar study in cats showed no loss of RBCs with the use of a syringe pump and HemoNate filter.[27] As a result of these studies, the author recommends that canine packed RBCs (pRBCs) be given through an in-line blood filter but not through a fluid pump. Feline pRBCs can be given using a syringe and HemoNate filter.

If available, leukoreduction (the process by which white blood cells [WBCs] are removed from an RBC unit) can be considered. Leukocytes in stored pRBCs can lead to release of inflammatory compounds such as histamine and plasminogen activator inhibitor-1, potentially predisposing to transfusion reaction.[28] The benefit of leukoreduction is that it can decrease the incidence of nonhemolytic transfusion reactions and the immunomodulation that has been seen after transfusion in some human patients.[28] Leukoreduction can be performed either before storage or at the time of administration, and is also available for purchase through commercial blood banks as leukoreduced pRBC (Hemosolutions, Colorado Springs, CO).

The process of leukoreduction is now more readily available for canine blood, and has been shown to be associated with smaller increases in WBCs, fibrinogen, and C-reactive protein levels in recipients than with than nonleukoreduced transfusions.[28] A pilot study was recently done with feline RBC; however, the use of the neonatal leukoreduction filters resulted in loss of 8 mL of blood and may not be justified at this time.[29]

BLOOD COMPONENTS

The appropriate use of blood components allows more specific treatment while avoiding the risks of giving the unnecessary parts of the blood.[30] Component therapy is a more efficient way of using blood resources, allowing 1 donated unit to be split into multiple products (which may then benefit more than 1 patient). For example, a chronically anemic FeLV-positive cat may only require RBCs rather than whole blood (WB), provided the patient is not coagulopathic or thrombocytopenic. Likewise, a coagulopathic patient secondary to long-acting anticoagulant toxicosis may not be clinically anemic, and may only require fresh frozen plasma (FFP) or frozen plasma (FP) rather than WB, thereby saving the RBCs for another patient.

Appropriate storage of blood components is also necessary to allow efficient and maximal use of blood products. For example, the storage of component therapy (eg, FFP and pRBCs) allows longer storage time (compared with WB alone).[31,32] Available blood products, storage times, and indications for use are summarized in **Table 2**.[33–35]

RBC PRODUCTS

RBCs are indicated for the treatment of anemia. Anemia is defined as a deficiency of RBCs or hemoglobin (Hb). Anemic animals are usually pale, exercise intolerant, weak, tachypneic, and potentially tachycardiac and hypotensive (consistent with hemorrhagic shock). These clinical signs of anemia are related to decreased oxygen delivery (Do_2), because Hb plays a significant role in delivering oxygen to cells. This is explained in the formula for Do_2:

$$Do_2 = \text{cardiac output} \times \text{oxygen content of blood } (Cao_2)$$

$$Cao_2 = [(Pao_2 \times 0.003) + (Sao_2 \times Hb \times 1.34)]$$

$$CO = \text{stroke volume} \times \text{heart rate}$$

Sao_2 is arterial oxygen concentration.

The transfusion trigger is the Hb level at which an animal's Do_2 has decreased enough that anaerobic metabolism occurs. In critically ill humans, transfusions are recommended at a Hb level of 7 g/dL (approximate hematocrit [HCT] of 21%) unless

Table 2
Summary of Blood Components

Blood Product	Definition	Composition	Stability	Indications for Use	Other Information	Dose
WB	Blood pulled from a donor with no processing	RBCs, WBCs, platelets, all components of plasma	In 1–6°C refrigerator, 28 d in CPDA-1, 30 d in ACD	Massive blood loss, need for multiple components	Platelets lose activity after refrigeration, must be used within 4–6 h if not refrigerated	Transfusion amount (mL) = (PCV$_{desired}$ − PCV$_{current}$)/PCV$_{donor}$ × blood volume (mL/kg) × wt (kg) Blood volume dog = 88 mL/kg, Blood volume cat = 66 mL/kg
Packed RBCs	RBCs centrifuged and most of the plasma removed	RBCs, may have some WBCs	In 1–6°C refrigerator: 20 d in CPDA-1, 35 d in CPDA-1 with Optisol or Nutricel, 37 d in CPDA-1 with Adsol 37 d in CPDA in 1–6°C refrigerator	Anemia	—	
Leukoreduced RBCs	Packed RBCs where WBC have been removed before storage	RBCs		Anemia; leukoreduction may reduce immunomodulation and nonhemolytic febrile reactions	—	
PRP	Plasma and platelets separated from RBCs using a soft spin	Platelets, plasma	5 d in gas-diffusible bags with constant agitation at 22°C	Severe thrombocytopenia or thrombocytopathia with active hemorrhage or need for an invasive procedure	—	1 unit per 10 kg
Platelet concentrate	Further centrifugation of PRP to have a smaller volume or platelets obtained via plateletpheresis	Platelets, plasma	5 d in gas-diffusible bags with constant agitation at 22°C	Severe thrombocytopenia or thrombocytopathia with active hemorrhage or need for an invasive procedure	—	1 unit per 10 kg

Product	Description	Contains	Storage	Indication	Dose
Frozen platelets	Platelet concentrate created by plateletpheresis and then frozen using DMSO for platelet stability	Platelets	6 mo at −20 to −30°C	Severe thrombocytopenia or thrombocytopathia with active hemorrhage or need for an invasive procedure	1 unit per 10 kg
Lyophilized platelets	Platelet concentrate created by plateletpheresis, aldehyde cross-linked for platelet stability and then lyophilized	Platelets	2 y in refrigerator	Severe thrombocytopenia or thrombocytopathia with active hemorrhage or need for an invasive procedure	Research product in development
FFP	Plasma separated from WB and frozen within 8 h; <1 y of age	Coagulation factors, anticoagulation factors such at antithrombin, alpha-macroglobulin, albumin	1 y in freezer maintained at −20 to −30°C	Coagulation disorders resulting in active hemorrhage or as prophylaxis before invasive surgery in an animal with a known significant clotting factor deficiency	Potential use for treatment of severe necrotizing pancreatitis, DIC
FP	Plasma separated from WB but not frozen completely within 8 h or plasma that has been frozen >1 y but <4 y	Contains stable coagulation factors II, VII, IX, X, albumin	5 y in freezer maintained at −20 to −30°C	Coagulation deficiencies, specifically of II, VII, IX, or X resulting in active hemorrhage	10–30 mL/kg, higher dose for vWF
Cryoprecipitate-poor plasma	Supernatant that remains after preparation of cryoprecipitate	Contains stable coagulation factors II, VII, IX, X, anticoagulant, and fibrinolytic factors, albumin	1 y from original collection date in freezer maintained at −20 to −30°C	Coagulation deficiencies of II, VII, IX, or X resulting in active hemorrhage that does not require vWF	10–15 mL/kg

—

(continued on next page)

Table 2
(continued)

Blood Product	Definition	Composition	Stability	Indications for Use	Other Information	Dose
Cryoprecipitate	The precipitate containing cold insoluble proteins, formed when FFP is slowly thawed and spun	Contains concentrated vWF, VIII, XIII, fibrinogen, and fibronectin	10 mo when stored at −20°C or colder	When active hemorrhage from specific deficiency in vWF and VIII, or as prophylaxis when invasive procedure needed for animal with known deficiency of one of these factors	—	1 unit per 10 kg
Albumin	Protein is extracted from pooled plasma	Albumin	3 y at 20–24°C	Treatment of hypotension or hypovolemia in the septic patient with severe hypoalbuminemia	Both canine and HSA available; only canine albumin should be used ideally in canine patients because of risk of reaction from human product	Albumin deficit = 0.3 × BW (kg) × 10 × (albumin desired − current albumin)
IVIG	Pooled IgG extracted from multiple human B9 donors	IgG	36 mo in refrigerator at 1–6°C	Treatment of immune disease	Monitor carefully for type I, III reactions	0.5 g/kg

Abbreviation: ACD, Acid-citrate-dextrose.

the patient has clinically significant heart disease, in which case a level of 10 g/dL (approximate HCT of 30%) is recommended.[36] Although the appropriate veterinary transfusion trigger has not been well studied or identified, animal data suggest that an HCT of 15% to 18% may be a reasonable guideline.[7,37] However, animals with low volume or poor contractility may require a higher Hb to maintain Do_2.

Fresh WB (FWB) has been the most common blood product traditionally used in veterinary medicine, because it is readily available to clinicians (often from an in-house donor or pet). WB is indicated when the patient is anemic, has a blood volume loss of more than 50%, or when the patient requires multiple components of blood (eg, RBC, clotting factors, platelets).[24] If WB is used before refrigeration, it is a good source of functional platelets.[38] One 500-mL unit of FWB obtained from a canine donor is estimated to contain 7×10^{10} platelets. Once refrigerated, platelet function decreases dramatically (discussed later). Recent work in human trauma has shown that maintaining the ratio of plasma, platelets, and RBCs close to 1:1:1 significantly improves the outcome in cases with large-volume blood loss.[39]

The amount of WB to administer can be calculated using the following formula[7]:

$$\text{Transfusion amount (mL)} = (PCV_{desired} - PCV_{current})/PCV_{donor} \times \text{blood volume (mL/kg)} \times \text{wt (kg)}$$

where PCV is packed cell volume.

pRBCs are indicated when blood volume is normal (eg, as shown clinically by a normal total protein) but the animal requires oxygen carrying capacity (eg, Hb). This is typically seen clinically when the anemia is caused by lack of production (eg, lack of erythropoietin, aplastic anemia), or a destructive process (eg, hemolysis).[24] Component therapy (eg, use of pRBC and FFP together) can be used to replace significant blood loss if the patient's platelet count is adequate and a WB donor is not available. The dose of pRBC can be calculated as listed for WB. When using pRBC with a PCV of approximately 60%, the formula: 1.5 mL × desired % increase in PCV × BW (kg), where *BW* is body weight, provides an accurate volume to administer.[40]

PLASMA PRODUCTS

Plasma contains albumin, globulins, clotting proteins, and anticoagulants. It can be stored and separated into many products. Indications for plasma use are debated in both human and veterinary medicine.[30,41] Plasma has been proved to be effective in actively bleeding patients with documented coagulation factor defects.[42] When dosing plasma products, a general guideline is 10 to 20 mL/kg. For example, a dose of 10 to 20 mL/kg of FFP is recommended for coagulopathic patients suffering from factor deficiency from vitamin K antagonist rodenticide toxicity,[35] whereas slightly higher doses (15–30 mL/kg) are needed to provide adequate factors to reverse coagulopathy from von Willebrand disease (vWD) or hemophilia A in dogs.[43]

The use of adequate dosing of plasma has also been proved, in humans, to be critical in preventing the dilutional coagulopathy that occurs with massive RBC transfusions.[39] As previously mentioned, studies in both civilian and military human patients with trauma have shown that 30-day survival is increased when maintaining a 1:1 ratio of plasma to RBC transfusion in massively transfused patients.[39,44–46]

Plasma is often administered to patients with increased coagulation parameters (but no active bleeding) before invasive procedures. However, there are no studies in human or veterinary medicine proving plasma's efficacy in prevention of hemorrhage.[42,47] Most human studies evaluating liver biopsies have found no association between coagulation times and the risk of bleeding.[48,49] One human study showed a mild increase in risk of hemorrhage with hyperbilirubinemia and a severely increased international normalized ratio (INR).[50] A single veterinary study showed that the risk of hemorrhage after liver biopsy was more associated with platelet count than either prothrombin (PT) or activated partial thromboplastin time (PTT). The author recommends that the use of prophylactic plasma only be reserved for those patients with significant coagulopathy or those with documented severe factor deficiency undergoing a significant procedure (eg, splenectomy).

The use of FFP for the treatment of both hypercoagulability and hypocoagulability associated with disseminated intravascular coagulation (DIC) is controversial.[30] A study of dogs with severe illness and decreased antithrombin (AT) levels showed maintenance of AT with administered FFP; however, AT levels were not maintained when FFP was given with concurrent heparin.[51] There have been no prospective studies of dose or timing of FFP administration with DIC.

Plasma has also been used in patients with severe pancreatitis to help replace alpha-macroglobulins and maintain albumin levels, because survival in humans is known to be decreased in patients with low alpha-macroglobulin.[52] However, no benefit was seen compared with the control group when plasma was given to human patients with pancreatitis, even though an increase in alpha-macroglobulin levels was seen.[53] However, the control group comprised patients receiving colloid support in the form of albumin; so it is unknown whether colloid support from the albumin may still be useful for patients with pancreatitis. In veterinary medicine, a recent canine retrospective study evaluated the use of FFP with pancreatitis[54]; no improvement in mortality was seen with plasma administration. However, albumin levels were not reported before or after treatment of either group.

Hypoalbuminemia is also a controversial indication for plasma transfusion. Low albumin levels have been correlated with increased mortality in both humans and animals.[55,56] Albumin plays a key role in the body, because it makes up 70% to 80% of colloid osmotic pressure (COP), acts as a primary carrier molecule (eg, for medications), is important for the removal of bacterial toxins and free radicals, acts as a buffer, helps maintain microvascular integrity, and reduces platelet aggregation.[55] Despite the numerous theoretic benefits, exogenous albumin supplementation has not been proved to improve survival in human or veterinary medicine. Several large meta-analyses have examined human trials of albumin administration and found no overall benefit.[57,58] In a large trial of 6997 people resuscitated with either crystalloids or 5% albumin, there was a trend toward worse outcome with the use of albumin in patients with trauma[59] and no benefit in patients with burns.[57] However, a current meta-analysis found evidence for benefit of resuscitation with an albumin-containing fluid in human patients with sepsis.[60]

If plasma is used to increase serum albumin, 22.5 mL/kg is needed to raise the serum albumin by 0.5 g/dL if there is no ongoing loss. However, in one canine study evaluating FFP transfusions, no increase in albumin level was seen with average administration rates of 15 to 18 mL/kg.[41] Concentrated albumin may be more effective in animals with severely low albumin and concurrent peripheral edema. Synthetic colloids may be as or more effective in raising the COP in hypoalbuminemic animals.

Available plasma products include FFP, FP, cryoprecipitate, cryoprecipitate-poor plasma (CPP), human serum albumin (HSA), canine albumin, and intravenous immunoglobulin (IVIG). Each is discussed later in further detail; readers are also referred to the article "Fluid Therapy for the Emergent Small Animal Patient" by Elisa elsewhere in this issue for additional information.

FFP is plasma that has been separated from RBCs and frozen within 8 hours of collection of the blood. It contains all the coagulation factors, along with anticoagulants, fibrinogen, fibronectin, albumin, and alpha-macroglobulin. FFP is considered fresh when frozen at −40°C for 1 year.[35] Coagulation factors are defined as either labile or nonlabile, based on their activity with storage. Labile clotting factors include factors V and VIII, whereas nonlabile factors generally include the vitamin K-dependent factors II, VII, IX, and X.

FP is plasma that has been separated from RBC and frozen greater than 8 hours after blood collection or when FFP is more than 12 months old but less than 5 years of age.[7] The labile coagulation factors and anticoagulants are not consistently active but the nonlabile coagulation factors (eg, vitamin K–dependent factors) are readily available, making it the transfusion treatment of choice for a coagulopathic patient secondary to long-acting anticoagulant rodenticide toxicosis. Likewise, it can potentially be used as source of albumin.

Cryoprecipitate is made by slow thawing and centrifugation of FFP. The supernatant is removed and the remaining slush/sediment, which contains cold insoluble proteins, is a concentrated form of factor VIII, von Willebrand factor (vWF), and fibrinogen. The cryoprecipitate can then be refrozen and is good for 10 months from the date of the initial blood draw.[61] Cryoprecipitate is the preferred treatment of prophylactic or active bleeding in dogs with hemophilia A or vWD.[43,62] Recommendations for dosing are 1 unit of cryoprecipitate for every 10 kg of body weight. Although FFP can also be used, the administration of cryoprecipitate allows a more concentrated amount of desirable factors versus the administration of much larger amounts of FFP to accomplish the same goal. Lyophilized (freeze-dried) canine cryoprecipitate is now commercially available (ABRI, Dixon, CA).

CPP is the supernatant removed in the process of making cryoprecipitate.[7] This plasma can be refrozen for 12 months and is a source of the nonlabile clotting factors II, VII, IX, and X; thus, CPP can be used to treat anticoagulant rodenticide toxicosis. It is also a source of albumin, although large amounts are required to increase the albumin. Dosing is similar to that for FFP or FP for coagulopathy.

Albumin can be extracted from plasma to make a concentrated product. Concentrated HSA has been used in both canine and feline patients with extremely low albumin levels (typically secondary to septic peritonitis, and so forth).[63–65] Doses for canine administration have been extrapolated from human medicine, and recommendations vary. A simple formula is 1.5 g/kg or the albumin deficit can be calculated as grams $= 10 \times$ (albumin desired – albumin current) $\times$ kg $\times 0.3$.[66] This volume should be started slowly to monitor for reactions and then slowly titrated based on the stability of the patient. Although several articles have shown safety with HSA in sick patients, 2 healthy dogs died when given HSA in a research trial; this was caused by severe type III hypersensitivity reactions and development of profound vasculitis and membranoproliferative glomerulonephritis.[67] In addition, a follow-up study showed that even sick, potentially immunocompromised canine patients developed significant antibodies to HSA after administration.[68] With the current availability of canine albumin, the use of a potentially antigenic human product is not recommended.

Canine albumin is available (ABRI, Dixon, CA) as a lyophilized product. Each bottle contains 5 g of albumin, and typically ranges from $125 to $175. Canine albumin dosing can be calculated as listed for human albumin. Canine albumin is generally considered to be safer than HSA because of less immunogenicity. Initial safety studies have shown no signs of reactions in 6 dogs who received the product weekly for 4 weeks.[69]

Human immunoglobulin (IVIG) is polyvalent immunoglobulin G (IgG) that has been extracted and pooled from the plasma from multiple donors. It has been used in veterinary medicine to treat multiple immune diseases, including immune-mediated thrombocytopenia (ITP), immune-mediated hemolytic anemia, nonregenerative anemias, cutaneous diseases, polyradiculoneuritis, myasthenia gravis, and sudden acquired retinal degeneration.[70–73] As with HSA, it is derived from humans, so antibody formation and type III hypersensitivity reactions are risks with its use in veterinary patients.[70] Type I hypersensitivity reactions and hypercoagulability are additional risks. Dosing for IVIG is extrapolated from human medicine, and is currently recommended at 0.5 g/kg.[70,72]

Specific clotting factors and anticoagulants are also extracted from human plasma and made into concentrates but these products are not yet used or produced in veterinary medicine. Examples include concentrates of factor VII, VIII, IX, and antithrombin.[74]

PLATELET PRODUCTS

Until recently, platelet transfusions were not viable, readily available options in veterinary medicine. Recent advances in platelet storage may make platelet transfusion more readily accessible to veterinarians, including the availability of lyophilized platelets. However, there are limited publications in veterinary medicine about triggers for prophylaxis or therapeutic efficacy of platelet products in actively bleeding patients.[75–78]

In humans, platelets are recommended for prophylaxis in any patient with a count less than 10,000/μL[74,79] and in patients who require an invasive procedure with counts less than 50,000/μL. Platelets are also recommended in patients with drug or hereditary impairments of platelet function that require an invasive procedure. In actively bleeding patients, the use of therapeutic platelet transfusions is also warranted with platelet counts less than 20,000/μL.[74,79] With ITP, the use of platelet transfusions is controversial because of the rapid destruction of any administered platelet unless the patient has evidence of life-threatening bleeding (eg, spinal cord bleed, bleeding into the brain).[74]

The risk of bleeding with severe thrombocytopenia is affected by the degree of anemia. RBCs scavenge nitric oxide, which leads to increases in platelet activity. In addition, high hematocrit values push platelets toward the endothelium and reduce sheer stress.[80] In cases of moderate thrombocytopenia and concurrent anemia, the risk of bleeding is potentially lessened with pRBC transfusion alone.

As previously discussed, FWB is the product most veterinarians have available to them to supply a limited number of platelets. A dose of 10 mL/kg of FWB is expected to raise the platelet count about 10,000/μLl, which is generally considered to be minimal; however, this may be life saving with severe thrombocytopenia.[75]

The advantage of FWB is that no platelets are lost, compared with component therapy production. In addition, the platelets are less activated than platelets obtained via centrifugation for concentrate.[76] FWB at room temperature is considered safe for use for 4 to 8 hours. Refrigeration of human platelets, either in WB or in platelet concentrate, rapidly leads to platelet aggregation and activation. In addition, refrigerated platelet survival is half that of platelets held at room temperature.[81] This effect is caused by clustering of the vWF receptors in response to temperature, leading to increased clearance by hepatic macrophages.[82] No studies have been done of canine refrigerated platelets to confirm whether a similar response occurs.[76] However, refrigeration of FWB should be avoided if used primarily for platelet transfusion.

Fresh platelet concentrate has traditionally been made by using a soft spin of WB, which separates the platelets into the plasma component. This technique allows appropriate allocation of component therapy and minimizes the volume or component of transfusion products that the patient may be receiving unnecessarily. After a soft spin, the plasma is expressed into a separate bag, and this plasma is then known as platelet-rich plasma (PRP). The PRP is spun again to create a platelet concentrate and the plasma is removed and stored as FFP.[7,74] One unit of platelet concentrate is the amount made from 1 unit (500 mL) of WB but contains fewer platelets. Studies have shown average in vivo platelet recovery of 80%.[83,84] The dose is normally calculated as 1 unit/10 kg.

Fresh platelet concentrate can also be made through plateletpheresis. In this process, blood is taken from the donor and split into components (using an apheresis machine). During plateletpheresis, platelets are retained and the remaining volume is returned to the donor. The process is time consuming for the donor; however, large amount of platelets can be collected in this manner (eg, typically $1–4 \times 10^{11}$ platelets). This amount is typically 4 to 6 times the amount collected in a centrifuged platelet concentrate. Plateletpheresis also allows maximum sterility of the product. In addition, during plateletpheresis, there is negligible WBC and RBC contamination, minimizing potential transfusion reaction. Fresh platelets must be stored in gas-soluble bags at room temperature with constant agitation to remain active. Bacterial contamination is a concern at room temperature and storage is limited to 5 days.[76,85,86]

Frozen platelet concentrate is made by stabilizing apheresed platelets with 6% Dimethyl sulfoxide (DMSO) or with 2% DMSO and Thrombosol.[83] Canine platelet recovery (after freezing with 6% DMSO at $-62°C$ [$-80°F$]) was shown to be 70% with a half-life of 2 days versus 3.5 days for fresh platelets.[87] The platelets were effective in halting active bleeding in thrombocytopenic dogs.[88] A more recent study comparing 6% DMSO with 2% DMSO and Thrombosol showed only 49% and 44% platelet recovery, respectively. Platelet half-life was confirmed to be about 2 days.[83] Frozen platelet concentrate with 6% DMSO is commercially available in veterinary medicine (ABRI, Dixon, CA). Dosing is recommended at 1 unit/10 kg of body weight given over 4 hours (see package insert for further information).

Lyophilized platelets (LYO) are an experimental product still undergoing research. Canine LYO are not yet commercially available but research is ongoing. Platelets are stabilized using a mild aldehyde cross-linking of membrane proteins and lipids, and then lyophilized and reconstituted with preservation of platelet structure and function. LYO can be stored for up to 24 months in the refrigerator, and can be reconstituted with saline immediately before use.[89] Research studies on LYO have shown that they bind to collagen, vWF and damaged endothelium. Receptors are activated normally and bind fibrinogen.[90] These platelets also retain the ability to increase procoagulant activity.[89] In a study of dogs on cardiac bypass, infusion of the LYO product led to improvement in venous bleeding time that was most pronounced at 20 to 30 minutes after infusion.[91]

A prospective, multicenter trial studied the use of fresh platelet concentrate (FRESH) and LYO in 37 dogs with active bleeding and thrombocytopenia. In this study, 22 dogs received LYO and 15 received FRESH. The incidence of transfusion reaction was low in both groups, and there was no difference in hospitalization time or mortality between the groups. The use of LYO seemed to be safe in dogs but larger studies are needed to study efficacy.[77] LYO products may also be used as hemostatic agents even if platelet numbers and function are normal. In a recent study, 20 swine were subjected to liver injury and then treated with either a placebo or LYO. Overall, 80% survived in the LYO group, whereas only 20% survived in the placebo group. One pig had evidence of thrombi in other locations on necropsy, indicating the need for further evaluation before these products are used in clinical patients.[92]

RISKS OF TRANSFUSION PRODUCTS

With administration of any type of blood product, the benefits and potential risks must be evaluated. Although potentially life saving, transfusions can result in acute or delayed reactions. Reactions have been reported to occur in 8% to 13% of pRBC transfusions in dogs and cats.[17,31] **Table 3** shows a list of non–immune-mediated and immune-related transfusion reactions.

Transfusion-associated circulatory overload (TACO) and nonhemolytic febrile reactions are the most common reactions seen in dogs and cats.[93,94] Most blood products cause significant oncotic pull, which is more pronounced with those containing albumin (eg, WB, FFP), which can be useful in animals that have severe peripheral edema or in animals that are severely hypotensive; however, volume overload with resultant pulmonary edema is a potential risk in those animals that are already normovolemic. Blood pressure should be monitored while administering blood products and patients should be appropriately monitored for signs of volume overload (eg, tachypnea, weight gain, hemodilution, serous nasal discharge, development of pulmonary edema or pleural effusion).

Nonhemolytic febrile reactions are defined as a temperature increase of 1 to 2°C within 1 to 2 hours of a transfusion. Nonhemolytic reactions are usually caused by antibody reactions against donor leukocyte or platelet antigens and are greatly reduced when leukoreduction filters are used before storage of blood. It is important to monitor patients carefully, because fever may also be an early indicator of a more severe reaction (eg, hemolytic reaction, sepsis). If a nonhemolytic febrile reaction is suspected, slowing of the transfusion or drug administration may be warranted.

Transfusion-related acute lung injury (TRALI) is the leading cause of transfusion-related mortality in human medicine. TRALI manifests clinically as respiratory distress with severe noncardiogenic edema within 24 hours of transfusion and is seen mostly in patients receiving multiple plasma transfusions.[94] In human medicine, the development of TRALI is associated with use of plasma from female donors, particularly those who are parturient. The use of plasma from male donors, plasma from women who have never been pregnant, or from plasma that has been screened for the presence of WBC antibodies greatly decreases the incidence of TRALI.[94,95] In veterinary medicine, it is unclear whether TRALI occurs. RBC alloantibodies do not seem to be increased in dogs with repeated pregnancies but WBC alloantibodies have not been studied.[96] The incidence of parturient canine blood donors is typically rare in veterinary medicine, so TRALI may also be rare.

Type I hypersensitivity can also occur with any type of blood product and includes pruritus and angioedema, and can progress to bronchoconstriction and hypotension.

Table 3	
Types of transfusion reactions	
Immunologic Reactions	**Nonimmunologic Reactions**
Allergic reactions (type I hypersensitivity)	Sepsis
Hemolytic reactions	Citrate toxicity: hypocalcemia
Nonhemolytic febrile reactions	TACO
TRALI	Hyperammonemia
TRIM	Hypothermia
Decreased RBC survival	Hypophosphatemia
—	Hyperkalemia
—	Infectious disease transmission

Abbreviations: TACO, transfusion-associated circulatory overload; TRALI, transfusion-related acute lung injury; TRIM, transfusion-related immunomodulation.

It has recently been found that humans with preexisting allergic conditions such as atopy seem to be more at risk.[94]

SUMMARY

Transfusion medicine may be life saving in the emergent or critically ill veterinary patient. Blood products are becoming readily available, and transfusions can be performed in many clinic settings. The appropriate use of transfusion medicine should balance the potential risks, albeit rare, associated with transfusions. Patients should be appropriately screened with blood typing and crossmatching before therapy, and component therapy should be used when possible. Ongoing research may provide even better cage-side typing, longer storage times for components, and a larger variety of products that are more specific for each species.

REFERENCES

1. Cotter SM. History of transfusion medicine. Adv Vet Sci Comp Med 1991;36:1–8.
2. Wardrop KJ, Reine N, Birkenheuer A, et al. Canine and feline blood donor screening for infectious disease. J Vet Intern Med 2005;19(1):135–42.
3. Hackett TB, Jensen WA, Lehman TL, et al. Prevalence of DNA of *Mycoplasma haemofelis*, '*Candidatus Mycoplasma haemominutum*,' *Anaplasma phagocytophilum*, and species of *Bartonella*, *Neorickettsia*, and *Ehrlichia* in cats used as blood donors in the United States. J Am Vet Med Assoc 2006;229(5):700–5.
4. Young LE, Ervin DM, Yuile CL. Hemolytic reactions produced in dogs by transfusion of incompatible dog blood and plasma; serologic and hematologic aspects. Blood 1949;4(11):1218–31.
5. Symons M, Bell K. Canine blood groups: description of 20 specificities. Anim Genet 1992;23:509–15.
6. Symons M, Bell K. Expansion of the canine A blood group system. Anim Genet 1991;22:227–35.
7. Day MJ, Barbara K, editors. BSAVA manual of canine and feline haematology and transfusion medicine. 2nd edition. Gloucester (United Kingdom): British Small Animal Veterinary Association; 2012.
8. Blais MC, Berman L, Oakley DA, et al. Canine Dal blood type: a red cell antigen lacking in some Dalmatians. J Vet Intern Med 2007;21(2):281–6.
9. Kessler RJ, Reese J, Chang D, et al. Dog erythrocyte antigens 1.1, 1.2, 3, 4, 7, and Dal blood typing and cross-matching by gel column technique. Vet Clin Pathol 2010;39(3):306–16.
10. Callan MB, Jones LT, Giger U. Hemolytic transfusion reactions in a dog with an alloantibody to a common antigen. J Vet Intern Med 1995;9(4):277–9.
11. Giger U, Gelens CJ, Callan MB, et al. An acute hemolytic transfusion reaction caused by dog erythrocyte antigen 1.1 incompatibility in a previously sensitized dog. J Am Vet Med Assoc 1995;206(9):1358–62.
12. Swisher SN, Young LE, Trabold N. In vitro and in vivo studies of the behavior of canine erythrocyte-isoantibody systems. Ann N Y Acad Sci 1962;97(1):15–25.
13. Seth M, Jackson KV, Winzelberg S, et al. Comparison of gel column, card, and cartridge techniques for dog erythrocyte antigen 1.1 blood typing. Am J Vet Res 2012;73(2):213–9.
14. Weinstein NM, Blais MC, Harris K, et al. A newly recognized blood group in domestic shorthair cats: the Mik red cell antigen. J Vet Intern Med 2007;21(2):287–92.

15. Malik R, Griffin DL, White JD, et al. The prevalence of feline A/B blood types in the Sydney region. Aust Vet J 2005;83(1–2):38–44.

16. Giger U, Kilrain CG, Filippich LJ, et al. Frequencies of feline blood groups in the United States. J Am Vet Med Assoc 1989;195(9):1230–2.

17. Klaser DA, Reine NJ, Hohenhaus AE. Red blood cell transfusions in cats: 126 cases (1999). J Am Vet Med Assoc 2005;226(6):920–3.

18. Giger U, Bucheler J, Patterson DF. Frequency and inheritance of A and B blood types in feline breeds of the United States. J Hered 1991;82(1):15–20.

19. Proverbio D, Spada E, Baggiani L, et al. Comparison of gel column agglutination with monoclonal antibodies and card agglutination methods for assessing the feline AB group system and a frequency study of feline blood types in northern Italy. Vet Clin Pathol 2011;40(1):32–9.

20. Giger U, Bucheler J. Transfusion of type-A and type-B blood to cats. J Am Vet Med Assoc 1991;198(3):411–8.

21. Tocci LJ. Transfusion medicine in small animal practice. Vet Clin North Am Small Anim Pract 2010;40:485–94.

22. Seth M, Jackson KV, Giger U. Comparison of five blood-typing methods for the feline AB blood group system. Am J Vet Res 2011;72(2):203–9.

23. Young LE, O'Brien WA, Swisher SN, et al. Blood groups in dogs – their significance to the veterinarian. Am J Vet Res 1952;13:207–13.

24. Lanevschi A, Wardrop KJ. Principles of transfusion medicine in small animals. Can Vet J 2001;42:447–54.

25. Novaretti MC, Jens E, Pagliarini T, et al. Comparison of conventional tube test technique and gel microcolumn assay for direct antiglobulin test: a large study. J Clin Lab Anal 2004;18(5):255–8.

26. McDevitt RI, Ruaux CG, Baltzer WI. Influence of transfusion technique on survival of autologous red blood cells in the dog. J Vet Emerg Crit Care 2011; 21(3):209–16.

27. Heikes B, Ruaux C. Syringe and aggregate filter administration does not affect survival of transfused autologous feline red blood cells. Paper presented at: ACVIM2012. New Orleans. Accessed May 30, 2012.

28. McMichael MA, Smith SA, Galligan A, et al. Effect of leukoreduction on Transfusion-induced inflammation in dogs. J Vet Intern Med 2010;24:1131–7.

29. Schavone J, Rozanski EA, Schaeffer J, et al. Leukoreduction of feline whole blood using a neonatal leukocyte reduction filter: a pilot evaluation. Paper presented at: ACVIM2012. New Orleans. Accessed June 2, 2012.

30. Logan JC, Callan MB, Drew K, et al. Clinical indications for use fresh frozen plasma in dogs: 74 dogs (October through December 1999). J Am Vet Med Assoc 2001;218(9):1449–55.

31. Kerl ME, Hohenhaus AE. Packed red blood cell transfusions in dogs: 131 cases (1989). J Am Vet Med Assoc 1993;202(9):1495–9.

32. Wardrop KJ. Selection of anticoagulant preservatives for canine and feline blood storage. Vet Clin North Am Small Anim Pract 1995;25(6):1263–76.

33. Wardrop KJ, Owen TJ, Meyers KM. Evaluation of an additive solution for preservation of canine red blood cells. J Vet Intern Med 1994;8:253–7.

34. Wardrop KJ, Tucker RL, Mugnai K. Evaluation of canine red blood cells stored in a saline, adenine, and glucose solution for 35 days. J Vet Intern Med 1997;11(1):5–8.

35. Brooks MB, Wardrop KJ. Stability of hemostatic proteins in canine fresh frozen plasma units. Vet Clin Pathol 2001;30(2):91–5.

36. Hebert PC, Wells G, Blajchman MA, et al. A multicenter, randomized, controlled clinical trial of transfusion requirements in critical care. Transfusion Requirements

in Critical Care Investigators, Canadian Critical Care Trials Group. N Engl J Med 1999;340(6):409–17.

37. Hardy JF. Should we reconsider triggers for red blood cell transfusion? Acta Anaesthesiol Belg 2003;54(4):287–95.

38. Tsuchiya R, Yagura H, Hachiya Y, et al. Aggregability and post-transfusion survival of canine platelets in stored whole blood. J Vet Med Sci 2003;65(8): 825–9.

39. Spinella PC, Perkins JG, Grathwohl KW, et al. Effect of plasma and red blood cell transfusions on survival in patients with combat related traumatic injuries. J Trauma 2008;64:S69–77.

40. Short JL, Diehl S, Seshadri R, et al. Accuracy of formulas used to predict post-transfusion packed cell volume rise in anemic dogs. J Vet Emerg Crit Care (San Antonio) 2012;22(4):428–34.

41. Snow SJ, Ari Jutkowitz L, Brown AJ. Trends in plasma transfusion at a veterinary teaching hospital: 308 patients (1996-1998 and 2006-2008). J Vet Emerg Crit Care (San Antonio) 2010;20(4):441–5.

42. Desborough M, Stanworth S. Plasma transfusion for bedside, radiologically guided, and operating room invasive procedures. Transfusion 2012;52(Suppl 1): 20S–9S.

43. Stokol T, Parry B. Efficacy of fresh-frozen plasma and cryoprecipitate in dogs with von Willebrand's disease or hemophilia A. J Vet Intern Med 1998;12(2): 84–92.

44. Holcomb JB, Wade CE, Michalek JE, et al. Increased plasma and platelet to red blood cell ratios improves outcome in 466 massively transfused civilian trauma patients. Ann Surg 2008;248(3):447–58.

45. Gunter OL Jr, Au BK, Isbell JM, et al. Optimizing outcomes in damage control resuscitation: identifying blood product ratios associated with improved survival. J Trauma 2008;65(3):527–34.

46. Shaz BH, Dente CJ, Nicholas J, et al. Increased number of coagulation products in relationship to red blood cell products transfused improves mortality in trauma patients. Transfusion 2010;50(2):493–500.

47. Stanworth SJ, Brunskill SJ, Hyde CJ, et al. Is fresh frozen plasma clinically effective? A systematic review of randomized controlled trials. Br J Haematol 2004; 126(1):139–52.

48. Ewe K. Bleeding after liver biopsy does not correlate with indices of peripheral coagulation. Dig Dis Sci 1981;26(5):388–93.

49. Caturelli E, Squillante MM, Andriulli A, et al. Fine-needle liver biopsy in patients with severely impaired coagulation. Liver 1993;13(5):270–3.

50. Gilmore IT, Burroughs A, Murray-Lyon IM, et al. Indications, methods, and outcomes of percutaneous liver biopsy in England and Wales: an audit by the British Society of Gastroenterology and the Royal College of Physicians of London. Gut 1995;36(3):437–41.

51. Rozanski EA, Hughes D, Giger U. The effect of heparin and fresh frozen plasma on plasma antithrombin III activity, prothrombin time and activated partial thromboplastin time in critically ill dogs. J Vet Emerg Crit Care 2001;11:15–21.

52. McMahon MJ, Bowen M, Mayer AD, et al. Relation of alpha 2-macroglobulin and other antiproteases to the clinical features of acute pancreatitis. Am J Surg 1984;147(1):164–70.

53. Leese T, Holliday M, Watkins M, et al. A multicentre controlled clinical trial of high-volume fresh frozen plasma therapy in prognostically severe acute pancreatitis. Ann R Coll Surg Engl 1991;73(4):207–14.

54. Weatherton LK, Streeter EM. Evaluation fresh frozen plasma administration in dogs with pancreatitis: 77 cases (1995-2005). J Vet Emerg Crit Care (San Antonio) 2009;19(6):617–22.

55. Mazzaferro EM, Rudloff E, Kirby R. The role of albumin replacement in the critically ill veterinary patient. J Vet Emerg Crit Care 2002;12(2):113–24.

56. Drobatz KJ, Macintire DK. Heat-induced illness in dogs: 53 cases. J Am Vet Med Assoc 1996;209(11):1894–9.

57. Perel P, Roberts I. Colloids versus crystalloids for fluid resuscitation in critically ill patients. Cochrane Database Syst Rev 2011;(3):CD000567.

58. Roberts I, Blackhall K, Alderson P, et al. Human albumin solution for resuscitation and volume expansion in critically ill patients. Cochrane Database Syst Rev 2011;(11):CD001208.

59. Finfer S, Bellomo R, Boyce N, et al. A comparison of albumin and saline for fluid resuscitation in the intensive care unit. N Engl J Med 2004;350(22):2247–56.

60. Delaney AP, Dan A, McCaffrey J, et al. The role of albumin as a resuscitation fluid for patients with sepsis: a systematic review and meta-analysis. Crit Care Med 2011;39(2):386–91.

61. Stokol T, Parry BW. Stability of von Willebrand factor and factor VIII in canine cryoprecipitate under various conditions of storage. Res Vet Sci 1995;59(2):152–5.

62. Ching YN, Meyers KM, Brassard JA, et al. Effect of cryoprecipitate and plasma on plasma von Willebrand factor multimeters and bleeding time in Doberman Pinschers with type-I von Willebrand's disease. Am J Vet Res 1994;55(1):102–10.

63. Trow AV, Rozanski EA, Delaforcade AM, et al. Evaluation use human albumin in critically ill dogs: 73 cases (2003-2006). J Am Vet Med Assoc 2008;233(4):607–12.

64. Matthews KA, Barry M. The use of 25% human serum albumin: outcome and efficacy in raising serum albumin and systemic blood pressure in critically ill dogs and cats. J Vet Emerg Crit Care 2005;15:110.

65. Vigano F, Perissinotto L, Bosco VR. Administration 5% human serum albumin in critically ill small animal patients with hypoalbuminemia: 418 dogs 170 cats (1994-2008). J Vet Emerg Crit Care (San Antonio) 2010;20(2):237–43.

66. Wingfield WE, Raffe MR. The veterinary ICU book. 1st edition. Jackson (WY): Teton NewMedia; 2002.

67. Francis AH, Martin LG, Haldorson GJ, et al. Adverse reactions suggestive of type III hypersensitivity in six healthy dogs given human albumin. J Am Vet Med Assoc 2007;230(6):873–9.

68. Martin LG, Luther TY, Alperin DC, et al. Serum antibodies against human albumin in critically ill and healthy dogs. J Am Vet Med Assoc 2008;232(7):1004–9.

69. Smith CL, Ramsey NB, Parr AM, et al. Evaluation of a novel canine albumin solution in normal beagles. Paper presented at: International Veterinary Emergency and Critical Care Symposium. Chicago, IL, September 9–13, 2009.

70. Spurlock NK, Prittie JE. A review of current indications, adverse effects, and administration recommendations for intravenous immunoglobulin. J Vet Emerg Crit Care (San Antonio) 2011;21(5):471–83.

71. Hirschvogel K, Jurina K, Steinberg TA, et al. Clinical course of acute canine polyradiculoneuritis following treatment with human IV immunoglobulin. J Am Anim Hosp Assoc 2012;48(5):299–309.

72. Bianco D, Armstrong PJ, Washabau RJ. A prospective, randomized, double-blinded, placebo-controlled study of human intravenous immunoglobulin for the acute management of presumptive primary immune-mediated thrombocytopenia in dogs. J Vet Intern Med 2009;23(5):1071–8.

73. Whelan MF, O'Toole TE, Chan DL, et al. Use of human immunoglobulin in addition to glucocorticoids for the initial treatment of dogs with immune-mediated hemolytic anemia. J Vet Emerg Crit Care (San Antonio) 2009;19(2):158–64.
74. Petrides M, Stack G, Cooling L, et al. Practical guide to transfusion medicine. Bethesda (MD): AABB Press; 2007.
75. Abrams-Ogg AC. Triggers for prophylactic use of platelet transfusions and optimal platelet dosing in thrombocytopenic dogs and cats. Vet Clin North Am Small Anim Pract 2003;33(6):1401–18.
76. Callan MB, Appleman EH, Sachais BS. Canine platelet transfusions. J Vet Emerg Crit Care (San Antonio) 2009;19(5):401–15.
77. Davidow EB, Brainard B, Martin LG, et al. Use of fresh platelet concentrate or lyophilized platelets in thrombocytopenic dogs with clinical signs of hemorrhage: a preliminary trial in 37 dogs. J Vet Emerg Crit Care (San Antonio) 2012;22(1):116–25.
78. Hux BD, Martin LG. Platelet transfusions: treatment options for hemorrhage secondary to thrombocytopenia. J Vet Emerg Crit Care (San Antonio) 2012;22(1): 73–80.
79. Callow CR, Swindell R, Randall W, et al. The frequency of bleeding complications in patients with haematological malignancy following the introduction of a stringent prophylactic platelet transfusion policy. Br J Haematol 2002;118(2):677–82.
80. Valeri CR, Khuri S, Ragno G. Nonsurgical bleeding diathesis in anemic thrombocytopenic patients: role of temperature, red blood cells, platelets, and plasma-clotting proteins. Transfusion 2007;47(Suppl 4):206S–48S.
81. Slichter SJ, Harker LA. Preparation and storage of platelet concentrates. Transfusion 1976;16(1):8–12.
82. Hoffmeister KM, Felbinger TW, Falet H, et al. The clearance mechanism of chilled blood platelets. Cell 2003;112(1):87–97.
83. Appleman EH, Sachais BS, Patel R, et al. Cryopreservation of canine platelets. J Vet Intern Med 2009;23(1):138–45.
84. Abrams-Ogg AC, Kruth SA, Carter RF, et al. Preparation and transfusion of canine platelet concentrates. Am J Vet Res 1993;54(4):635–42.
85. Allyson K, Abrams-Ogg AC, Johnstone IB. Room temperature storage and cryopreservation of canine platelet concentrates. Am J Vet Res 1997;58(11): 1338–47.
86. Murphy S, Kahn RA, Holme S, et al. Improved storage of platelets for transfusion in a new container. Blood 1982;60(1):194–200.
87. Valeri CR, Feingold H, Marchionni LD. A simple method for freezing human platelets using 6 per cent dimethylsulfoxide and storage at -80 degrees C. Blood 1974;43(1):131–6.
88. Valeri CR, Feingold H, Melaragno AJ, et al. Cryopreservation of dog platelets with dimethyl sulfoxide: therapeutic effectiveness of cryopreserved platelets in the treatment of thrombocytopenic dogs, and the effect of platelet storage at -80 degrees C. Cryobiology 1986;23(5):387–94.
89. Bode AP, Fischer TH. Lyophilized platelets: fifty years in the making. Artif Cells Blood Substit Immobil Biotechnol 2007;35(1):125–33.
90. Read MS, Reddick RL, Bode AP, et al. Preservation of hemostatic and structural properties of rehydrated lyophilized platelets: potential for long-term storage of dried platelets for transfusion. Proc Natl Acad Sci U S A 1995;92(2):397–401.
91. Bode AP, Lust RM, Read MS, et al. Correction of the bleeding time with lyophilized platelet infusions in dogs on cardiopulmonary bypass. Clin Appl Thromb Hemost 2008;14(1):38–54.

92. Hawksworth JS, Elster EA, Fryer D, et al. Evaluation of lyophilized platelets as an infusible hemostatic agent in experimental non-compressible hemorrhage in swine. J Thromb Haemost 2009;7(10):1663–71.

93. Narick C, Triulzi DJ, Yazer MH. Transfusion-associated circulatory overload after plasma transfusion. Transfusion 2012;52(1):160–5.

94. Pandey S, Vyas GN. Adverse effects of plasma transfusion. Transfusion 2012; 52(Suppl):65S–79S.

95. Arinsburg SA, Skerret DL, Karp JK, et al. Conversion to low transfusion-related acute lung injury (TRALI)-risk plasma significantly reduces TRALI. Transfusion 2012;52:946–52.

96. Blais MC, Rozanski EA, Hale AS, et al. Lack of evidence of pregnancy-induced alloantibodies in dogs. J Vet Intern Med 2009;23(3):462–5.

Emergency Management and Treatment of the Poisoned Small Animal Patient

Justine A. Lee, DVM

KEYWORDS

- Toxicology • Poisoning • Charcoal • Decontamination • Antidote • Toxicosis
- Emetics

KEY POINTS

- Clinicians should be aware of the importance of history, triage, decontamination, and emergency management of the poisoned patient.
- Knowledge of the underlying mechanism of action, the pharmacokinetics, and the toxic dose of the toxicant are imperative in determining appropriate decontamination and therapy for the patient.
- Particular attention to the cardiorespiratory system, central nervous system, and gastrointestinal tract are important in the poisoned patient.

Accidental poisoning of pets occurs frequently because of the availability of toxicants in the household, the kitchen, the yard, and the garden, and because of the prevalence of over-the-counter and prescription medications. As a result, emergency clinicians commonly encounter poisoned patients. Management of the acutely poisoned patient includes initial telephone triage, appropriate communication and history gathering from the pet owner, thorough physical examination, initial stabilization, decontamination (if appropriate), and treatment to ensure the best outcome.

When managing the poisoning patient, it is imperative to understand the toxicant's mechanism of action, the pharmacokinetics (ie, absorption, distribution, metabolism, and excretion), and whether a potentially toxic dose was ingested. Consultation with an animal poison helpline is often recommended, particularly if the underlying toxicant is not well recognized by the clinician, if the toxicant has a narrow margin of safety (eg, baclofen, macrocyclic lactones, calcium channel blockers, cholecalciferol), or if it is an unknown human medication (eg, calcipotriene, 5-fluorouracil).

Disclosure: The author has nothing to disclose.
Pet Poison Helpline, a division of SafetyCall International, PPLC, 3600 American Boulevard West, Suite 725, Minneapolis, MN 55431, USA
E-mail address: jlee@safetycall.com

Vet Clin Small Anim 43 (2013) 757–771
http://dx.doi.org/10.1016/j.cvsm.2013.03.010 **vetsmall.theclinics.com**
0195-5616/13/$ – see front matter © 2013 Elsevier Inc. All rights reserved.

OBTAINING AN APPROPRIATE HISTORY

With the poisoned patient, a specific toxicologic history should be obtained to determine what the active ingredient (AI) is, whether the toxicant or dosage ingested was poisonous, when the ingestion or poisoning occurred, whether any home antidotes were administered (eg, milk, salt), or whether the patient developed any clinical signs at home. Once presented to the veterinary clinic, poisoned patients should be appropriately triaged by the veterinary staff; they cannot sit and wait in the waiting room, because the time to decontamination may have passed. In addition, veterinarians should appropriately assess and triage the poisoned patient on presentation, focusing on airway, breathing, circulation, and dysfunction (ABCDs). Readers are directed to the article "Monitoring of the Emergent Small Animal Patient" elsewhere in this issue for more information.

Following initial triage, appropriate next steps include:

- Verification of the spelling of the product and confirmation of the AI.
- Evaluation of the prescription vial label to verify whether it is a sustained-release (SR), extended-release (XR), or long-acting (LA) product. These initials follow the name of the drug on the vial. If the vial is not available, the pet owner should be counseled to call the pharmacy for further information (including amount dispensed, AI, and drug strength).
- Evaluation of whether the pet owner has already attempted emesis induction and, if so, with what emetic agent.
- Stabilization of the patient based on triage and physical examination findings (eg, temperature, heart rate, pulse rate, pulse quality).

Additional important questions to include as part of a thorough toxicology history are listed in **Table 1**.

WHEN TO DECONTAMINATE

The goal of decontamination is to inhibit or minimize further toxicant absorption and to promote excretion or elimination of the toxicant from the body.[1,2] Decontamination can only be performed within a narrow window of time for most substances; therefore, it is important to obtain a thorough history and time since exposure to identify whether or not decontamination is medically appropriate. Decontamination categories may include ocular, dermal, inhalation, injection, gastrointestinal (GI), forced diuresis, and surgical removal to prevent absorption or enhance elimination of the toxicant.[1,2]

One of the primary ways of decontaminating veterinary patients is via emesis induction. However, veterinarians should be aware of which circumstances are appropriate or contraindicated for GI decontamination (eg, emesis induction, gastric lavage). **Box 1** and **Table 2** show indications for emesis induction and gastric lavage.

With decontamination, whether performed at home or by the veterinarian, the appropriate emetic agent should always be used. There are currently no safe, effective emetic agents for pet owners to use at home in cats. Hydrogen peroxide is not recommended in cats, because it can cause a severe hemorrhagic esophagitis and/or gastritis. Instead, cats should have emesis induction performed by the veterinarian with the use of alpha$_2$-adrenergic agonists (eg, xylazine, dexmedetomidine).[2] In dogs, the use of hydrogen peroxide can be recommended for at-home emesis for pet owners; however, the use of salt, mustard, liquid dish soap, or syrup of ipecac is no longer recommended.[2] In the clinical setting, hydrogen peroxide and/or apomorphine are the emetics of choice for dogs,[2] and are of similar efficacy.[3] A summary of appropriate emetic agents is given in **Table 3**.

Table 1
Obtaining an appropriate toxicology history

Questions to Ask Pet Owners on Presentation	Pet Owners Should be Appropriately Consulted to Do the Following:	Triage
What was the product ingested? Do you know the AI?	To safely remove their pet from the area of poisoning so additional ingestion does not occur	Airway
Did you give your pet anything at home (eg, hydrogen peroxide, milk) when you found out it was poisoned?	To not give any home remedies found circulating on the Internet (eg, milk, peanut butter, oil, grease, salt)	Breathing
How many total tablets could have been ingested? What was the minimum and maximum amount that your pet could have been exposed to?	To not induce emesis without first consulting a veterinarian or an animal poison control helpline	Circulation
Was this an extended-release or SR product? Was there an extra letter behind the brand name (eg, Claritin vs Claritin-D)?	To bring the pill vial, bait station, or container so that the veterinarian can assess the bottle for verification of the product name	Dysfunction
When did your pet get into this?	To call the original pharmacy to find out how many total pills were prescribed, and attempt to back-count how many were taken/ingested	—
Has your pet shown any clinical signs yet?	To seek immediate veterinary attention if considered toxic	—

Abbreviations: AI, active ingredient; SR, sustained-release.

Gastric lavage, although rarely performed in veterinary poisoned patients, is also considered a mainstay therapy for GI decontamination. The use of gastric lavage may be warranted, particularly with certain toxicants and in those patients that are already symptomatic (see **Box 1**). The goal of gastric lavage is to remove gastric contents when emesis induction is unproductive or contraindicated. In human studies, if gastric lavage was performed within 15 to 20 minutes after toxicant ingestion, recoveries were minimal (38% and 29%, respectively).[1,4–6] If lavage was performed 60 minutes after ingestion, only 8.6% to 13% was recovered.[1,4–6] Because most poisoned

Box 1
Indications for gastric lavage

Massive ingestions that may result in a foreign body obstruction (eg, bone meal, blood meal, kitty litter

Massive ingestions that may result in a medical bezoar (eg, iron capsules, aspirin, large ingestions of vitamins, massive wads of xylitol-containing gum)

Drugs approaching the lethal dose for 50% of animals (LD_{50})

Drugs with a narrow margin of safety or those that result in severe clinical signs (eg, calcium channel blockers, β-blockers, cholecalciferol, organophosphates, baclofen, macrocyclic lactones, metaldehyde)

Table 2
Emesis induction: indications and contraindications

When Emesis Should be Performed	When Emesis Should not be Performed
With recent ingestion (<1 h) in an asymptomatic patient	With corrosive toxicant ingestion (eg, lime-removal products, ultrableach, batteries, oven cleaning chemicals)
With unknown time of ingestion in an asymptomatic patient	With hydrocarbon toxicant ingestion (eg, tikki-torch oil, gasoline, kerosene)
When products known to stay in the stomach for a long time are ingested (eg, grapes, raisins, chocolate, xylitol gum)	In symptomatic patients (eg, tremoring, agitation, seizuring, hyperthermic, hypoglycemic, weak, collapsed)
—	In patients with underlying disease predisposing them toward aspiration pneumonia (eg, megaesophagus, history of aspiration pneumonia, laryngeal paralysis)

patients present to the veterinary clinic after 1 hour, the clinical usefulness of gastric lavage is debated.[1]

However, gastric lavage is generally considered to be more effective at removing gastric contents than emesis alone. In veterinary medicine, it is often less commonly performed because of labor intensiveness; it requires intravenous (IV) catheter placement, sedation, intubation with an appropriately inflated endotracheal tube (ETT), gavage, charcoal administration, techniques to prevent aspiration (eg, head elevation, antiemetic therapy), and extubation. Despite its labor intensiveness, the use of gastric lavage is indicated in symptomatic patients that are showing clinical signs predisposing them toward aspiration pneumonia (eg, excessively sedate, unconscious, tremoring, seizuring) and that still need controlled decontamination (eg, metaldehyde, organophosphates). Gastric lavage is also indicated when the toxicant or ingested material can potentially cause a bezoar or concretion (eg, bone meal, iron tablets, large amounts of chocolate, tremorgenic mycotoxins) or foreign body, when the

Table 3
Suggested emetic agents, dosing, and species

Emetic Agent	Where It Works	Dose	Indicated for this Species Only
Hydrogen peroxide 3%	Local gastric irritant	1–5 mL/kg PO, up to 2 times; maximum of 50 mL/dog	Dogs
Apomorphine	CRTZ	0.03 mg/kg IV; 0.04 mg/kg IM; crushed tablet subconjunctivally (typically 6.25-mg tablets)	Dogs
Xylazine	Centrally acting	0.44 mg/kg IM (reverse with yohimbine after emesis)	Cats

Abbreviations: CRTZ, chemoreceptor trigger zone; IM, intramuscular; IV, intravenous; PO, by mouth.

Emetic agents no longer recommended: table salt (sodium chloride), liquid dishwashing detergent, or 7% syrup of ipecac.

toxicant ingested approaches the LD_{50} (eg, calcium channel blockers, β-blockers, baclofen, organophosphate), or when the toxicant has a narrow margin of safety (see **Box 1**).[2]

Complications of gastric lavage include aspiration pneumonia, risks of sedation, hypoxemia secondary to aspiration pneumonia, or hypoventilation from sedation, or mechanical injury to the mouth, oropharynx, esophagus, or stomach. Contraindications for gastric lavage include:

- A corrosive agent, if esophagus or gastric perforation can occur with orogastric tube placement
- A hydrocarbon agent that may easily be aspirated into the pulmonary parenchyma because of its low viscosity
- Sharp objects ingested (eg, sewing needles)

Many veterinarians are not comfortable performing the procedure, but it can easily be accomplished when organized with the appropriate supplies in a team-oriented approach. **Box 2** shows a step-by-step procedural outline of how to perform gastric lavage.

ACTIVATED CHARCOAL (AC)

After an appropriate history, triage, and physical examination have been performed, the patient should be decontaminated, if appropriate. The second step of decontamination is the administration of activated charcoal (AC) with a cathartic, if appropriate. AC should only be administered to the poisoned patient when warranted and medically appropriate. It should not be given when the toxicant does not reliably bind to AC (eg, heavy metals, xylitol, ethylene glycol, alcohols)[1,2] or when it is contraindicated to administer AC (eg, salt toxicosis, corrosives, hydrocarbons).[1,2] Also, symptomatic patients who are at risk for aspiration pneumonia (eg, decreased gag reflex) should not be administered AC orally. In addition, the administration of AC with a cathartic should be cautiously used in dehydrated patients, because of the potential (albeit rare) risk of hypernatremia secondary to free water loss in the GI tract (GIT).[2,7]

To be most effective, AC should ideally be given as soon as possible after toxic ingestion. In veterinary medicine, this is almost impossible because of driving time (to the clinic), lapsed time since ingestion, time to triage, and the amount of time it takes to physically deliver AC (eg, syringe feeding, orogastric tube).[8] As a result, administration of AC is often delayed up to an hour or more. Because time since ingestion is often unknown (eg, pet owner coming home from work to find the pet poisoned), decontamination (including emesis and administration of AC) is often a benign course of action, provided the patient is not already symptomatic. As always, when administering any drug, it is important that benefits outweigh the risks, and that complications be prevented, when possible. In veterinary medicine, administration of AC with a cathartic as long as 6 hours out may still be beneficial with certain types of toxicosis, particularly if the product is a delayed-release (eg, extended release or SR) toxicant or if it undergoes enterohepatic recirculation (discussed later).[2,8]

Although human medicine has moved away from administration of AC with poisoned patients,[7] the aggressive use of AC in veterinary medicine is still warranted, because this is often the last line of defense in adequately decontaminating patients.[8] Certain modalities of therapy (eg, antidotes [such as fomepizole, pralidoxime chloride (2-PAM), digoxin-specific antibody fragments], plasmaparesis, hemodialysis, mechanical ventilation), along with financial limitations of pet owners, limit veterinarians' ability to treat poisoned pets aggressively compared with human medicine; as a result,

---

Box 2
How to perform gastric lavage

1. Begin by preparing all materials in an organized fashion: white tape; mouth gag; sterile lubrication; gauze; warm lavage fluid in a bucket (tap water); bilge or stomach pump; funnel; step stool; sedatives predrawn and appropriately labeled; sterile endotracheal tube (ETT) with a high-volume, low-pressure cuff; material to secure and tie in the ETT; IV catheter supplies; anesthesia machine; activated charcoal (AC) predrawn in 60-mL syringes ready for administration; and sedation reversal agents if necessary.

2. Place IV catheter; sedate and intubate with ETT. Secure ETT in place and connect to oxygen with or without inhalant anesthesia source. Inflate ETT cuff to prevent aspiration of gastric contents or lavage fluid. Place the patient in right lateral recumbency or sternal position.

3. Premeasure an appropriately sized orogastric tube to the last rib and mark this line with white tape; this will be the maximum distance to insert the tube.

4. Lubricate the orogastric tube, and pass the tube into the stomach using gentle, twisting motions. Insufflating the tube by blowing may help inflate the esophagus with air and further assist with passage of the tube into the stomach.

5. Confirm orogastric tube placement by:

   a. Abdominal palpation of the orogastric tube

   b. Insufflation into the orogastric tube and simultaneous auscultation for bubbles or gurgling sounds within the stomach

   c. Palpation of the neck for 2 tubelike structures (eg, one tube being the trachea and the other tube being the tube palpated within the esophagus)

6. Infuse tepid or warm water by gravity flow via funnel, bilge pump, or stomach pump. The volume of the stomach is approximately 60 to 90 mL/kg, therefore copious amounts of fluid can be used to gavage. Fluid recovery (by gravity) should be directed into an empty bucket.

7. The stomach should be palpated frequently during lavage to prevent over-distension of the stomach. Frequent massaging or agitation of the stomach during lavage also assists in breaking up gastric contents; this should allow small material to be removed via gastric lavage.

8. Several lavage cycles (approximately 5–10) should be performed to maximize decontamination of the stomach. Most of the gavage liquid should be removed before AC administration. The gastric lavage fluid should be examined for the presence of plant material or pills, and can be saved for toxicologic testing, if appropriate.

9. Before removal of the orogastric tube, the appropriate amount of AC (with a cathartic for the first dose) should be instilled. The charcoal contents can then be flushed further into the orogastric tube with water or by blowing forcefully into the tube.

10. Before removal of the orogastric tube, it is imperative that the tube be kinked to prevent remaining tube contents from being aspirated. Once kinked, the tube should be removed quickly in a sweeping movement.

11. The patient should continue to be intubated until a gag reflex is present. Positioning the patient in sternal recumbency with the head elevated may help prevent aspiration.

---

the continued use of decontamination in veterinary medicine is still warranted as a first line of defense.[8] Current recommended dosing for single-dose AC is 1 to 5 g of AC/kg with a cathartic (eg, sorbitol) to promote transit time through the GIT.[2,8] Contraindications for AC administration are listed in **Table 4**.

Table 4
Contraindications for administration of AC

Contraindications for Administration of AC	
Central nervous system depression (decreased level of consciousness)	Diminished gag reflex or compromised airway (increased risk of aspiration pneumonia)
Time frame for benefits of AC are exceeded (eg, late stage presenting with clinical signs already present)	Toxicants that do not reliably bind, including ethylene glycol, xylitol, and heavy metals
Ingestion of corrosive/caustic agents	Ingestion of hydrocarbons
Dehydration or hypovolemia	Ingestions of salt (eg, paintballs, homemade play dough, ocean water, table salt)
GI obstruction or perforation	Ileus/GI stasis
Imminent endoscopy or surgery	Hyperosmolar states (eg, renal disease, diabetes mellitus, psychogenic polydipsia, diabetes insipidus)
Hypernatremia	Underlying medical condition predisposing to aspiration pneumonia (eg, laryngeal paralysis, megaesophagus, upper airway disease)

Abbreviations: AC, Activated charcoal; GI, gastrointestinal.

MULTIDOSE AC

Human studies have found that multidose AC significantly decreases the serum half-life of certain drugs, including antidepressants, theophylline, digitoxin, and phenobarbital.[7] Although veterinary studies are lacking, there is likely an added benefit from using multi-dose AC, provided the patient is well hydrated and monitored appropriately. Certain situations or toxicities, including drugs that undergo enterohepatic recirculation; drugs that diffuse from the systemic circulation back into the GIT down the concentration gradient; or ingestion of SR, XR, or LA release products, require multidose administration of AC.[1,2,8] Keep in mind that, when administering multiple doses of AC to a patient, additional doses of charcoal ideally should not contain a cathartic (eg, sorbitol), because of increased potential risks for dehydration and secondary significant hypernatremia. Current recommended dosing for multiple doses of AC is 1 to 2 g of AC without a cathartic per kilogram of body weight, by mouth every 4 to 6 hours for 24 hours.[2]

DIAGNOSTIC TESTING

In the poisoned patient, appropriate diagnostic testing may include a complete blood count, biochemistry panel, venous blood gas analysis (VBG), electrolytes, urinalysis, prothrombin time, or activated partial thromboplastin time, packed cell volume (PCV), total solids (TS), and blood glucose. Additional diagnostics may include radiographs and specific toxicant testing (eg, ethylene glycol test). Pretreatment blood samples should be drawn before administration of any therapy because of the potential risk of contamination of samples. For example, the administration of IV diazepam or oral administration of AC may result in a false-positive ethylene glycol test because of the presence of propylene glycol or sorbitol, respectively. The use of isopropyl alcohol at the venipuncture site may cause a false-positive ethylene glycol test, depending on which type of test is used. Appropriate interpretation of clinicopathologic testing should be used.

TREATMENT

In veterinary toxicology, there are only a few toxicants that have a specific antidote (eg, fomepizole, 2-PAM, vitamin K_1) available. As a result, symptomatic and supportive care is imperative in the poisoned patient, and considered the mainstay therapy once decontamination (including emesis induction, gastric lavage, administration of AC) has been performed. There are 7 broad categories for treatment of the poisoned patient[9]:

1. Fluid therapy
2. GI support
3. Central nervous system (CNS) support
4. Sedatives/reversal agents
5. Hepatoprotectants
6. Miscellaneous
7. Antidotal therapy

Fluid Therapy

Fluid therapy is 1 of the cornerstone therapies of emergency management for the poisoned patient. Fluid therapy is warranted in the poisoned patient to help with the following[9]:

- To maintain perfusion at a cellular level
- To correct or prevent dehydration
- To aid in detoxification by increasing renal excretion of toxicants by forced diuresis
- To vasodilate the renal vessels (particularly with nephrotoxicants such as nonsteroidal antiinflammatory drugs [NSAIDs], lilies, grapes, raisins)
- To correct electrolyte imbalances
- To treat hypotension (particularly with toxicants like β-blockers, calcium channel blockers, angiotensin-converting enzyme (ACE) inhibitors that may result in profound decreases in cardiac output)
- To treat hypoproteinemia secondary to protein loss (eg, long-acting anticoagulants) with the use of synthetic colloids (eg, hydroxyethyl starch) (Please see the article "Fluid therapy: Crystalloids, Colloids and Albumin Products" elsewhere in this issue for more information.)
- To treat decreased oxygen delivery with blood or plasma transfusions if indicated (eg, anemia secondary to GI blood loss from NSAIDs or coagulopathy from long-acting anticoagulants)

In general, a balanced, maintenance, isotonic crystalloid (eg, Lactated Ringers Solution, Normosol-R) can be used. In a healthy patient, fluid rates of 4 to 8 mL/kg/h can be used to force renal clearance of the toxicant. Neonates have a higher maintenance fluid rate (80–100 mL/kg/d), and fluid rates should be adjusted accordingly. Patients with cardiac disease, respiratory disease, or those who have ingested toxins that may increase the patient's risk toward pulmonary edema (eg, tricyclic antidepressants [TCA], phosphide rodenticides) should have judicious fluid administration tailored to the patient's condition.

Patients treated with fluid therapy should be appropriately monitored for hydration status by assessing for weight gain (or loss), hemodilution (PCV/TS), azotemia (for evidence of prerenal azotemia), or urine specific gravity while on IV fluid therapy. Evidence of hypersthenuria (cat >1.040; dog >1.025) in the hospitalized patient on fluid therapy is consistent with continued dehydration, and aggressive fluid therapy is warranted.[9]

The use of artificial colloids (eg, hydroxyethyl starch) should be considered for those patients that have a low colloid osmotic pressure (normal reference range 18–20 mm Hg). Colloids are large molecules that stay in the intravascular space for a long time (ie, they do not easily sieve across the vascular membrane). In general, patients that are hypoproteinemic (TS <6 g/dL) or persistently hypotensive may benefit from the addition of a colloid (eg, hydroxyethyl starch boluses at 5 mL/kg, followed by a constant rate infusion (CRI) of 1 mL/kg/h).

GI Support

The use of antiemetics, antacids, antiulcer drugs, and gastric pH altering medications are often of benefit in the poisoned patient. Antiemetics are warranted in those patients that had emesis induction performed; the duration of emetic effects from both apomorphine and hydrogen peroxide can be as long as 27 to 42 minutes,[3] and administration of antiemetics aids in patient comfort, alleviates adverse effects from emetic agents, and prevents vomition of AC administered later. Antiemetics are also warranted when certain toxicants that result in profound GI signs (eg, gastric irritation, nausea, gastric distension, vomiting) are ingested (eg, zinc phosphide rodenticides, medical bezoars). Patients exposed to toxicants known to result in gastric ulceration (eg, veterinary NSAIDs, human NSAIDs, corrosive toxicants) should also be treated with antacids, antiulcer medication, and gastric pH altering medications. See **Table 5** for appropriate dosing of GI drug therapy for the poisoned patient.

CNS Support

In the poisoned patient, either stimulatory (eg, agitation, tremors, seizures) or sedatory (eg, severe sedation, coma, drowsiness) clinical signs may be seen with certain toxicants. Prescription medications such as attention deficit disorder (ADD)/attention-deficit/hyperactivity disorder (ADHD) drugs (eg, amphetamines), selective serotonin reuptake inhibitor (SSRI) antidepressants, and sleep aids may result in either stimulatory or sedatory signs. Certain muscle relaxants (eg, baclofen), pain medications, and sedatives (eg, opioids) may cause severe sedation. Appropriate anticonvulsant therapy should be used for petit mal or grand mal seizures, whereas muscle relaxants (eg, methocarbamol) should be used for toxicants causing tremors (eg, pyrethrin

Table 5		
Suggested GI medication dosing (canine)		
Maropitant	1 mg/kg SQ q 24 h	Antiemetic
Ondansetron	0.1–0.3 mg/kg PO, IV q 8–12 h	Antiemetic
Dolasetron	0.6–1 mg/kg PO, SQ, IV q 24 h	Antiemetic
Metoclopramide	0.1–0.5 mg/kg PO, SQ, IM q 6 h or 1–2 mg/kg/d as CRI IV	Antiemetic
Famotidine	0.5–1 mg/kg PO, SQ, IV q 12–24 h	H₂ blockers
Ranitidine	0.5–2 mg/kg, PO, SQ, IV q 8–12 h	H₂ blockers
Cimetidine	5–10 mg/kg PO, IV q 6–8 h	H₂ blockers
Omeprazole	0.5–1 mg/kg PO q 24 h	Proton-pump inhibitor
Pantoprazole	1 mg/kg IV q 24 h	Proton-pump inhibitor
Sucralfate	100–1 g PO q 8 h	Antiulcer

Abbreviations: constant rate infusion, CRI; IV, intravenous; IM, intramuscular; PO, by mouth; q, every; SQ, subcutaneous.

toxicosis in cats, SSRIs, amphetamines, compost toxicosis). See **Table 6** for appropriate dosing for CNS drugs.

Sedatives/Reversal Agents

In patients showing severe anxiety, tachycardia, or hypertension, the use of anxiolytic drugs is indicated. These clinical signs are consistent with serotonin syndrome, and is seen as result of ingestion of SSRI antidepressants or ADD/ADHD medications. The use of phenothiazines (eg, acepromazine, chlorpromazine) is warranted in these conditions. Likewise, in patients showing paradoxic CNS stimulation from the accidental ingestion of sleep aids (eg, zolpidem), the use of benzodiazepines as a sedative is contraindicated; instead, the use of phenothiazines should be considered. Flumazenil may be considered as a reversal agent for benzodiazepines or nonbenzodiazepinelike drugs in severely affected patients (eg, respiratory depression). For comatose patients, the use of the opioid reversal naloxone may be beneficial for opioid or baclofen toxicosis.

Hepatoprotectants

The use of hepatoprotectants such as S-adenosylmethionine (SAMe) or N-acetylcysteine (NAC) can be considered for hepatotoxicants such as acetaminophen, xylitol, blue-green algae, sago palm (eg, *Cycad*), NSAIDs, and *Amanita* mushrooms The benign nutraceutical SAMe acts as a methyl donor and generates sulfur-containing

Table 6
Appropriate neurologic medication dosing

Phenobarbital	4 mg/kg, IV q 4 h × 4 doses to load; additional doses may be necessary	Anticonvulsants
Diazepam	0.25–0.5 mg/kg IV, PRN to effect, followed by CRI if indicated	Anticonvulsants Sedative[a]
Levetiracetam	20 mg/kg PO, IV q 8 h	Anticonvulsants
Propofol	1–6 mg/kg IV slow, PRN to effect, followed by CRI at 0.1–0.6 mg/kg/min PRN	Anticonvulsants
Inhalant therapy (eg, sevoflurane, isoflurane)	To effect by mask or via endotracheal tube	General anesthetic to control seizures
Methocarbamol	55–220 mg/kg, IV, PO, PRN to effect	For the treatment of tremors; as a muscle relaxant
Naloxone	0.01–0.02 mg/kg IV, SQ, IM	Opioid reversal
Acepromazine	Dog: 0.05–0.2 mg/kg, IM, IV, SQ PRN to effect. In general, no more than 3 mg total per dog is recommended	Sedative
Butorphanol	0.1–1 mg/kg PO, SQ, IM, IV to effect PRN	Sedative
Chlorpromazine	Dog: 0.5 mg/kg, IV, IM, SQ PRN to effect	Sedative

Abbreviations: constant rate infusion, CRI; IV, intravenous; IM, intramuscular; PO, by mouth; PRN, as needed; q, every; SQ, subcutaneous.
[a] Contraindicated with SSRI, benzodiazepine or nonbenzodiazepine toxicosis (eg, sleep aids).

compounds that are important for conjugation reactions used in detoxification and as a precursor to glutathione.[10] NAC acts as the antidote for acetaminophen (eg, Tylenol) toxicosis by providing an alternate substrate for conjugation when acetaminophen is metabolized; NAC also acts as a glutathione source.[10]

Miscellaneous

Other miscellaneous therapies often used for the treatment of the poisoned patient include the use of β-blockers (for severe tachycardia associated with SSRI, amphetamine, chocolate toxicosis, and so forth); IV lipid emulsion (which acts as a lipid sink for fat-soluble toxins such as calcium channel blockers, macrocyclic lactones, cholecalciferol, baclofen)[11]; and vitamin K₁ therapy (for long-acting anticoagulant toxicosis). Readers are referred to a toxicology resource for additional information on these topics. **Table 7** shows the dosing for miscellaneous other drugs commonly used with poisoned patients.

Antidotal Therapy

Appropriate antidote (eg, fomepizole, 2-PAM, naloxone) therapy should be promptly initiated with the appropriate toxicant; however, keep in mind that most toxicants do not have a readily available antidote. The reader is referred to an appropriate toxicology resource for further information specific to antidotes.[12] See **Table 7** for antidotal dosing for the poisoned patient.

Table 7
Suggested miscellaneous drugs and antidotes used for the poisoned patient

Cyproheptadine	Dogs: 1.1 mg/kg q 4–6 h PO or rectal PRN Cats: 2–4 mg total dose q 4–6 h PO or rectal PRN	Serotonin antagonist for use with toxicants causing serotonin syndrome (eg, SSRI, TCAs, amphetamines)
NAC	140–280 mg/kg IV, PO initial loading dose, followed by 70 mg/kg IV, PO q 6 h for 7–17 doses. Dilute as appropriate	Hepatoprotectant (glutathione source)
SAMe	20 mg/kg/d PO q 24 h on an empty stomach × 14–30 d	Hepatoprotectant and antioxidant (glutathione source)
Ascorbic acid (vitamin C)	30 mg/kg PO q 6 h	Antioxidant
Fomepizole	Dogs: 20 mg/kg IV; at 12 h, 15 mg/kg IV; at 24 h, 15 mg/kg IV; at 36 h,5 mg/kg Cats: 125 mg/kg IV; at 12, 24, 36 h, 31.25 mg/kg IV	Synthetic alcohol dehydrogenase inhibitor for ethylene glycol poisoning
Atropine	Dogs: 0.1–0.5 mg/kg IV, IM, SQ PRN Cats: 0.2–2 mg/kg IV, SC, IM PRN	Antimuscarinic antidote for organophosphate toxicosis
2-PAM	20 mg/kg IM, SQ q 8–12 h	Cholinesterase reactivator for the treatment of organophosphate toxicosis

Abbreviations: IV, intravenous; IM, intramuscular; NAC, N-acetylcysteine; PAM, pralidoxime chloride; PO, by mouth; PRN, as needed; q, every; SAM, S-adenosylmethionine; SSRI, selective serotonin reuptake inhibitor; SQ, subcutaneous; TCA, tricyclic antidepressants.

Table 8
Monitoring of the poisoned patient

Monitoring Parameter	Important with Key Toxicants	Parameters for Concern

ECG[a]	SSRI
	Amphetamines
	Caffeine/theobromine
	Beta-agonists (eg, albuterol)
	Calcium channel blockers
	Beta-blockers
	Digoxin
	Opioids
	Lamotrigine
	Cardiac glycoside-containing plants
	Bufo toads
	Amitraz
		Bradycardiac (dog, HR <50 bpm;
		  cat HR <120 bpm)
		Tachycardiac (dog, HR >180 bpm;
		  cat HR >240 bpm)
		Presence of arrhythmias
		Presence of R-on-T phenomenon
		Ventricular premature contractions
		Corresponding pulse deficits,
		  hypotension, or abnormal
		  perfusion parameters

BP	SSRI antidepressants Amphetamines Calcium channel blockers Beta-blockers Cardiac glycoside-containing plants *Bufo* toads Beta-agonists (eg, albuterol) Diuretics ACE-inhibitors Sedatives (eg, baclofen, opioids)	Hypotension (systolic <90 mm Hg) Hypertension (systolic >180 mm Hg)

CVP	Nephrotoxicants (eg, lilies,
	  grapes/raisins) resulting in
	  oliguric or anuric renal failure
	Cardiopulmonary disease
	  predisposing toward volume
	  overload
		CVP <0 or >10 cm H_2O (normal
		  reference range 0–5 cm H_2O)

UOP	Nephrotoxicants (eg, lilies,
	  grapes/raisins) resulting in
	  oliguric or anuric renal failure
	Cardiac medications (eg, calcium
	  channel blockers, β-blockers)
	  potentially resulting in decreased
	  cardiac output and therefore
	  decreased renal flow
		Normal UOP: 1–2 mL/kg/h
		Oliguric: 0.5 mL/kg/h
		Anuric: <0.5 mL/kg/h

Pulse oximetry	Toxicants affecting pulmonary
	  function (eg, long-acting
	  anticoagulants, zinc phosphide
	  rodenticides, essential oils,
	  hydrocarbons)
		Pulse oximetry reading <92%,
		  indicating moderate to severe
		  hypoxemia

ET_{CO_2}	Toxicants resulting in severe
	  hypercapnea (hypoventilation)
	  such as macrocyclic lactones
	  (eg, ivermectin, moxidectin),
	  muscle relaxants (eg, baclofen),
	  anticonvulsants (eg, phenobarbital,
	  gabapentin, pentobarbital),
	  opioids (eg, fentanyl), and
	  benzodiazepines or
	  nonbenzodiazepines
	  (eg, sleep aids)
		Gradient between ET_{CO_2} and P_{CO_2}
		  is typically <5 mm Hg
		ET_{CO_2} >40–50 mm Hg suggests
		  severe hypercapnea and
		  hypoventilation

VBG	Toxicants resulting in the presence of
	  a metabolic acidosis (eg, ethylene
	  glycol, amphetamines, salicylates)
		pH <7.35
		BE <−5 mm Hg
		HCO_3 <20 mm Hg

(continued on next page)

Table 8 (continued)		
Monitoring Parameter	**Important with Key Toxicants**	**Parameters for Concern**
ABG	Toxicants affecting pulmonary function (eg, long-acting anticoagulants, zinc phosphide rodenticides, essential oils, hydrocarbons)	P_{O_2} <80 mm Hg P_{CO_2} <25 or >50 mm Hg

Abbreviations: ABG, arterial blood gas; BP, blood pressure; BE, base excess; bpm, beats per minute; CVP, central venous pressure; ECG, electrocardiogram; ET_{CO_2}, end-tidal carbon dioxide; HR, heart rate; UOP, urine output; VBG, venous blood gas; SSRI, selective serotonin reuptake inhibitor.
[a] See **Table 9** for suggested cardiac medication dosing if indicated.
Data from Refs.[9,13,14]

Table 9 Suggested cardiac medication dosing		
Atropine	0.02–0.04 mg/kg SQ, IM, IV PRN	For the treatment of bradycardia
Glycopyrrolate	0.01–0.02 mg/kg SQ, IM; or 0.005 mg/kg IV, PRN	For the treatment of bradycardia
Lidocaine	Dog: 2–8 mg/kg IV bolus, then 25–80 μg/kg/min IV CRI Cat: 0.25–0.5 mg/kg IV bolus, then 10–20 μg/kg/min IV CRI (use with caution in cats because of the risk of neurotoxicity)	For the treatment of ventricular tachycardia
Procainamide	Dog: 2–4 mg/kg IV bolus, repeated to maximum cumulative dosage of 20 mg/kg, then 10–40 μg/kg/min IV CRI Cat: 1–2 mg/kg IV slowly followed by 10–20 μg/kg/min IV CRI	For the treatment of ventricular tachycardia
Verapamil	Dog: 0.05 mg/kg IV, then repeat up to a total dose of 0.15 mg/kg Cat: 0.025 mg/kg IV slowly, then repeat up to a total dose of 0.15 mg/kg	Calcium channel blocker used for the treatment of supraventricular tachycardia
Esmolol	250–500 μg/kg IV slowly over 2 min, then 10–200 μg/kg/min CRI	Beta-blocker, for the treatment of tachycardia
Propranolol	Dog: 0.02 mg/kg IV slowly, up to 0.1 mg/kg IV or 0.1–0.2 mg/kg PO q 8 h Cat: 0.02 mg/kg IV slowly, up to 0.1 mg/kg IV or 2.5 mg total dose per cat q 8–12 h	Beta-blocker, for the treatment of tachycardia
Diltiazem	Dog: 0.05–0.15 mg/kg slowly IV, up to 0.1–0.3 mg/kg total or 0.5–2 mg/kg PO q 8 h Cat: 0.25 mg/kg IV bolus over 2 min, up to a total dose of 0.75 mg/kg or 1–2.5 mg/kg PO q 8 h (standard release)	Calcium channel blocker, for the treatment of tachycardia
Amlodipine	Dog: 0.1–0.5 mg/kg, PO q 12–24 h PRN to effect Cat: 0.625 mg total per cat, PO q 24 h PRN to effect Use cautiously in patients with cardiac or hepatic disease. Do not use in hypotensive patients or those with toxicants that may result in hypotension (eg, calcium channel blockers, β-blockers)	Calcium channel blocker, for the treatment of tachycardia
Hydralazine	Dog: 0.5–3 mg/kg, PO q 12 h to effect Cat: 2.5 mg total per cat, PO q 12–24 h to effect	Vasodilator

Abbreviations: constant rate infusion, CRI; IV, intravenous; IM, intramuscular; PO, by mouth; PRN, as needed; q, every.
Bradycardia defined as: dog, HR <50 bpm; cat, HR <120 bpm.
Tachycardiac defined as: dog, HR >180 bpm; cat, HR >240 bpm.

Monitoring of the Poisoned Patient

Appropriate monitoring of the critically ill poisoned patient may necessitate monitoring of continuous electrocardiogram (ECG), blood pressure (BP), central venous pressure (CVP), urine output (UOP), pulse oximetry, end-tidal carbon dioxide ($ETco_2$), and venous blood gas (VBG) or arterial (ABG) blood gas analysis. For more details, the reader is referred to **Tables 8** and **9**, the article elsewhere in this issue, and pertinent emergency critical care resources.[9,13,14]

SUMMARY

Clinicians should be aware of the importance of history, triage, decontamination, and emergency management of the poisoned patient. Knowledge of the underlying mechanism of action, the pharmacokinetics, and the toxic dose of the toxicant are imperative in determining appropriate decontamination and therapy for the patient. Particular attention to the cardiorespiratory system, CNS, and GIT are important in the poisoned patient.

REFERENCES

1. Peterson ME. Toxicological decontamination. In: Peterson ME, Talcott PA, editors. Small animal toxicology. St Louis (MO): Elsevier Saunders; 2006. p. 127–41.
2. Lee JA. Decontamination of the poisoned patient. In: Osweiler GD, Hovda LR, Brutlag AG, Lee JA, editors. Blackwell's five-minute veterinary consult clinical companion: small animal toxicology. Iowa City (IA): Wiley-Blackwell; 2011. p. 5–19.
3. Khan SA, Mclean MK, Slater M, et al. Effectiveness and adverse effects of the use of apomorphine and 3% hydrogen peroxide solution to induce emesis in dogs. J Am Vet Med Assoc 2012;241(9):1179–84.
4. Arnold FJ, Hodges JB Jr, Barta RA Jr. Evaluation of the efficacy of lavage and induced emesis in treatment of salicylate poisoning. Pediatrics 1959;23:286–301.
5. Abdallah AH, Tye A. A comparison of the efficacy of emetic drugs and stomach lavage. Am J Dis Child 1967;113:571–5.
6. Corby DG, Lisciandro RC, Lehman RW, et al. The efficiency of methods used to evacuate the stomach after acute ingestion. Pediatrics 1967;40:871–4.
7. American Academy of Clinical Toxicology. Position paper: single-dose activated charcoal. Clin Toxicol 2005;43:61–87.
8. Lee JA. Complications and controversies of decontamination: activated charcoal - to use or not to use. In: Proceedings of the American College of Veterinary Internal Medicine Conference. Anaheim (CA): 2010. p. 677.
9. Lee JA. Emergency management of the poisoned patient. In: Osweiler GD, Hovda LR, Brutlag AG, Lee JA, editors. Blackwell's five-minute veterinary consult clinical companion: small animal toxicology. Iowa City (IA): Wiley-Blackwell; 2011. p. 20–38.
10. Plumb DC. Plumb's veterinary drug handbook. 7th edition. Ames (IA): Wiley-Blackwell; 2011.
11. Fernandez AL, Lee JA, Rahilly L, et al. The use of intravenous lipid emulsions as an antidote in veterinary toxicology: a review. J Vet Emerg Crit Care 2011;21(4): 309–20.
12. Hovda LR. Antidotes and other useful drugs. In: Osweiler GD, Hovda LR, Brutlag AG, Lee JA, editors. Blackwell's five-minute veterinary consult clinical companion: small animal toxicology. Iowa City (IA): Wiley-Blackwell; 2011. p. 39–49.

13. Waddell LS, Brown AJ. Hemodynamic monitoring. In: Silverstein D, Hopper K, editors. Small animal critical care medicine. St Louis (MO): Elsevier Saunders; 2009. p. 859–64.
14. Sorell-Raschi L. Blood gas and oximetry monitoring. In: Silverstein D, Hopper K, editors. Small animal critical care medicine. St Louis (MO): Elsevier Saunders; 2009. p. 878–82.

The Use of Ultrasound for Dogs and Cats in the Emergency Room
AFAST and TFAST

Søren R. Boysen, DVM[a],*, Gregory R. Lisciandro, DVM[b]

KEYWORDS

• FAST • AFAST • TFAST • Vet Blue • Ultrasound • Emergency • Trauma

KEY POINTS

• AFAST with the abdominal fluid score (AFS) should be repeated at 4 hours in stable patients and sooner in unstable patients.
• An increase in the AFS over time suggests ongoing intra-abdominal hemorrhage.
• A decreasing AFS may be used to monitor resolution (because most cases resolve within 48 hours after bleeding ceases).
• TFAST has high sensitivity and specificity for the rapid diagnosis of pneumothorax (PTX); and the search for the lung point for assessing the degree of PTX as partial versus massive helping determine its clinical significance.
• The detection of pneumothorax (PTX) using TFAST is helpful in blunt and penetrating trauma, and has better sensitivity in patients that are breathing slow and deep.
• To aid in diagnosis of pleural and pericardial effusions, the sonographer should adhere to the axiom that "one view is no view" and clinically use at least two views (eg, using pericardial site [PCS] and DH views) while imaging.

INTRODUCTION TO FOCUSED ASSESSMENT WITH SONOGRAPHY FOR TRAUMA

Since the early 1990s, focused assessment with sonography for trauma (FAST) has been studied extensively in humans, and has become the initial diagnostic test of choice for the assessment of free fluid (eg, typically indicates hemorrhage) in the peritoneal, pleural, and pericardial spaces in unstable patients suffering blunt trauma.[1]

Funding Sources: None.
Conflict of Interest: None.
[a] Department of Veterinary Clinical and Diagnostic Sciences, Faculty of Veterinary Medicine, University of Calgary, 3280 Hospital Drive Northwest, Calgary, Alberta T2N 4Z6, Canada;
[b] Hill Country Veterinary Specialists, Emergency Pet Center, Inc, San Antonio, TX 78259, USA
* Corresponding author.
E-mail address: srboysen@ucalgary.ca

Vet Clin Small Anim 43 (2013) 773–797
http://dx.doi.org/10.1016/j.cvsm.2013.03.011   vetsmall.theclinics.com
0195-5616/13/$ – see front matter © 2013 Elsevier Inc. All rights reserved.

It has been used to assess patients with penetrating injury and to detect retroperitoneal, solid organ, and hollow viscous injuries,[1] and has been used serially with and without abdominal fluid scoring systems.[2] The advent of FAST in veterinary medicine is in its infancy. Preliminary studies show it has clinical use in diagnosing and managing intra-abdominal injury, especially when used serially and when identifiable free fluid is quantified.[3,4] To differentiate thoracic FAST from abdominal FAST examinations in dogs and cats, the two have been referred to as TFAST and AFAST, respectively. The AFAST examination is analogous to the FAST examination in human medicine and the two terms are used throughout this article when referring to veterinary and human studies, respectively.

AFAST FOR BLUNT TRAUMA: DETECTION OF FREE FLUID

The AFAST examination is an ideal initial screening test for early recognition of intra-peritoneal blood because it is rapid, noninvasive, safe, portable, and can be repeated if the patient's status changes.[3–5] The purpose of AFAST is to rapidly identify free fluid in the peritoneal space (and less frequently the pleural and pericardial spaces) of patients with trauma, particularly in those patients that are unstable.[3–5] It should be performed as soon as possible following the triage examination after the patient enters the intensive care unit, concurrent with other therapies and diagnostics.[2,4] Multiple human studies have demonstrated that the FAST examination is very sensitive and specific at detecting blunt trauma-induced injury as evidenced by free abdominal fluid, comparable with more invasive or expensive tests, such as diagnostic peritoneal lavage and computed tomography.[2,6] Furthermore, the sensitivity and specificity of the FAST examination for detection of free fluid remains high even when performed by nonradiologists.[2,7,8] Human and veterinary studies have demonstrated that radiographic serosal detail is not sensitive or specific at detecting abdominal fluid following blunt trauma.[4,9] For these reasons, the FAST examination has become the initial imaging test of choice for blunt trauma in human emergency medicine, is part of the advanced trauma life support protocol, and is part of the American College of Emergency Physicians Use of Emergency Ultrasound Guidelines.[10]

Two prospective veterinary studies have confirmed the value of AFAST in detecting free abdominal fluid after blunt trauma in dogs.[3,4] One of these studies also demonstrated the value of performing serial AFAST examinations and an abdominal fluid score (AFS).[4] The serial AFAST examination allows detection of delayed accumulations of abdominal fluid not apparent on the initial AFAST scan and has been used to detect changes in the quantity of abdominal fluid over time when combined with the AFS.[4] The AFS has also been shown to correlate well with markers of injury (eg, alanine aminotransferase, blood lactate) and the need for blood transfusion, especially when evaluated serially.[4] In bluntly traumatized dogs, the AFS semiquantitates the degree of intra-abdominal blood loss. In dogs without pre-existing anemia, AFS of one or two is unlikely to develop anemia (barring other sites of hemorrhage). In contrast, dogs with AFS of three or four frequently become anemic with 25% of this subset developing hematocrit values less than 25%. However, a recent abstract failed to show similar findings of an AFS in cats.[11] With the success of AFAST and the use of serial AFAST and AFS scores in dogs, the authors have developed algorithms that incorporate AFAST and the AFS to help direct diagnostic and therapeutic decisions in dogs suffering from blunt trauma (**Fig. 1**). The use of the AFS in small animal patients with regards to its integration into trauma algorithms, value as an end-point of resuscitation, ability to localize organ injury, and ability to direct fluid therapy or surgical intervention requires further investigation.

Application of AFAST and AFS in Blunt Trauma

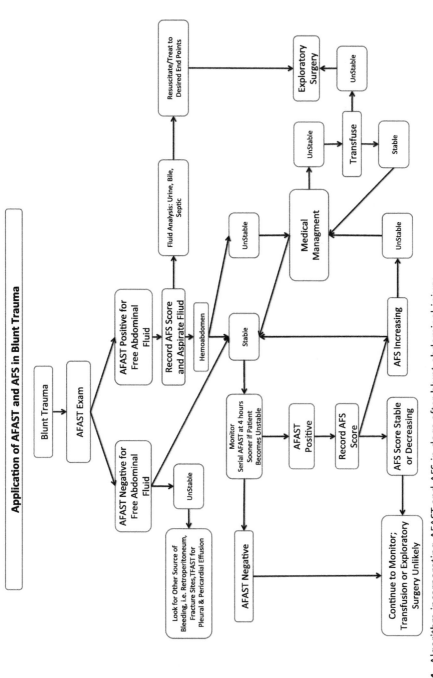

Fig. 1. Algorithm incorporating AFAST and AFS in dogs after blunt abdominal injury.

AFAST FOR BLUNT TRAUMA: DETERMINING THE CAUSE OF INJURY

Hemoabdomen and uroabdomen are two of the most frequent intra-abdominal injuries reported in dogs suffering from abdominal trauma.[3,4,12,13] Because these injuries typically result in free fluid accumulation, both are easily detectable through AFAST examination and have been confirmed in dogs after blunt trauma, centesis, and fluid analysis.[3,4] Because it is not possible to differentiate blood from urine or other fluid types on abdominal ultrasound, fine-needle aspiration and fluid analysis is recommended in patients that are AFAST positive.[3-5] The success of centesis is increased with the use of ultrasound guidance compared with blind techniques.[14] In addition, centesis could help differentiate less common conditions, such as traumatic biliary and intestinal tract rupture, if detected on initial or serial AFAST examinations by facilitating sample collection for stat fluid analysis and cytology.[3]

In small animals, splenic and hepatic injuries are the most common causes of intra-peritoneal hemorrhage.[15,16] Human studies demonstrate that FAST has a limited role in the detection of solid organ injury. The sensitivity for sonographic detection of hepatic and splenic injury after blunt trauma varies from 41% to 80%, depending on the organ affected, location of the lesion, organ size, and presence of overlying bowel and gastrointestinal gas.[17-19] Contrast-enhanced ultrasound has increased the ability of ultrasound to detect solid organ injury in human patients with trauma, with sensitivity and specificity of 96.4% and 98%, respectively.[20] The use of contrast-enhanced ultra-sonography after trauma in veterinary patients remains to be determined. Challenges in the detection of solid organ injury include greater expertise needed to detect parenchymal changes that indicate solid organ injury and the added time needed to evaluate organs in detail.

The detection of retroperitoneal injury has also demonstrated low sensitivity in human FAST studies.[21,22] Serial FAST examinations may improve detection of solid and retroperitoneal injury; however, missed injuries may still occur, and computed tomography scans are currently recommended in humans with negative FAST examinations suspected of solid organ or retroperitoneal injury.[21-23] In veterinary medicine, the AFAST examination has not been evaluated for the detection of solid organ or retroperitoneal injury after blunt abdominal trauma.

AFAST FOR PENETRATING TRAUMA

Human studies evaluating the FAST examination indicate that it is less sensitive at detecting intra-abdominal injury in cases of penetrating trauma.[24-26] In particular, bowel injuries, which are common in penetrating trauma, are not readily detected on initial sonographic evaluation. Penetrating abdominal trauma in humans often results in localized injury. The FAST examination omits large portions of the abdomen so it does not reliably exclude localized injury. However, it should be noted that humans with penetrating abdominal injury and positive FAST examinations are usually referred for emergency exploratory laparotomy.[24-26] Therefore, a positive FAST examination still has use; however, intra-abdominal injury after penetrating trauma cannot be ruled out based on a negative FAST examination.[24,26] Serial FAST examinations in humans (12-24 hours posttrauma) improve the sensitivity of FAST at detecting intestinal injury after trauma.[27] Keep in mind that the mechanism of injury after penetrating trauma differs between humans and veterinary patients because bite wounds comprise a large number of veterinary penetrating trauma cases compared with projectile penetrating trauma in most humans cases. The role of the AFAST and serial AFAST examinations in projectile and nonprojectile penetrating abdominal trauma in veterinary patients requires further investigation.

AFAST AND AFS SCANNING TECHNIQUE

The purpose of the FAST examination is the detection of free fluid indicating injury. The AFAST examination involves visualizing the diaphragm, liver, gallbladder, spleen, kidneys, intestinal loops, and urinary bladder for the detection of free fluid in the peritoneal cavity. Free fluid is anechoic (black on ultrasound) and tends to collect in the most dependent areas as triangles surrounded by organs (**Figs. 2–5**).

Changing the depth of the scan at the subxiphoid location allows evaluation of the area distal to the diaphragm as far as the level of the heart (see **Fig. 2**). This allows detection of free fluid in the pleural and pericardial spaces during the AFAST examination (**Fig. 6**). However, the sensitivity and specificity of detecting free fluid in the pleural and pericardial spaces by the subxiphoid view has not yet been evaluated in dogs or cats.

The basic four-view protocol provides the foundation for the AFAST examination (**Fig. 7**). The technique has been validated in right and left lateral recumbency in dogs.[3,4] Currently, there are no studies investigating if either position has greater accuracy than the other. At this time, either left or right lateral recumbency can be used and may be decided by the position in which the animal presents (eg, animals that present in left lateral recumbency can be scanned in left lateral to minimize stress to the patient with movement or manipulation). However, if given the choice (eg, the patient presents in sternal recumbency or is ambulatory) there may be theoretical advantages of choosing one side over the other, depending on the objectives of the examiner.[5] Right lateral recumbency may be preferred if standardized electrocardiography evaluation of the patient is desired; if the volume status of the patient is to be echographically evaluated (eg, using an echocardiography table); or if the left retroperitoneal space is to be evaluated in detail.[4,5] Right lateral recumbency may also be preferred to prevent iatrogenic puncture of the spleen when performing centesis, although this should be less of a concern if ultrasound guidance is used.[4,5] Left lateral recumbency may be preferred if the right retroperitoneal space is to be evaluated. Certain injuries, such as flail chest, fractures, or injury to the vertebral column, may also dictate the FAST examination position.[4] Dorsal recumbency is not typically recommended because thoracic injury is common after blunt trauma and pulmonary function may deteriorate when patients with significant thoracic injury are placed in dorsal recumbency.[3,4] Also, the AFS system has not been validated in dorsal recumbency.[4]

The median time to perform AFAST in dogs is reported to be 3 to 6 minutes using the four standard views, consisting of the (1) subxiphoid view to evaluate the

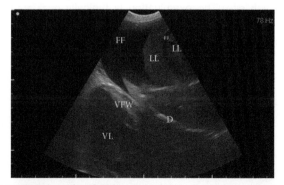

Fig. 2. Positive AFAST at the subxiphoid or DH view demonstrating anechoic free fluid (FF) between the liver lobes (LL) and diaphragm (D). The heart can be seen in the far field distal to the diaphragm as indicated by the ventricular free wall (VFW) and the ventricular lumen (VL). In this case the pleural and pericardial space are negative for free fluid.

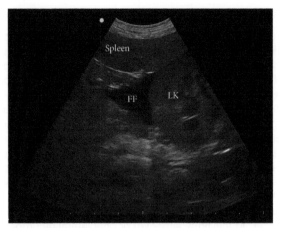

Fig. 3. Positive AFAST at the left flank or SR view demonstrating an anechoic accumulation of free fluid (FF) between the spleen (S) and left kidney (LK).

hepatodiaphragmatic interface, gallbladder region, pericardial sac, and pleural spaces; (2) a left flank view to assess the splenorenal (SR) interface and areas between the spleen and body wall; (3) a midline bladder view to assess the apex of the bladder; and (4) the right flank view to assess the hepatorenal (HR) interface and areas between intestinal loops, right kidney, and the body wall (see **Fig. 7**).[3,4] The time to complete the examination in dogs did not include evaluation of the pleural or pericardial spaces by the subxiphoid view; evaluation of free fluid in these sites may potentially prolong the examination. To assist sonographers in associating the AFAST examination with underlying anatomic structures, these four sites have been named the diaphragmaticohepatic (DH), SR, cystocolic (CC), and HR sites, respectively (see **Fig. 7**).[4,5] An advantage of consistently evaluating the underlying organs at each site during the AFAST examination is that incidental findings may be detected, which have been discovered in up to 7.8% of people undergoing FAST examinations.[28]

The order in which the scan is completed will not likely affect the ability to detect injury, but a systematic approach that identifies target organs consistently will likely expedite the process and assist examiners in becoming familiar with the anatomy associated with each site. The examination is typically evaluated in a clockwise

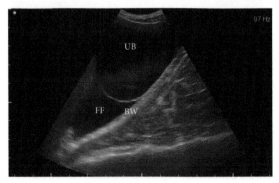

Fig. 4. Positive AFAST at the bladder or CC view showing a triangular accumulation of anechoic free fluid (FF) between the urinary bladder (UB) and the body wall (BW).

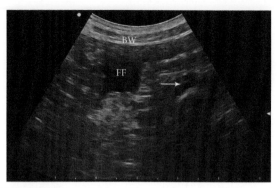

Fig. 5. Positive AFAST at the right flank or HR view demonstrating anechoic free fluid (FF) between loops of intestine (*arrow*) the body wall (BW) and omentum.

rotation, moving from the subxiphoid, to the non–gravity-dependent flank, to bladder, to gravity-dependent flank.[4] At each site, the ultrasound probe can be moved a few inches in several directions and fanned through an angle of 45 degrees until target organs are identified.[3] The subxiphoid or DH site is a good initial starting point because it allows the gallbladder to be identified.[3–5] The gallbladder can be visualized by tilting the probe to the right of midline, and adjusting the gain until the fluid-filled gallbladder appears anechoic.

The initial veterinary AFAST study used two ultrasonographic planes at each site: longitudinal and transverse.[3] This study demonstrated strong agreement between the two planes with only 1 of 400 sites scanned showing discrepancy in results. A subsequent veterinary study evaluated the four sites in only one plane, typically the longitudinal plane, which took less time to perform (eg, 3 minutes median time vs 6 minutes).[4] With comprehensive ultrasound studies, it is recommended to scan organs in two different planes, each plane at a 90 degree angle to the other. However, the AFAST examination can be effectively performed with limited scanning planes because the goal is to detect the presence of free fluid and not to do a comprehensive

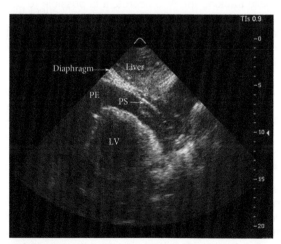

Fig. 6. Positive AFAST for pericardial effusion (PE) identified as anechoic fluid surrounding the left ventricle (LV) by the subxiphoid or DH view. The pericardial sac (PS) is seen in the far field distal to the liver and diaphragm.

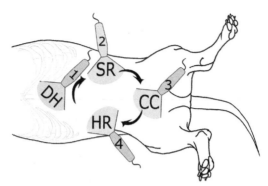

Fig. 7. The AFAST examination, shown here in right lateral recumbency, involves four views of the abdomen: (1) the diaphragmaticohepatic view by placing the probe at the subxiphoid, (2) the splenorenal view by placing the probe at the left flank, (3) the cystocolic view by placing the probe on midline over the bladder, and (4) the hepatorenal view by placing the probe at the right flank. At each site, the ultrasound probe is moved a few inches in several directions and fanned through an angle of 45 degrees until target organs are identified. CC, cystocolic; DH, diaphragmaticohepatic; HR, hepatorenal; SR, splenorenal. (*From* Lisciandro GR. Abdominal and thoracic focused assessment with sonography for trauma, triage, and monitoring in small animals. J Vet Emerg Crit Care 2011;21(2):108; with permission.)

survey of involved organs. However, with equivocal results, evaluating multiple planes may help confirm the presence of free fluid. If solid organ or retroperitoneal injury assessment is desired, then multiple planes at each site may improve detection of such injuries. It should be stressed that detection of solid organ and retroperitoneal injury is not the initial goal of the AFAST examination.

The AFS is easily accomplished by recording the number of sites (among the four standard views) in which free fluid is detected with the animal in lateral recumbency (eg, AFS 0, negative all sites; AFS 1, positive in one site; AFS 2, positive in any two sites; AFS 3, positive in any three sites; AFS 4, positive in all four sites) (**Table 1**).[4] By recording and serially tracking the AFS scores, it is possible to document the progression or resolution of intra-abdominal hemorrhage, which in conjunction with other clinical examination findings, may help direct therapeutic clinical decisions (see **Fig. 1**). Serial AFAST examinations should be performed every 4 hours, or more frequently if clinical findings (eg, deterioration in hemodynamic status) dictate otherwise.[4,29] In Lisciandro and colleagues,[5] AFS was performed in right and left lateral recumbency in dogs and cats; however, it is unknown if patient position, with respect to organ injury, affects the AFS score. Further investigation of the AFS in regards to patient position and clinical decision-making in dogs and cats is warranted.

AFAST BEYOND BLUNT ABDOMINAL TRAUMA-INDUCED INJURY

The subxiphoid site of the FAST examination in humans is sensitive and specific for identification of pleural and pericardial effusions.[30,31] Two studies in dogs presenting for trauma have identified the presence of pleural fluid by the subxiphoid view.[3,4] The authors have detected pleural effusions in dogs with trauma and pericardial effusions in dogs without trauma by the subxiphoid view, and the sensitivity and specificity of this view at detecting pleural and pericardial effusion in dogs and cats is currently being investigated (application of the DH view, either during TFAST or AFAST in

Table 1			
Abdominal focused assessment with sonography for trauma, triage, and tracking (AFAST[3]) template for medical records			
Patient positioning	Right or left lateral recumbency		
Gallbladder	Present or absent, contour (normal or not) and wall (normal or not)		
Urinary bladder	Present or absent, contour (normal or not) and wall (normal or not)		
Diaphragmaticohepatic view	Pleural fluid	Present or absent (mild, moderate, severe) or indeterminate	
	Pericardial fluid	Present or absent (mild, moderate, severe) or indeterminate	
	Hepatic veins	Unremarkable or distended or indeterminate	
Positive or negative at the four views (0 negative, 1 positive)			
Diaphragmaticohepatic site	0 or 1		
Splenorenal site	0 or 1		
Cystocolic site	0 or 1		
Hepatorenal site	0 or 1		
Abdominal fluid score: 0–4 (0 negative all quadrants to a maximum score of 4 positive all quadrants)			
Comments: _____.			
The AFAST[3] examination is an ultrasound scan used to detect the presence of free abdominal fluid and other conditions to better direct resuscitation efforts and patient care. AFAST[3] allows indirect assessment for evidence of intra-abdominal injury or disease and intrathoracic injury or disease. The AFAST[3] examination is not intended to replace a formal abdominal ultrasound.			

Data from Lisciandro GR, Lagutchik MS, Mann KA, et al. Evaluation of an abdominal fluid scoring system determined using abdominal focused assessment with sonography for trauma in 101 dogs with motor vehicle trauma. J Vet Emerg Crit Care 2009;19(5):426–37.

detecting pericardial effusion and cardiac tamponade; Greg Lisciandro, unpublished data, 2012). Given the subxiphoid view is part of the standard AFAST examination, it is recommended to continue to evaluate the pleural and pericardial spaces of patients with trauma for the presence of fluid by this view.

In humans, the application of bed-side emergency ultrasound performed by non-radiologists has expanded from the simple detection of free fluid in patients with trauma to the detection of numerous intra-abdominal pathology from a variety of causes in critically ill patients without trauma.[10,32–34] In veterinary medicine, the AFAST examination readily lends itself to the identification of injuries beyond trauma, and the AFAST examination has been applied to patients without trauma for the detection of free abdominal fluid and other intra-abdominal pathology, especially in cardiovascularly unstable patients.[5,35] To emphasize the importance of the AFAST examination in triage of patients without trauma and its importance of following patients serially, it has been referred to as the "AFAST[3]"examination to include the three "T's" of trauma, triage, and tracking (eg, monitoring).[5] To this extent, it has been used to assess patient volume status by evaluating the width of the caudal vena cava and hepatic veins.[5] However, there are no published clinical studies that have investigated the use of the AFAST examination at diagnosing non–trauma-related internal injury when performed by nonradiologists in veterinary medicine.

In summary, many abdominal injuries are not readily detectable on physical examination despite the fact some are serious enough to result in hypoperfusion and shock. Rapid assessment of the abdomen to detect occult or potentially lethal injuries should be a high priority in all unstable patients in which the underlying cause is not readily apparent. In humans, FAST examination has proved useful for detecting trauma and non–trauma-related injury in the abdominal, pleural, and pericardial spaces. Preliminary studies in dogs suggest that the AFAST examination has value in assessing the presence of abdominal injuries, and possibly pleural and pericardial injuries in patients with trauma. The AFAST examination may also prove valuable at detecting non–trauma-related injuries in unstable veterinary patients (eg, hemoabdomen secondary to neoplasia). Finally, the AFAST examination is not an extensive examination of all internal organs but rather a focused examination looking at specific sites of the abdomen to try and answer specific questions: Is free fluid indicative of internal injury present? How much fluid is present? What does this fluid signify? Is the quantity of fluid static, increasing, or decreasing over time?

TFAST FOR BLUNT AND PENETRATING TRAUMA: DETECTION OF FREE AIR AND FREE FLUID

The clinical use of the novel veterinary TFAST scan was documented in a large prospective study of 145 dogs incurring both blunt and penetrating trauma.[36] The primary objective was to determine the accuracy, sensitivity, and specificity of using TFAST for the rapid detection of pneumothorax (PTX), dubbed the most preventable cause of death in traumatized people.[26,37] Secondary objectives included the detection of other injuries, including those within the pleural and pericardial spaces and involving the thoracic wall. The sensitivity and specificity for the detection of PTX by the most experienced sonographer was greater than 95% (using thoracic radiography as the gold standard), thus proving that thoracic ultrasound could be used as a first-line screening test in blunt and penetrating trauma.[36]

More recently, the clinical uses for TFAST have extended beyond trauma (as similar with AFAST). The original TFAST acronym has since evolved into TFAST[3].[5] Patient care and clinical course are potentially improved by rapidly detecting conditions and complications in various subsets of patients using TFAST[3] as an extension of the physical examination including nontrauma, postinterventional, and postsurgical at risk (pleural effusions [hemothorax, pyothorax] and PTX) cases.[1,38–40] As a result of correlating TFAST lung findings with thoracic radiographs (TXRs), a more comprehensive novel lung surveillance called the Vet Blue Lung Scan that extends beyond the TFAST[3] chest tube site (CTS) is currently being evaluated with favorable results (Vet Blue is reliable in veterinary patients; Greg Lisciandro, unpublished data, 2012). The Vet Blue Lung Scan, nicknamed Vet Blue ("blue" for cyanosis, and "BLUE" for bedside lung ultrasound examination[41]), is a rapid point-of-care lung ultrasound scan used as a first-line screening evaluation in respiratory distressed or respiratory compromised veterinary patients (discussed later). In the properly trained physician, lung ultrasound has been shown to exceed chest auscultation and supine chest radiography in sensitivity and specificity for PTX, pleural effusion, lung consolidation, and interstitial syndrome in human patients.[40–46]

These abbreviated ultrasound techniques may be mastered by the nonradiologist veterinarian and serve to rapidly detect life-threatening and potentially life-threatening conditions and complications in hospitalized veterinary patients that have historically been either missed (occult) by traditional means of physical examination, laboratory, and radiographic findings or incurred delay in arranging formal ultrasound studies. By using these abbreviated ultrasound techniques to rapidly answer clinical questions, clinical course is positively affected.[4,5,36,38,41,47,48]

PERFORMING THE TFAST[3] EXAMINATION: NOW A FIVE-POINT SCAN

The TFAST[3] examination consists of five points or areas to scan: the stationary horizontally probe-positioned CTS view; the two bilateral dynamically spotlighted PCS views; and the DH view (part of both AFAST[3] and TFAST[3]) (**Fig. 8**). The CTS is best used to exclude PTX and survey for lung pathology, whereas the PCS view is used to detect the presence of pleural and pericardial fluid. Additionally, the right PCS view may be used for volume status assessment (by the left ventricular short-axis view) and to evaluate the aortic/left atrial ratio (which is important in patients suspected to have left-sided heart failure or cardiac disease). The DH view is advantageous over the PCS views because of the acoustic window into the pleural and pericardial spaces through the liver and gallbladder. To differentiate between pleural and pericardial fluid, multiple views (eg, right and left PCS and the DH views) prevent potentially catastrophic mistakes of misidentifying an enlarged right ventricle for pleural effusion or pericardial effusion, and for the presence or absence of cardiac tamponade (see **Fig. 6**).

PATIENT PREPARATION AND POSITIONING FOR TFAST[3] AND VET BLUE

Fur does not need to be shaved for the TFAST[3] and Vet Blue techniques; rather, the fur can be parted for probe-to-skin contact with the use of alcohol and acoustic coupling gel. By not shaving, the cosmetic appearance of the patient is preserved and imaging quality is sufficient with newer ultrasound machines. Alcohol should not be used if electrical defibrillation is anticipated.

For positioning, either right or left lateral recumbency may be used in nonrespiratory patients with all but the opposing CTS. To make the latter side accessible, the patient can be moved into sternal for the final view. For patients with respiratory compromise, sternal recumbency should be used. Right lateral may be preferable because it is standard positioning for electrocardiographic and echocardiographic evaluation (see AFAST). Because most patients are evaluated with AFAST[3] and TFAST[3] (referred to

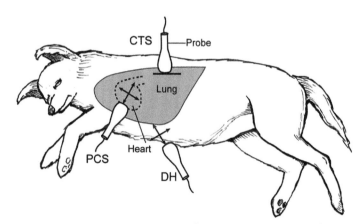

Fig. 8. Depiction of the revised five-point TFAST[3] protocol. (*From* Lisciandro GR. Abdominal and thoracic focused assessment with sonography for trauma, triage, and monitoring in small animals. J Vet Emerg Crit Care 2011;21(2):113; with permission.)

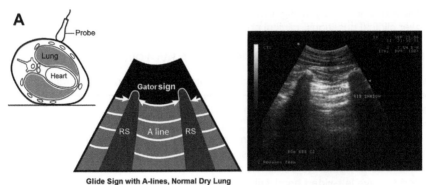

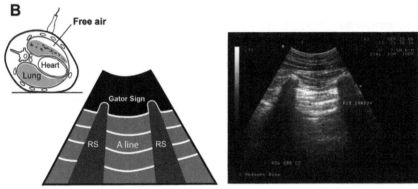

Fig. 9. The glide sign and pneumothorax at the chest tube site. (*A*) Normal CTS view orientation for TFAST[3]. The "gator sign" composed of adjacent ribs with the pulmonary–pleural interface interposed between, is likened to a submerged alligator peering from the water's surface with the eyes as rib heads, and the bridge of the nose in between the eyes representing the pleural- pulmonary interface (PP-line). Along the PP-line, the presence of a glide sign indicates normal apposition of lung against the thoracic wall, thus ruling out PTX. The *bold white arrows* indicate motion to-and-fro during inspiration and expiration, analogous to the cursor of an Etch-a-Sketch moving back and forth through the same line. (*Bold line with arrows*, glide sign). (*B*) CTS view illustrating PTX, where the glide sign is absent, as a real-time finding, depicted by lack of arrows along the pulmonary–pleural interface. Note that A-lines are present in PTX and non-PTX cases. *A* and *B* are identical still B mode ultrasound images to illustrate that a normal pulmonary–pleural interface is indistinguishable from the presence of PTX, and the real-time dynamic presence or absence of the glide sign is the distinguishing feature. (*C*) CTS view illustrating ultrasound lung rockets (ULRs) also called B-lines (previously referred to a comet-tail artifacts) that are defined as laser-like hyperechoic lines that do not fade and extend from the pulmonary-pleural interface to the far field and oscillate (*bold arrows*) swinging like a pendulum with inspiration and expiration. Their presence rules out PTX. A-line, air reverberation artifact; RS, rib shadow. (*From* Lisciandro GR. Abdominal and thoracic focused assessment with sonography for trauma, triage, and monitoring in small animals. J Vet Emerg Crit Care 2011;21(2):114; with permission.)

as combo FAST [CFAST]) the authors find it most efficient to perform six of eight of the views while the patient is in lateral with similar ultrasound settings.[11] Dorsal recumbency should never be used for several important reasons including the high risk to compromised patients (see AFAST).

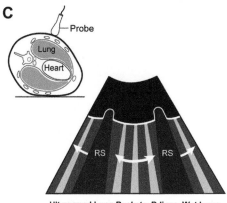

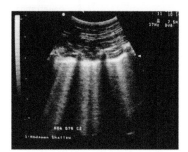

Ultrasound Lung Rockets, B-lines, Wet Lung

Fig. 9. (continued)

THE DIAGNOSIS OF PTX: THE TFAST[3] CTS

The normal to-and-fro motion of the lung sliding along the thoracic wall is called the glide sign.[49] The pulmonary-pleural interface (PP-line) is not to be confused by the distally positioned equidistant reverberation artifacts A-lines (air reverberation artifact) that parallel and extend from the PP-line. When using B-mode, standard two-dimensional ultrasound, still images are the same for a glide sign and PTX because the presence of the glide sign along the PP-line may only be appreciated in real-time (**Fig. 9**A and B). Additionally, the presence of ultrasound lung rockets (ULRs) or B-lines exclude PTX. ULRs, now called B-lines in a recent consensus statement,[46] are defined as hyperechoic (bright) laser-like streaks that do not fade extending through the far field obliterating A-lines. ULRs must also swing like a pendulum, a to-and-fro motion with inspiration and expiration (see **Fig. 9**C). The presence of the glide sign or the presence of ULRs excludes PTX at that respective point on the thoracic wall; thus, by imaging the highest point on the thorax, PTX is best ruled out.[50] An algorithm to diagnose pneumothorax has been developed (see **Fig. 10**).

USING THE LUNG POINT FOR THE DEGREE OF PTX: PARTIAL VERSUS MASSIVE

Historically, the ultrasound diagnosis of PTX has been incorrectly considered an all-or-none phenomenon; however, it is possible to determine the degree of PTX by identifying the location at which collapsed lung recontacts the thoracic wall called the "lung point." To find the lung point the ultrasound probe is positioned sequentially from dorsal to ventral, searching for the presence of either a glide sign or ULRs (evidence that aerated lung is recontacting the thoracic wall). The distance from the CTS to the lung point may be used to subjectively assess the degree of a partial PTX and help determine its clinical relevance.[5,51,52] In the absence of the lung point, a massive PTX is present or the scan is indeterminate (**Fig. 11**).

THE DIAGNOSIS OF LUNG CONTUSIONS

The presence of wet lung (ULRs) in patients with trauma at the TFAST[3] CTS view represents lung contusions until proved otherwise.[53] By extending the TFAST[3] examination using Vet Blue (see below), the severity of lung contusions may be subjectively assessed by recording the number of ULRs at each of the Vet Blue regional lung views. In addition, by using Vet Blue, the detection of occult lung contusions based

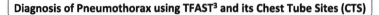

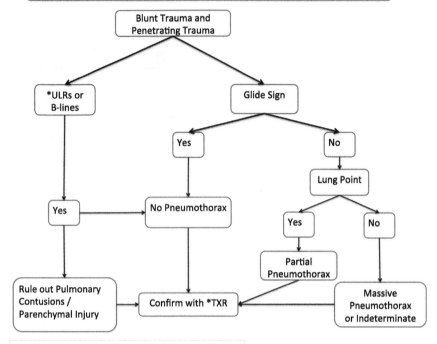

Fig. 10. TFAST diagnosis of pneumothorax using TFAST[3] and its chest tube sites.

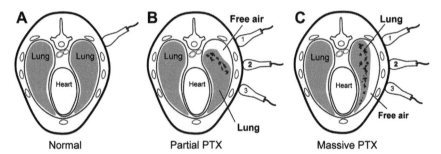

Fig. 11. Depiction of cross-sectional thoraces illustrating the search for the lung point. Cross-sectional canine thoraces depicting the quantification of the degree of PTX as partial or massive by searching for the lung point with the patient positioned in sternal recumbency (safer than lateral recumbency in compromised patients). In the absence of the glide sign or ULRs, the probe is moved sequentially in a ventral manner as numerically labeled from dorsal to ventral. (*A*) Normal thorax in which pneumothorax has been excluded. (*B*) PTX has been identified at position 1 and the lung point at position 2 suggests the pneumothorax to be partial. (*C*) PTX has been identified and a lung point is nonexistent at any of the three probe positions, suggesting massive pneumothorax. (*From* Lisciandro GR. Abdominal and thoracic focused assessment with sonography for trauma, triage, and monitoring in small animals. J Vet Emerg Crit Care 2011;21(2):115; with permission.)

on the limitations of the TFAST[3] CTS view (a single site) is possible by the more extensive regionally based lung scan (three more sites, four total per hemithorax). Because of the simplicity and short duration of the Vet Blue regional lung scan (<90 seconds), it should be considered an extension of TFAST[3] and used routinely. Moreover, the resolution of lung contusions may be tracked using serial Vet Blue examinations.

THE DIAGNOSIS OF CHEST WALL PATHOLOGY: THE STEP SIGN

The step sign is defined as an inconsistency from the normal expected linear continuity along the PP-line.[5] The observance of the step sign should arouse clinical suspicion for thoracic wall injury, such as intercostal tears, rib fractures, flail chest, subcostal hematoma, hemothorax, and so forth.[5,36] In nontrauma subsets of patients, the step sign may represent types of pleural effusion, lung consolidation, or lung masses (**Fig. 12**). The step sign may be misinterpreted (eg, as a false-positive) if the probe is placed too far caudally on the thoracic wall where the lung, diaphragm, and thoracic wall dynamically come into close proximity.[5,36]

THE DIAGNOSIS OF PLEURAL AND PERICARDIAL EFFUSION

Ultrasound is well established in being superior to physical examination and radiography for the detection of free fluid in the pleural and pericardial space, and is arguably the gold standard for the diagnosis of pericardial effusion.[1,42,54,55] The PCS views are gravity-dependent and can be used for detecting either type of effusion. The DH view (also part of AFAST) is considered the most sensitive view in human protocols, and should be used because of the acoustic window provided into the pleural and pericardial spaces.[1,55] Multiple views improve the probability of an accurate assessment, while lowering the probability of mistaking normal structures for pathology. Ideally, a PCS view and the TFAST[3] DH view should be used, adhering to the axiom that "one view is no view" (**Fig. 13**).

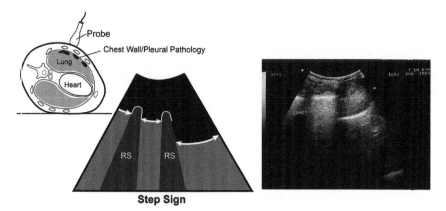

Step Sign

Fig. 12. The step sign. CTS view illustrating the step sign where the glide sign deviates from the expected normal linear continuity of the pulmonary–pleural interface indicated by the offset arrows. Observation of a step sign suggests thoracic trauma, such as partial PTX, hemothorax, rib fractures, intercostals muscle tear, pulmonary contusions, and diaphragmatic hernia. In nontrauma the step sign may represent areas of lung consolidation or masses. A-line, air reverberation artifact; RS, rib shadow. (*From* Lisciandro GR, Lagutchik MS, Mann KA, et al. Evaluation of a thoracic focused assessment with sonography for trauma (TFAST) protocol to detect pneumothorax and concurrent thoracic injury in 145 traumatized dogs. J Vet Emerg Crit Care 2008;18:261; with permission.)

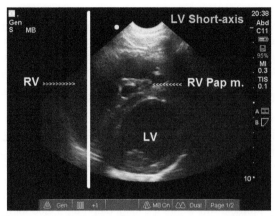

Fig. 13. The pitfall of the pericardial site. Shown is a B mode image of a short-axis view of a canine heart illustrating that by not recognizing normal heart anatomy, the right ventricle may be mistaken for an effusion and its distorted papillary muscle as a mass or other pathology. The *vertical line* emphasizes that by focusing too closely (if the sonographer was only looking at the field to the right of the *vertical line*) an error may be made; however, by zooming away or increasing depth (including the image to the left of the *vertical line* [or the entire B mode image depicted]), the normal anatomy is better appreciated. The image shows the classic left ventricular short-axis "mushroom" view for subjective volume assessment. LV, left ventricle; RV, right ventricle; RV Pap m., right ventricular papillary muscle.

THE DIAGNOSIS OF CARDIAC TAMPONADE

The diagnosis of cardiac tamponade is made when the intrapericardial pressure exceeds right atrial and ventricular pressure, causing their outer walls to paradoxically move inward (eg, collapse) during the cardiac cycle. Generally, in real-time ultrasound imaging, this life-threatening condition may be easily recognized by the nonradiologist veterinarian using TFAST[3]. It behooves the veterinarian incorporating the FAST[3] protocols into their practice to review the causes and treatment of pericardial effusion, including left atrial tears secondary to mitral valve disease in dogs, hemorrhage from right atrial neoplasia, heart base tumors, idiopathic pericardial effusion, and hemorrhage caused by anticoagulant rodenticide toxicity. In comparing 2005 (pre-TFAST[3]) cases with 2011 (post-AFAST[3] and TFAST[3]) cases at the author's practice (GRL) the incidence in detecting pericardial effusion was dramatic (eg, 2 cases vs 24, annual caseload approximately 11,000). Moreover, of the 24 cases, 21 (88%) of 24 were recognized by the DH view, either during TFAST[3] or AFAST[3], and approximately 50% had pericardiocentesis performed because of the diagnosis of cardiac tamponade (many tamponade cases diagnosed via the DH view) (application of the DH view, either during TFAST[3] or AFAST[3] in detecting pericardial effusion and cardiac tamponade; unpublished data, Greg Lisciandro, 2012).

THE VET BLUE LUNG SCAN

In human patients, lung ultrasound has been shown to be superior to chest auscultation and supine radiography for the detection of PTX, interstitial syndrome, and lung consolidation, and has most recently become an important facet of pulmonary and emergency and critical care medicine.[41,43,44,46,56,57] Vet Blue is a rapid point-of-care lung ultrasound scan used as a first-line screening evaluation in respiratory-distressed or respiratory-compromised veterinary patients. The Vet Blue is primarily based on the easily recognizable concept of wet (ULRs) versus dry lung (glide sign and A-lines) (see **Fig. 9**A, C). Normally, in dogs and cats without respiratory disease, ULRs (wet lung) are infrequently detected, and when present, are found in low numbers (one or two ULRs) at a single Vet Blue site (Vet Blue is reliable in veterinary patients; unpublished data, Greg Lisciandro, 2012). Most nonrespiratory dogs and cats have no or infrequent ULRs at any Vet Blue site (**Fig. 14**A and B).

The potentially practice-changing advantage of Vet Blue for the small animal practitioner is that often, patient instability or lack of immediate technical support delays radiographic imaging (which is the historical diagnostic mainstay for veterinarians). As a result, clinical decisions have been traditionally based on insensitive information including patient history, thoracic auscultation, and the characterization of breathing patterns.[58,59] By adding Vet Blue as an extension of TFAST[3] or as a standalone technique, the attending veterinarian has an additional rapid, point-of-care modality for diagnosing lung conditions and anticipating TXR findings; thus, directing more evidence-based therapeutic decisions to the patient's benefit. Moreover, lung ultrasound is unaffected by environmental and patient noise and its imaging is a more objective evaluation (vs the art of thoracic auscultation).

The Vet Blue format should also be considered as an applicable survey for the same T[3] scenarios assigned to AFAST[3] and TFAST[3] (trauma, triage, and tracking [monitoring]). The use of Vet Blue may be advantageous (because of rapid scan, point-of-care testing, minimal restraint, radiation-sparing, and so forth) and effectively monitored (by serial examinations) throughout the patient's therapy surveying the thorax with the ultrasound probe similar as with a stethoscope.[60]

THE USE OF VET BLUE AND LUNG ULTRASOUND: PRINCIPLES AND ASSUMPTIONS

The wet lung (ULRs) versus dry lung concept works well for the rapid inclusion or exclusion of lung contusions in patients with trauma and cardiogenic and noncardiogenic causes of pulmonary edema in nontrauma subsets of patients. In human medicine, this highly sensitive technique is very effectively used as a bedside test in people to confidently rule out cardiogenic pulmonary edema when lung fields are dry; based on the author's experience, Vet Blue proves reliable in veterinary patients (Vet Blue is reliable in veterinary patients; unpublished data, Greg Lisciandro, 2012).[44,46,47,57]

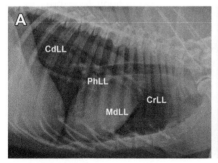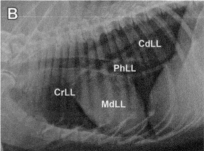

Fig. 14. The Vet Blue Lung Scan. Illustrated here are right (*A*) and left (*B*) hemithoraces. Vet Blue is performed with the probe positioned the same as that of the TFAST[3] CTS view and should be considered as an extension of TFAST[3] and a standalone technique for more comprehensive lung surveillance. The lung is evaluated at regional lung locations as follows: caudodorsal lung lobe region (CdLL) (same as the TFAST[3] CTS view); perihilar lung lobe region (PhLL); middle lung lobe region (MdLL); and cranial lung lobe region (CrLL). The maximum number of ULRs over a single intercostal space at each respective site is recorded.

Equally as important, the recognition of interstitial edema by lung ultrasound precedes alveolar edema (as evidenced by less serious [ULRs] vs more serious lung consolidation, respectively).[44,47,48,50,57] Because lung ultrasound seems to be more sensitive than physical examination findings and TXR, the incorporation of Vet Blue as lung surveillance is beneficial. This may also allow more rapid therapeutic intervention, and thus limit more serious progression to lung failure, as shown in humans.[41,44,46,47,50,57] Finally, it should be noted that several limitations of Vet Blue exist: lung conditions must have reached the anatomic periphery (and thus be accessible by ultrasound visualization); and recognition that lesions located deep within the lung lobes will be missed because ultrasound cannot penetrate or image through aerated lung.[44,46,50] However, in acute respiratory distress, the wet-to-dry lung principles prove very helpful in categorizing causes of acute respiratory distress with high sensitivity and specificity in human patients.[41,43,44,46,47,50,57] By the very achievable goal of learning the recognition of wet versus dry lung, the nonradiologist sonographer begins to recognize additional signs of ultrasonographically detectable lung pathology (discussed later).

THE USE OF REGIONALLY BASED VET BLUE FINDINGS: DIAGNOSING AND MONITORING LUNG CONDITIONS

Many acute non–trauma-associated respiratory conditions have classic distribution patterns of wet versus dry lung (**Fig. 15**). For example, dogs with early stages of left-sided heart failure or volume overload (other than Doberman Pinschers with

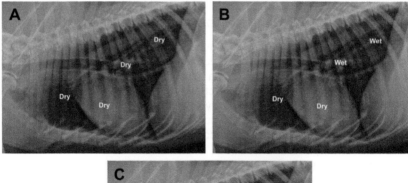

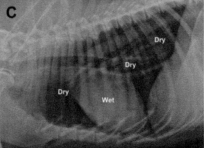

Fig. 15. The basic Vet Blue patterns. Each depicts examples of the distribution of expected findings in acute respiratory distress. (*A*) The finding of dry lung all regions (glide sign with A-lines) effectively rules out any clinically significant degree of cardiogenic or noncardiogenic forms of pulmonary edema and suggests other respiratory and nonrespiratory causes. (*B*) The finding of wet lungs in the dorsal lung regions strongly suggests the presence of cardiogenic and noncardiogenic pulmonary edema (referred to as interstitial syndrome). (*C*) The finding of wet fields isolated to the ventral regions suggests acute pneumonia.

dilated cardiomyopathy) typically have ULRs at the caudodorsal and perihilar lung regions and dry lungs ventrally at the middle and cranial lung lobe regions. The same pattern seems to hold true for acute noncardiogenic pulmonary edema (NCPE) from neurogenic causes, electrocution, or choking or other causes (eg, drowning, acute lung injury, respiratory distress syndrome).

Conversely, ventral wet lung patterns are more suggestive of pneumonias. For example, consider a dog presenting that may have aspirated after choking on an upper airway foreign body. The cause of respiratory distress (or respiratory concerns, if seemingly asymptomatic) may be aspiration pneumonia, NCPE, or both. Each of these scenarios may be expediently addressed using Vet Blue (potentially preempting the need for TXR, particularly if financial constraints exist). If this dog has wet lungs (ULRs) only identified at the right middle lung lobe region, the major cause of its respiratory distress is more likely to be acute aspiration (eg, wet lungs at the classically affected lung lobe) rather than NCPE. If this same dog has a ULR distribution at the caudodorsal and perihilar lung regions, it is more likely to have NCPE; however, the same dog may have Vet Blue findings supportive of both conditions. Finally, if this dog has dry lungs in all fields, then these complications are potentially ruled-out, especially when Vet Blue is used in serial fashion. Because therapy is much different for aspiration pneumonia than NCPE (and no therapy is needed for their nonexistence), a simple Vet Blue examination rapidly and expediently puts the clinician on potentially the correct therapeutic path. However, other differential diagnoses must be considered in patients presenting with respiratory distress when dry lungs are observed in all fields, including feline asthma, upper airway disease, pulmonary thromboembolism, and nonrespiratory causes of distress (eg, nonrespiratory "lookalikes," such as high fever/pyrexia, cardiac tamponade, hypovolemia, anemia, and severe metabolic acidosis).

THE FUTURE OF SMALL ANIMAL LUNG ULTRASOUND

The wet (ULRs or B-lines) versus dry lung (glide sign or A-lines) concept is easily mastered by the nonradiologist veterinarian. In more chronic conditions (and some acute), additional lung ultrasound signs are seen. These signs are suspected by recognizing deviations from the normal linear continuity of the PP-line (previously referred to as step signs). Lung consolidation may appear as subsets of the step sign and include newly defined terminology by the author including the shred sign, tissue sign, and nodule sign, full definitions of which are beyond the scope of this review but similar to propositions in human medicine.[56]

THE USE OF TFAST[3] AND VET BLUE: CARDIOVASCULAR ASSESSMENT

TFAST[3] and Vet Blue can also be used for cardiovascular assessment during resuscitation, and monitoring for complications associated with fluid therapy.[47,57] A subjective cardiovascular assessment may be made by looking at the left ventricular short-axis (right TFAST[3] PCS [mushroom view]) for volume status and contractility, the caudodorsal and perihilar lung regions of Vet Blue for wet lung (evidence of pulmonary edema), and caudal vena caval size and hepatic venous distention (the DH view) for preload assessment and detection of volume overload (**Fig. 16**).[1]

THE USE OF GLOBAL FAST[3]: MONITORING HOSPITALIZED, CRITICALLY ILL PATIENTS, AND AT-RISK PATIENTS

By combining these three focused ultrasound techniques (referred to as global FAST[3] or GFAST[3]) as an extension of the cursory ultrasound (AFAST[3], TFAST[3]) and the

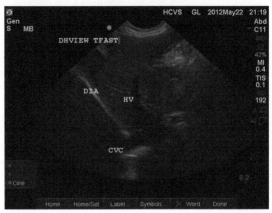

Fig. 16. The use of AFAST[3], TFAST[3], and Vet Blue for cardiovascular status. By combining the right TFAST[3] PCS view for contractility and left ventricular filling (short-axis "mushroom" view) (see **Fig. 13**), and Vet Blue for the presence or absence of cardiogenic pulmonary edema (ULRs) (see **Fig. 9**A, C), the DH view of both AFAST[3] and TFAST[3] for caudal vena caval (CVC) size and degrees of hepatic venous distention (HV) for preload and right-sided cardiac status, the veterinarian can noninvasively subjectively evaluate overall cardiovascular status of the veterinary patient. DIA, diaphragm.

Table 2	
Thoracic focused assessment with sonography for trauma, triage, and tracking (TFAST[3]) template for medical records	
CTS glide sign[a]	Present (normal): no pneumothorax *or* Absent: pneumothorax
CTS lung rockets[a]	Present (no PTX): interstitial lung fluid (edema, hemorrhage) *or* Absent: no interstitial lung fluid (edema, hemorrhage)
CTS step sign[a]	Present: concurrent thoracic wall trauma (rib fractures, hematoma, intercostal muscle tear) or pleural space disease is suspected or nontraumatic lung conditions *or* Absent: no concurrent thoracic wall trauma or pleural space disease is suspected
PCS view[a]	Absent: no pleural *or* pericardial fluid Present: pleural *or* pericardial fluid *or* both (mild, moderate, or severe)
Cardiac tamponade	Absent Present Indeterminate
LV filling (short-axis)	Adequate, suggesting normovolemia *or* Inadequate, suggesting hypovolemia *or* Indeterminate
Diaphragmaticohepatic view: there is no apparent pericardial or pleural fluid present *or* there is pericardial effusion (mild, moderate, severe) or pleural effusion (mild, moderate, severe)	
Comments: _____.	

Abbreviations: CTS, chest tube site; LV, left ventricle; PCS, pericardial sac; PTX, pneumothorax.

The TFAST[3] examination is an ultrasound scan used to help detect chest wall, lung, and pleural and pericardial space problems as a screening test to better direct resuscitation efforts and patient care. TFAST[3] is not necessarily intended to replace chest radiographs or formal echocardiography.

[a] Right and left sides are listed in templates for the CTS and PCS views.

Data from Lisciandro GR, Lagutchik MS, Man KA, et al. Evaluation of a thoracic focused assessment with sonography for trauma (TFAST) protocol to detect pneumothorax and concurrent thoracic injury in 145 traumatized dogs. J Vet Emerg Crit Care 2008;18(3):258–69.

Table 3	
The Vet Blue Lung Scan template for medical records	
Record the maximum number of ULRs over a single intercostals space (0, 1, 2, 3, >3) at each respective Vet Blue site in the order of caudodorsal, perihilar, middle and cranial lung lobe regions.	
Left hemithorax (Cd, Ph, Md, Cr)	(x, x, x, x)
Right hemithorax (Cd, Ph, Md, Cr)	(x, x, x, x)
Case examples	
Dry all fields	Left (0, 0, 0, 0)
	Right (0, 0, 0, 0)
Wet fields dorsally	Left (>3, >3, 0, 0)
	Right (2, >3, 0, 0)
Wet field ventrally	Left (0, 0, 0, 0)
	Right (0, 0, >3, 0)
Comments: _____.	

Abbreviations: Cd, caudodorsal lung lobe region; Cr, cranial lung lobe region; Md, middle lung lobe region; Ph, perihilar lung lobe region.

The Vet Blue Lung Scan is a lung ultrasound examination used to help detect and monitor lung conditions; and not necessarily intended to replace thoracic radiographs or formal non-thoracic ultrasound or echocardiography.

"modern stethoscope" (Vet Blue), the nonradiologist veterinarian has the ability to rapidly and expediently arrive at a more probable working diagnoses, decrease morbidity because of delay of diagnosis, avoid mistreating otherwise occult conditions, and improve patient care.[60] These global techniques survey four spaces (eg, peritoneal, retroperitoneal, pleural, and pericardial) in addition to the lung. By using these FAST techniques, the veterinarian may positively direct therapy with evidence-based medicine in the emergent setting or as a cage-side, point-of-care test in hospitalized at-risk or critically ill veterinary patients.

TEMPLATES FOR MEDICAL RECORDS AND TERMINOLOGY

Technique standardization for the AFAST[3], TFAST[3], and Vet Blue examinations is key for veterinarians to not only effectively communicate findings, but also to be able to evaluate the proficiency and clinical use of these ultrasound examinations. These objectives are best met through the use of standardized templates. Included in **Table 1**; **Tables 2** and **3** are suggested goal-directed templates for each of the three ultrasound scans, which may be modified according to the veterinarian's skills. The semantic renaming of abdominal FAST[3] to AFAST[3], thoracic FAST[3] to TFAST[3], the combination of AFAST[3] and TFAST[3] as CFAST[3], and lastly the most comprehensive scan of CFAST[3] and Vet Blue as GFAST[3]' is suggested to avoid the confusing slew of acronyms in human medicine.[5]

SUMMARY

By combining AFAST[3], TFAST[3], and Vet Blue (to global FAST[3] or GFAST[3]), the non-radiologist veterinarian now has reliable, brief ultrasonographic examinations to better direct, diagnose, and monitor therapy that is achievable with minimal training. In addition, these diagnostic tests can help the clinician diagnose potentially serious, life-threatening conditions through the use of point-of care, radiation-sparing tests within minutes on the triage table or during hospitalization of emergent and critically ill veterinary patients.

REFERENCES

1. Matsushima K, Frankel H. Beyond focused assessment with sonography for trauma: ultrasound creep in the trauma resuscitation area and beyond. Curr Opin Crit Care 2011;17:606–12.
2. Nordenholz KE, Rubin MA, Gluarte CG, et al. Ultrasound in the evaluation and management of blunt abdominal trauma. Ann Emerg Med 1997;29:357–66.
3. Boysen SR, Rozanski EA, Tidwell AS, et al. Evaluation of focused assessment with sonography for trauma protocol to detect abdominal fluid in dogs involved in motor vehicle accidents. J Am Vet Med Assoc 2004;225(8):1198–204.
4. Lisciandro GR, Lagutchik MS, Mann KA, et al. Evaluation of an abdominal fluid scoring system determined using abdominal focused assessment with sonography for trauma in 101 dogs with motor vehicle trauma. J Vet Emerg Crit Care 2009;19(5):426–37.
5. Lisciandro GR. Abdominal and thoracic focused assessment with sonography for trauma, triage, and monitoring in small animals. J Vet Emerg Crit Care 2011;21(2):104–22.
6. Richards JR, McGahan JP, Pali MJ, et al. Sonographic detection of blunt hepatic trauma: hemoperitoneum and parenchymal patterns of injury. J Trauma 1999;17: 117–20.
7. Ma OJ, Kefer MP, Mateer JR, et al. Evaluation of hemoperitoneum using a single versus multiple view ultrasonographic examination. Acad Emerg Med 1995;2: 581–6.
8. Shackford SR, Rogers FB, Osler TM, et al. Focused abdominal sonogram for trauma: the learning curve of nonradiologist clinicians in detecting hemoperitoneum. J Trauma 1999;46:553–64.
9. Sondertrom CA, DuPriest RW, Crowley RA. Pitfalls of peritoneal lavage in blunt abdominal trauma. Surg Gynecol Obstet 1980;151:513–8.
10. American College of Emergency Physicians. American College of Emergency Physicians. ACEP emergency ultrasound guidelines-2001. Ann Emerg Med 2001;38:470–81.
11. Lisciandro G. Evaluation of initial and serial combination focused assessment with sonography for trauma (CFAST) examination of the thorax (TFAST) and abdomen (AFAST) with the application of an abdominal fluid scoring system in 49 traumatized cats. J Vet Emerg Crit Care 2012;22(2):S11.
12. Streeter EM, Rozanski EA, Laforcade-Buress A, et al. Evaluation of vehicular trauma in dogs: 239 cases (January-December 2001). J Am Vet Med Assoc 2009;235(4):405–8.
13. Simpson S, Syring R, Otto CM. Severe blunt trauma in dogs: 235 cases (1997-2003). J Vet Emerg Crit Care 2009;19(6):588–602.
14. Nazeer SR, Dewbre H, Miller AH. Ultrasound-assisted paracentesis performed by emergency physicians vs the traditional technique: a prospective, randomized study. Am J Emerg Med 2005;23:363–7.
15. Kolata RJ, Dudley EJ. Motor vehicle accidents in urban dogs: a study of 600 cases. J Am Vet Med Assoc 1975;167:938–41.
16. Mongil CM, Drobatz KJ, Hendricks JC. Traumatic hemoperitoneum in 28 cases: a retrospective review. J Am Anim Hosp Assoc 1995;31:217–22.

17. Rothlin MA, Naf R, Amgwerd M, et al. Ultrasound in blunt abdominal and thoracic trauma. J Trauma 1993;34:488–95.
18. Korner M, Krotz MM, Degenhart C, et al. Current role of emergency US in patients with major trauma. Radiographics 2008;28:225–42.
19. Cokkinos D, Anypa E, Stefanidis P, et al. Contrast-enhanced ultrasound for imaging blunt abdominal trauma: indications, description of the technique and imaging review. Ultraschall Med 2012;33:60–7.
20. Valentino M, Ansaloni L, Catena F, et al. Contrast-enhanced ultrasonography in blunt abdominal trauma: considerations after 5 years of experience. Radiol Med 2009;114:1080–93.
21. Miller M, Pasquale M, Bromberg W, et al. Not so FAST. J Trauma 2003;54(1):52–9.
22. Poletti PA, Kinkel K, Vermeulen B, et al. Blunt abdominal trauma: should US be used to detect both free fluid and organ injuries? Radiology 2003;227:95–103.
23. Shanmurganathan K, Mirvis SE, Sherbourne CD, et al. Hemoperitoneum as the sole indicator of abdominal visceral injuries: a potential limitation of screening abdominal US for trauma. Radiology 1999;212:423–30.
24. Boulanger BR, Kearney PA, Tsuei B, et al. The routine use of sonography in penetrating torso injury is beneficial. J Trauma 2001;51:320–5.
25. Udobi KF, Rodriguez A, Chiu WC, et al. Role of ultrasonography in penetrating abdominal trauma: a prospective clinical study. J Trauma 2001;50:475–9.
26. Kirkpatrick AW, Sirois M, Ball C, et al. The hand-held ultrasound examination for penetrating abdominal trauma. Am J Surg 2004;187:660–5.
27. Mohammadi A, Ghasemi-Rad M. Evaluation of gastrointestinal injury in blunt abdominal trauma "FAST is not reliable": the role of repeated ultrasonography. World J Emerg Surg 2012;7(1):2.
28. Sgourakis G, Lanitis S, Zacharioudakis C, et al. Incidental findings in trauma patients during focused assessment with sonography for trauma. Am Surg 2012; 78(3):366–72.
29. Pathan A. Role of ultrasound in the evaluation of blunt abdominal trauma. J Liaquat Univ Med Health Sci 2005;4(1):23–8.
30. Tayal VS, Beatty MA, Marx JA, et al. FAST (focused assessment with sonography in trauma) accurate for cardiac and intraperitoneal injury in penetrating anterior chest trauma. J Ultrasound Med 2004;23(4):467–72.
31. Rozycki GS, Ballard RB, Feliciano DV, et al. Surgeon-performed ultrasound for the assessment of truncal injuries: lessons learned from 1540 patients. Ann Surg 1998;228(4):557–67.
32. Yen K, Gorelick MH. Ultrasound applications for the pediatric emergency department: a review of the current literature. Pediatr Emerg Care 2002;18(3):226–34.
33. Legome E, Pancu D. Future applications for emergency ultrasound. Emerg Med Clin North Am 2004;22:817–27.
34. Ballard R, Rozycki GS, Knudson MM, et al. The surgeons' use of ultrasound in the acute setting. Surg Clin North Am 1998;78(2):337–64.
35. Panagiotis M. Use of ultrasonography by veterinary surgeons in small animal clinical emergencies. Ultrasound 2012;20:77–81.
36. Lisciandro GR, Lagutchik MS, Man KA, et al. Evaluation of a thoracic focused assessment with sonography for trauma (TFAST) protocol to detect pneumothorax and concurrent thoracic injury in 145 traumatized dogs. J Vet Emerg Crit Care 2008;18(3):258–69.
37. Kirkpatrick AW, Nicolaou S, Rowan K, et al. Thoracic sonography for pneumothorax: the clinical evaluation of an operational space medicine spin-off. Acta Astronaut 2005;56:831–8.

38. Rozycki GS, Pennington SD, Feliciano DV. Surgeon-performed ultrasound in the critical care setting: its use as an extension of the physical examination to detect pleural effusion. J Trauma 2001;50:636–42.
39. Lichtenstein DA. Ultrasound in the management of thoracic disease. Crit Care Med 2007;35(S5):S250–61.
40. Reibig A, Kroegel C. Accuracy of transthoracic sonography in excluding post-interventional pneumothorax and hydrothorax: comparison to chest radiography. Eur J Radiol 2005;53:463–70.
41. Lichtestein DA, Meziere GA. Relevance of lung ultrasound in the diagnosis of acute respiratory failure: the BLUE protocol. Chest 2008;134(1):117–25.
42. Brooks A, Davies B, Smethhurst M, et al. Emergency ultrasound in the acute assessment of haemothorax. Emerg Med 2004;21:44–6.
43. Lichtenstein DA, Lascos N, Meziere GA, et al. Ultrasound diagnosis of alveolar consolidation in the critically ill. Intensive Care Med 2004;30:276–81.
44. Lichtenstein DA, Meziere GA, Lagoueyte J, et al. A-Lines and B-Lines. Lung ultrasound as a bedside tool for predicting pulmonary artery occlusion pressure in the critically ill. Chest 2009;136(4):1014–20.
45. Ball CG, Kirkpatrick AW, Laupland KB, et al. Factors related to the failure of radiographic recognition of occult posttraumatic pneumothoraces. Am J Surg 2005;189:550–6.
46. Volpicelli G, Elbarbary M, Blaivas M, et al. International evidence-based recommendations for point-of-care lung ultrasound. Intensive Care Med 2012;38: 577–91.
47. Lichtenstein D, Karakitsos D. Integrating lung ultrasound in the hemodynamic evaluation of acute circulatory failure (the fluid administration limited by lung sonography protocol). J Crit Care 2012;27(5):533.e11–9.
48. Ollerton JE, Sugrue M, Balogh Z, et al. Prospective study to evaluate the influence of FAST on trauma patient management. J Trauma 2006;60:785–91.
49. Nyland TC, Matton JS. Thorax. In: Nyland TC, Matton JS, editors. Small animal diagnostic ultrasound. 2nd edition. Philadelphia: WB Saunders Company; 2002. p. 335.
50. Soldati G, Sher S, Testa A. Lung and ultrasound: time to "reflect." Eur Rev Med Pharmacol Sci 2011;15(2):223–7.
51. Sargsyan AE, Hamilton DR, Nicolau S, et al. Ultrasound evaluation of the magnitude of pneumothorax: a new concept. Am Surg 2001;67:232–5.
52. Lichtenstein D, Meziere G, Biderman P, et al. The "lung point": an ultrasound sign specific to pneumothorax. Intensive Care Med 2000;26:1434–40.
53. Soldati G, Testa A, Silva FR, et al. Chest ultrasonography in lung contusion. Chest 2006;130(2):533–8.
54. Ball CG, Williams BH, Wyrzykowski AD, et al. A caveat to the performance of pericardial ultrasound in patients with penetrating cardiac wounds. J Trauma 2009;67(5):1123–4.
55. Chelly MR, Marguiles DR, Mandavia D, et al. The evolving role of FAST scan for the diagnosis of pericardial fluid. J Trauma 2004;56:915–7.
56. Lichtenstein D. Should lung ultrasonography be more widely used in the assessment of acute respiratory disease? Expert Rev Respir Med 2010;4(5):533–8.
57. Lichtenstein D. Fluid administration limited by lung sonography: the place of lung ultrasound in assessment of acute circulatory failure (the FALLS-protocol). Expert Rev Respir Med 2012;6(2):155–62.
58. Sigrist NE, Doherr MG, Spreng DE. Clinical findings and diagnostic value of post-traumatic thoracic radiographs in dogs and cats with blunt trauma. J Vet Emerg Crit Care 2004;14:259–68.

59. Sigrist NE, Adamik KN, Doherr MG, et al. Evaluation of respiratory parameters at presentation as clinical indicators of the respiratory localization in dogs and cats with respiratory distress. J Vet Emerg Crit Care 2011;21(1):13–23.
60. Filly RA. Ultrasound: the stethoscope of the future, alas. Radiology 1988;167:400.

Management of Respiratory Emergencies in Small Animals

Catherine Sumner, DVM[a], Elizabeth Rozanski, DVM[b],*

KEYWORDS

- Upper airway • Respiratory distress • Cough • Pulmonary edema • Oxygen
- Ventilation • Pleural effusion

KEY POINTS

- Respiratory distress is a common presenting complaint for animals brought to the emergency room, and it is important for clinicians to feel comfortable diagnosing and treating these animals.
- Prompt recognition of the localization of the source of respiratory distress, based on history, pattern recognition, and physical examination findings, will help to determine the underlying cause and is key to determining an appropriate therapeutic course.
- Careful handling, minimizing stress, and rapid and focused treatment are crucial in the management of all patients in respiratory distress.

Respiratory distress is a common presenting complaint for dogs and cats in the emergency room and may develop during hospitalization for noncardiopulmonary disease as well. Appropriate management and a favorable outcome require rapid recognition, assessment of the underlying cause, and timely interventions. This article focuses on current recommendations for emergent diagnostics and management of dogs and cats either presenting to the emergency room with respiratory distress or developing respiratory distress while hospitalized.

The initial approach to a patient with respiratory distress involves localization of the affected region(s) of the airway, lungs, or pleural space, and creation of an initial list of differential diagnoses based on patient history, signalment, and physical examination findings.

Localization is key in determining the best step in management. Respiratory dysfunction occurs because of difficulty in getting oxygen into the lungs (eg, upper airway obstruction, pleural effusion, or lower airway disease) or with difficulty in gas exchange (eg, abnormalities at the alveolar-capillary membrane caused by edema, neoplasia, or hemorrhage).

[a] Emergency and Critical Care Section, Tufts VETS, 525 South Street, Walpole, MA 02081, USA;
[b] Department of Clinical Sciences, Tufts University Cummings School of Veterinary Medicine, 200 Westboro Road, North Grafton, MA 01536, USA
* Corresponding author.
E-mail address: elizabeth.rozanski@tufts.edu

Vet Clin Small Anim 43 (2013) 799–815
http://dx.doi.org/10.1016/j.cvsm.2013.03.005
0195-5616/13/$ – see front matter © 2013 Elsevier Inc. All rights reserved.

vetsmall.theclinics.com

UPPER AIRWAY DISEASE

Normal upper airway physiology reflects negative pressure ventilation; this involves a drop in pressure in the lumen of the upper airway during inspiration, which permits room air to move into the lungs down the pressure gradient. Increased resistance, resulting from narrowing of the upper airway lumen, requires increased inspiratory pressure for equivalent flow rate and clinically may be recognized as loud or stridorous breathing. Increased resistance may be associated with a fixed and/or dynamic obstruction. Specific sites commonly associated with upper airway obstruction include the larynx (eg, due to paralysis, collapse, or masses), the nasopharynx (eg, due to abnormalities in the soft palate or pharyngeal tissues), the cervical trachea, and the nasal passages (**Fig. 1**). Brachycephalic dogs and cats are at increased risk of upper airway obstruction because of their abnormal anatomy, and older large-breed dogs are at increased risk of laryngeal paralysis.

LOWER AIRWAY DISEASE

Lower airway diseases include bronchial disease, such as feline lower airway disease ("asthma") and canine chronic bronchitis. Lower airway disease may present as an emergency in cats with moderate to severe bronchoconstriction, and dogs can present for increased coughing and wheezing. Respiratory distress from lower airway disease is associated with expiratory airflow obstruction. During inspiration, the airways are open, but often collapse or narrow during expiration, resulting in increased expiratory effort and often an expiratory "push" on physical examination. Many dogs with lower airway disease/chronic bronchitis are overweight or obese (**Fig. 2**). Eosinophilic bronchopneumopathy (or bronchitis), commonly seen in northern-breed dogs,

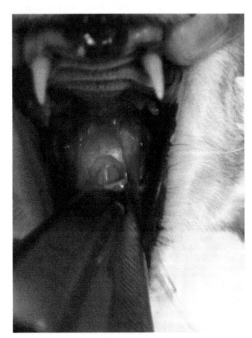

Fig. 1. A 10-year-old Maine coon cat with a laryngeal squamous cell carcinoma evident on laryngeal examination.

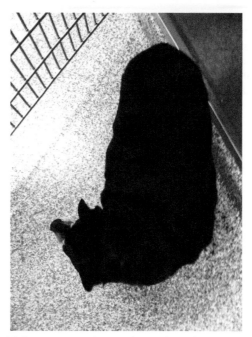

Fig. 2. Many dogs with lower airway disease/chronic bronchitis are overweight or obese.

may also result in lower airway disease. Eosinophilic bronchopneumopathy is associated with coughing, gagging, and a marked bronchial pattern. Tracheal wash cytology is strongly eosinophilic, and concurrent peripheral eosinophilia may or may not be present.

PULMONARY PARENCHYMAL DISEASE

Pulmonary parenchymal diseases include cardiogenic and noncardiogenic pulmonary edema, pneumonia, pulmonary contusions, hemorrhage, interstitial disease, and neoplasia. Parenchymal diseases are characterized by decreased pulmonary compliance, or the development of "stiff" lungs, that require higher inspiratory pressures to reach the same tidal volume.[1] Inspiratory and expiratory efforts may both be increased. Specifically, there is often fluid in the alveolar space, resulting in collapse of the alveoli, or thickening of the alveolar-capillary membrane, which decreases the efficiency of gas exchange.

PLEURAL SPACE DISEASE

Pleural effusion or pneumothorax may result in respiratory distress because of compression of the lungs and relative limitation of lung expansion. The pleural space may develop pathology due to air, pure or modified transudates, exudates, or solid tissue (eg, neoplasia, organs) filling the pleural cavity and resulting in decreasing ability of the lungs to expand and to ventilate. Pleural effusion is not a final diagnosis, and may develop from several different conditions. Common underlying etiologies include trauma, which may result in pneumothorax or diaphragmatic hernia, right-sided or biventricular heart failure, neoplasia, or infection (pyothorax). Anticoagulant rodenticide intoxication may result in a hemorrhagic pleural effusion, and it may be accompanied by mediastinal and pericardial hemorrhage as well. Traditionally, pleural space disease has been reported to result in a restrictive pattern of breathing, characterized by fast and shallow breaths. Paradoxic chest wall movement has also been associated with pleural space disease; however, in a recent study of respiratory parameters of animals in respiratory distress, it was found that a fast and shallow breathing pattern was not associated with pleural space disease in dogs and cats, whereas an asynchronous or inverse breathing pattern was associated with pleural space disease.[2]

PROFILING AND PATTERN RECOGNITION

Profiling and pattern recognition is a commonly used, but underappreciated, technique when evaluating the patient with respiratory distress. Profiling, when applied to animals, simply reflects the recognition that some ages and breeds of pets are more likely to be affected with a specific disease than another. For example, a geriatric Labrador retriever may be much more likely affected with laryngeal paralysis than an English bulldog puppy, which is more commonly affected with pneumonia. Profiling and pattern recognition may help direct the clinician to a more likely diagnosis, but clearly a complete assessment of each individual pet is warranted. **Table 1** provides a list of breeds of dogs and cats with common clinical respiratory problems.

Table 1
Specific breeds of dogs and cats may be more commonly affected by certain respiratory conditions; this is a short list of the common diseases seen in the authors' practice

Breed of Dog	Common Respiratory Problem
Yorkshire terrier	Tracheal collapse
Toy poodle	Tracheal collapse; chronic bronchitis; chronic valvular heart disease
Norwich terrier	Brachycephalic airway syndrome; laryngeal collapse
Pug	Brachycephalic airway syndrome
Cocker spaniel	Bronchiectasis; chronic bronchitis
West Highland white terrier	Interstitial lung disease (pulmonary fibrosis), chronic bronchitis
Labrador retriever	Laryngeal paralysis
Bulldog	Brachycephalic airway syndrome
Golden retriever	Spontaneous pneumothorax
Northern breeds (husky/malamutes)	Spontaneous pneumothorax; eosinophilic bronchopneumopathy
Doberman pinscher	Cardiogenic pulmonary edema secondary to dilated cardiomyopathy
Young puppies	Noncardiogenic pulmonary edema secondary to electric cord injury, and so forth; long-acting anticoagulant rodenticide; *Bordetella bronchiseptica* pneumonia
Hunting breeds	Pyothorax; blastomycosis in endemic areas
Young cats	Nasopharyneal polyps; upper respiratory infection
Pointed cats (Siamese/Himalayan)	Allergic airway disease ("asthma")

PERTINENT HISTORY

Obtaining an appropriate, thorough history is imperative in the patient with respiratory distress. Identifying the duration and progression of clinical signs (eg, coughing, vomiting, anorexia, febrile), any prior therapies, current medications (eg, prednisone), previous medical problems, history of recent anesthesia or sedation, potential exposures to toxicants, any environmental changes, and other underlying indicators of metabolic disease (eg, polyuria/polydipsia) is important. Some animals with respiratory distress may have chronic pulmonary disease with acute exacerbations.

Cats with lower respiratory disease may have a history of "trying to cough up hairballs," although no hairball ever materializes. Smaller dogs with congestive heart failure (CHF) typically have a long-standing heart murmur, and often a recent history of weight (muscle) loss. Dogs or cats that have sustained trauma should be monitored closely for pneumothorax or progressive pulmonary contusions.

For dogs that develop respiratory distress during hospitalization, common causes include aspiration pneumonia, fluid overload, pulmonary thromboembolism, and, less commonly, acute lung injury/acute respiratory distress syndrome. Cats that develop respiratory distress while hospitalized are most often diagnosed with fluid overload.

INITIAL ASSESSMENT AND ACTION STEPS

After initial patient evaluation, the history, signalment, and patient profile should lead the clinician to the most likely anatomic localization of respiratory distress, and help the clinician create a list of differential diagnoses. Although stressful handling may not be tolerated in animals in respiratory distress, particularly cats, it is also important to recognize that simple observation is rarely therapeutic. Major action steps for a patient with respiratory distress include the following:

1. Supplemental oxygen therapy
2. Sedation/Anxiolytic therapy
3. Control of hyperthermia
4. Thoracocentesis (if indicated)/thoracostomy tube placement
5. Pharmacologic therapy specific for the underlying disease
6. Assessment of oxygenation (pulse oximetry/arterial blood gas analysis)
7. Tracheostomy (if upper airway obstruction cannot be relieved)
8. Intubation and positive pressure ventilation (PPV) for imminent respiratory failure
9. Thoracic radiographs, ultrasound, or echocardiography. Note that diagnostic imaging of any form is *never* therapeutic; however, detection of the specific underlying pathology may permit the clinician to proceed with targeted therapy, which increases the potential of therapeutic benefit. Imaging may be brief, and include an ultrasound scan for effusion (thoracic focused assessment with sonography [TFAST]), a single radiograph view, or an assessment of the left atrial size via rapid echocardiography. More extensive imaging should be pursued only when the patient has been stabilized.
10. Laboratory evaluation (eg, venous or arterial blood gas, packed cell volume, total solids, coagulation testing)

Supplemental Oxygen Therapy

Oxygen therapy should be initiated promptly in all patients presenting in respiratory distress; however, keep in mind that patients with pleural space disease or upper airway obstruction will benefit more from therapeutic intervention (eg, thoracocentesis, sedation for relief of airway obstruction), and should always have an initial brief assessment done before placement in an oxygen cage to exclude a more definitively treatable cause of distress. Initially, oxygen can be administered via flow-by oxygen, an oxygen cage, an oxygen mask, or via an oxygen hood. Longer-term oxygen therapy can be administered via oxygen cage, nasal oxygen cannulas, transtracheal oxygen, or intubation and administration of PPV. The approximate Fio_2 achieved with different methods of oxygen administration is shown in **Table 2**.[3,4] Keep in mind that benefit of nasal oxygen cannulas is reduced in panting dogs, and an alternate form of oxygen supplementation should be used.

Sedation/Anxiolytic Therapy

Sedation is most often used to ameliorate the dynamic component of upper respiratory obstruction associated with laryngeal paralysis, tracheal collapse, or brachycephalic airway syndrome. Low-dose acepromazine and/or butorphanol can be used. Recent anecdotal evidence has suggested that either doxepin or trazodone may be useful for laryngeal paralysis; however, there are no clinical trials supporting this. Diazepam or midazolam may also be used in combination with butorphanol; however, benzodiazepines alone are not effective at sedating dogs, and should therefore not be used as a single agent. Excessive respiratory effort leads to increased energy expenditure and may contribute to hyperthermia and/or respiratory failure, resulting in a vicious cycle and an exacerbation of clinical signs.

It is challenging to decide whether to use sedation in animals with nondynamic respiratory distress, such as heart failure, and must be weighed carefully; if sedation is administered, the patient should be closely monitored for respiratory depression or exhaustion. Patients with imminent respiratory failure (eg, exhibiting air hunger, orthopnea, respiratory exhaustion) that fail to respond to therapy should ideally be sedated, intubated, and administered PPV; this will provide a protected airway, patient comfort, and allows the clinician the ability to perform diagnostics in a more controlled manner and without patient discomfort or stress. Additionally, the use of PPV may provide a humane option during the decision making on a patient's ongoing care.

Control of Hyperthermia

Upper respiratory disease may result in severe hyperthermia, which will further contribute to respiratory distress. **Fig. 3** shows a pug with severe upper airway obstruction, who had a rectal temperature higher than 110°F (>43.3°C). Prompt active cooling, with room temperature intravenous (IV) fluids, fans, alcohol to the footpads,

Table 2	
The approximate Fio_2 achieved with different methods of oxygen administration	
Oxygen Administration Technique	**Mean Fio_2 Achieved (%)**
Oxygen cage	21–60
Flow-by oxygen	24–45
Face mask, loose fitting	35–55
Oxygen hood	30–50
Unilateral nasal catheter	30–50
Bilateral nasal catheter	30–70
Intratracheal catheter	40–60
Positive pressure ventilation	21–100

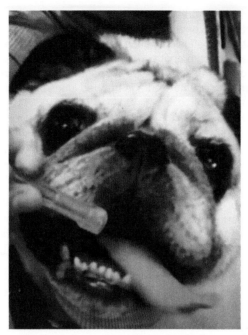

Fig. 3. A pug with severe upper airway obstruction, that had a rectal temperature higher than 110°F (>43.3°C). Prompt active cooling with room temperature IV fluids, fans, alcohol to the footpads, cool towels to the body, and so forth is imperative to prevent secondary DIC and multiple organ failure.

cool towels to the body, and so forth, is imperative to prevent secondary disseminated intravascular coagulation (DIC) and multiple organ failure. Cooling measures should be discontinued at a temperature of 103.5°F (39.7°C). Sedation and/or intubation to relieve the upper airway obstruction may also be warranted, and may help control hyperthermia.

Thoracocentesis

Removal of pneumothorax or pleural effusion is therapeutic in alleviating clinical signs of dyspnea. In animals with moderate to severe distress, thoracocentesis *before* imaging is warranted, as one cannot evaluate cardiac size, presence of metastasis, or mass lesions easily when pleural effusion is present. Dogs with pleural effusion and anemia should be evaluated for anticoagulant rodenticide *before* thoracocentesis. The recent emergence of limited-use ultrasound scanning in the emergency room (TFAST) will aid the clinician in appropriately treating the dyspneic patient (see the article "Emergency Management and Treatment of the Poisoned Small Animal Patient" elsewhere in this issue, for more information).

Thoracocentesis is performed between the seventh and ninth intercostal spaces, ideally avoiding the caudal edge of the rib due to the location of the vessels and nerves. In smaller animals, a butterfly catheter is typically adequate, whereas in larger animals, an 18-gauge to 20-gauge, 1.0-inch to 1.5-inch needle or catheter may be required. The mediastinum in cats and dogs is less robust than in people, and may be fenestrated or incomplete; thus, recording volumes from the right or the left side may reflect only which side was tapped first, rather than the underlying pathology.

Rarely, complications from thoracocentesis may occur, including hemorrhage, cardiac puncture, or iatrogenic pneumothorax. The latter may occur more frequently in animals with long-standing effusions, such as chylothorax or with hyperinflated lung (eg, asthma). Iatrogenic pneumothorax develops due to either laceration of the pleura overlying the lungs, or the creation of excessive negative pressure in the pleural space, which may cause "ripping" of the pleura in trapped lungs rather than reexpansion of the lungs to fill the pleural space.[5]

Thoracostomy tube placement may be necessary for management of pleural space disease. In an emergency setting, this is most commonly needed to treat pneumothorax, as large-volume pneumothorax can reform much more quickly than pleural effusions. In patients requiring more than 3 to 4 therapeutic, large-volume thoracocentesis procedures within a 24-hour period, placement of either unilateral or bilateral thoraocostomy tube placement should be strongly considered.

In the vast majority of cases, placement of a thoracostomy tube should be done with the patient under general anesthesia and intubated for control of the airway and PPV. In rare cases in which the patient is unconscious or moribund, thoracostomy tubes may be placed without general anesthesia. See **Box 1** for a brief guideline on thoracostomy tube placement.

Red rubber catheters or trocar catheters can be used for thoracostomy tubes. More recently, a thoracostomy tube has been developed that is placed using the modified Seldinger technique, which uses a smaller tube and may be placed more

---

Box 1
Guidelines for placement of a thoracostomy tube

1. Determine clinical need.
2. Assemble needed technical help and supplies. Supplies needed include
   a. Sterile drape and supplies for aseptic preparation of the skin
   b. Sterile instruments and suture material
   c. Desired chest tube (eg, Argyle, red rubber)
3. Anesthetize and monitor the patient. Rarely, local analgesics are sufficient.
4. Place the patient in sternal or lateral recumbency. If placing bilateral tubes, sternal is advised; otherwise clinician preference.
5. Clip and prepare the site.
6. Drape the site.
7. Have an assistant pull the skin forward.
8. Make a small incision (<1 cm) into the skin and underlying musculature at approximately the 10th intercostal space.
9. Alert the individual monitoring anesthesia that entry into chest is imminent.
10. Place the chest tube through the incision into the chest.
11. Have the assistant release the skin, this creates a tunnel for the tube.
12. Aspirate the tube to ensure patency.
13. Securely suture the tube to the patient.
14. Place an adherent dressing if desired over the insertion site.
15. Confirm placement radiographically.

quickly, under sedation, and appears more comfortable for patients (Mila International, Lexington, KY).

Pharmacologic Therapy Specific for the Underlying Disease

The use of specific pharmacologic therapy is often considered essential in the patient with respiratory distress. Appropriate, titrated use of specific drugs is warranted, depending on the underlying disease process and pathophysiology of disease. Important pharmacologic drugs include antibiotics, diuretics, vasodilators, glucocorticoids, bronchodilators, and inhalation therapy.

Broad-spectrum antibiotics are warranted for the treatment of bacterial pneumonia or pyothorax. Appropriate antibiotics should be based on results of culture and sensitivity data, including ampicillin-fluoroquinolones or cefazolin-gentamicin–metronidazole. In some cases, a Gram stain may be useful to guide preliminary therapy. For young, rapidly growing neonates, the use of certain antibiotics may be relatively contraindicated (eg, tetracyclines, fluoroquinolones), and potential adverse effects should be discussed with the pet owner.

For animals with suspected hospital-acquired infections, antibiotics should be chosen based on known hospital resistance patterns. Hospital-acquired infections (HAI) should be suspected in dogs with a new fever or cough developing 48 hours or more after hospital admission, and they should be treated with antibiotics that have known efficacy against HAI.

Diuretics, including furosemide (2–8 mg/kg IV every 2–8 hours) or torsemide (0.2–0.8 mg/kg IV) are the mainstay therapy for patients with pulmonary edema due to CHF or potentially, noncardiogenic pulmonary edema. By removing excessive body water (eg, circulating blood volume and subsequently pulmonary edema), and reducing preload, they will relieve clinical signs of respiratory distress. In dogs, the intermittent use of 2 to 4 mg/kg of furosemide (IV or intramuscularly) every 1 to 2 hours in fulminant CHF, in conjunction with cage rest and supplemental oxygen, should result in improvement in respiratory rate and effort, typically within a few hours. Cats are may be treated similarly, although they be more prone to volume depletion and weakness. Continuous rate infusions (CRI) of diuretics have been used occasionally, but more recent human studies show no better outcomes with a CRI than with intermittent bolus injections.[6] Diuretics are occasionally used without a definitive diagnosis of CHF, particularly in cats considered too unstable for more definitive imaging (radiographs or echocardiogram). Excessive use of diuretics is associated with volume contraction, electrolyte disturbances, including hypokalemia, and metabolic alkalosis. Additionally, prerenal azotemia may develop. Although a single dose of a diuretic is unlikely to be harmful, excessive use in the patient without a definitive diagnosis should be avoided.

Vasodilators are also useful in treatment of CHF and include either topical nitroglycerin (venodilator) or IV nitroprusside (a balanced vasodilator). There is limited evidence of the efficacy of topical nitroglycerin in dogs and cats, although it remains a popular therapeutic option. Nitroprusside is given by continuous-rate infusion and as very effective vasodilator it may be associated with severe hypotension. Nitroprusside must be given by an infusion pump, with a covered IV line to prevent degradation, and in a small volume of 5% dextrose in water (D5W), such as 1 to 2 mL per hour (Fig. 4). As an infusion, the line must not be flushed, as severe hypotension may result. Additionally, long-term therapy is associated with the potential for thiocyanate or cyanide toxicity. Frequent blood pressure monitoring is commonly advocated during use of nitroprusside, and if possible, is ideal. However, in many animals with severe CHF, the amount of time required to noninvasively determine blood pressure may be

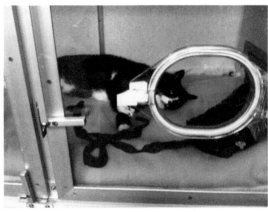

Fig. 4. Nitroprusside must be given by an infusion pump, with a covered IV line to prevent degradation, and in a small volume of D5W, such as 1 to 2 mL/h.

counterproductive. Palpation of pulses may be substituted, and any patient receiving nitroprusside should be carefully monitored. The starting dose of nitroprusside is 0.5 to 1.0 μg/kg per minute; this may be titrated up every 15 minutes by 0.5 to 1.0 μg/kg per minute until 10.0 μg/kg per minute is reached, although most animals are improved by 2.0 to 3.0 μg/kg per minute.

Glucocorticoids are useful for the treatment of inflammatory lower airway disease, and tracheal collapse. In the short term, glucocorticoids also may be useful in laryngeal paralysis with arytenoid inflammation, and with brachycephalic airway syndrome with pharyngeal or laryngeal swelling. Airway inflammation is associated with airway narrowing, which increases airway resistance, worsens cough, and perpetuates inflammation. Cats with suspected lower airway disease will typically respond very quickly to dexamethasone (2–4 mg/cat) or prednisone/prednisolone. Most cats convert prednisone to prednisolone; however, a small subset of cats do not, and, thus, if possible, prednisolone should be substituted for prednisone. Dogs with tracheal collapse and chronic bronchitis will also respond rapidly to glucocorticoids. Long-term high doses of glucocorticoids are associated with side effects, similar to Cushing disease, including lethargy, polyuria/polydipsia, polyphagia, hepatomegaly, muscle weakness, poor fur growth, and diabetes. Although cats are overall more tolerant of glucocorticoid therapy, diabetes and CHF have been reported, particularly in conjunction with reposital products. Glucocorticoids should be tapered to the lowest possible dose, and consideration should be given for the use of inhaled glucocorticoids if low-dose glucocorticoids are inadequate to control clinical signs.

Bronchodilators include theophylline and β-2 agonists, such as terbutaline or albuterol (salbutamol outside the United States). Bronchodilators are not effective in tracheal collapse, although they may be useful in some lower airway diseases in dogs.

Inhaled Therapy

In human medicine, inhaled corticosteroids (ICs) are the mainstay for people with asthma and other inflammatory airway diseases. Advantages of ICs include avoidance of systemic side effects of oral glucocorticoids. ICs have been proposed in both cats and dogs with moderate to severe lower airway disease that are steroid responsive. The appeal of ICs includes targeting therapy to the lungs, and avoidance of the bulk of the systemic side effects. The "Internet presence" of the use of ICs in dogs and particularly cats is strong, including the site www.fritzthebrave.com, which provides guidelines for the cat with lower airway disease. It is important that the clinician is familiar with ICs, and is able to discuss both pros and cons logically with clients.

Because of the lack of voluntary cooperation in cats and dogs, administration of inhaled medication requires the use of a face mask and spacer. Although several models are available, [Trudell Medical, London, Ontario Canada (http://www.trudellmed.com/animal-health)] has the most widely used products with the Aerokat and Aerodawg chambers.

The nasal cavities of both dogs and cats are much more complex than the human nasal cavity. This permits more aerosolized drug to settle out in the nasal passage rather than being delivered specifically to the lungs. A study by Schulman and colleagues,[7] using a similar device with aerosolized radiopharmaceuticals, demonstrated that there was deposition of the radiopharmaceutical to the lung, although in three-fourths of the cats there was also evidence that some of the radiopharmaceutical was present in the stomach, suggesting that the aerosol had been subsequently swallowed.

ICs have also been found to affect the hypothalamic pituitary axis in a study by Cohn and colleagues,[8] although there were limited effects on the immune system. The diabetogenic effect of ICs has not been evaluated to date in cats, although systemic glucocorticoids are well known to facilitate the development of diabetes mellitus. As mentioned earlier, administration of ICs requires the use of a face mask and spacer. Although some animals, particularly dogs, may be trained quite easily to accept the facemask, in other pets it may take a period of acclimation to have the acceptance of the mask and treatment.

There are several IC preparations available, including fluticasone (Flovent), beclomethasone (QVAR), budensonide (Pulmicort), ciclesonide (Alvesco), and mometasone (Asmanex). There is no generic product available yet. All ICs are expensive, with beclomethasone dipropionate HFA (QVAR) usually the least expensive. Most descriptions of small animal use have focused on fluticasone. The optimal dosing of ICs is unknown in dogs and cats. One study in cats supported a starting fluticasone dose of 44 μg per cat twice a day, whereas some anecdotal studies suggest 110 μg per cat twice daily up to a maximum of 440 μg twice daily. Most commonly, oral glucocorticoid therapy is continued for about 10 to 14 days with a tapering overlap. In dogs, a starting dose of 110 μg (up to 10 kg), 220 μg (10–25 kg), and 440 μg (>25 kg) may be considered. ICs were initially available in metered dose inhalers (MDIs) with the propellant chlorofluorocarbons (CFCs). However, because of evolving concerns about the effect on the ozone layer, CFCs have been phased out. MDIs are available using other ozone-safe propellants, or as a dry powder. The dry powder preparations are also available but are NOT useful in animals because of the voluntary effort required to use the product. There are also products (eg, Advair) that combine fluticasone and the long-acting β-2 agonist salmeterol; one recent study by Leemans and colleagues[9] showed improved efficacy in an experimental model of feline asthma.

To date, there have been no studies specifically evaluating any advantages of ICs over oral prednisone in dogs or cats with naturally occurring airway disease; however, it is prudent for the advanced practitioner to be familiar with inhaled medications. The advantages of inhaled medications may include fewer systemic effects, and limitations of potential complications. It is rare for a cat or dog to respond well to ICs if they have not shown an improvement with oral steroids. Thus, if the pet is not clearly improved with oral prednisone (or prednisolone in cats), it is quite unlikely they will do well on ICs. On the other hand, if a pet does well on steroids, but the side effects are poorly tolerated, or if another risk factor, such as diabetes or CHF is present, it is a very reasonable plan to transition to ICs. Clients should learn of the options of inhaled medication from their primary care veterinarian, who can effectively counsel them on their specific pet. Inhaled glucocorticoids are rarely started as an emergency therapy.

Other medications may also be administered by aerosol; these include bronchodilators, antibiotics, and saline. Older textbooks suggest the use of N-acetylcysteine (NAC) as a nebulized agent to decrease the viscosity of mucus; however, recent evidence supports that nebulized NAC may cause bronchoconstriction or even death.[10]

Tracheostomy

Although not commonly performed in the emergency setting, a tracheostomy can be life-saving in patients with upper airway obstruction that fail to respond to medical management (eg, sedation, supplemental oxygen therapy, inability to intubate orally) or in cases of complete airway occlusion. With complete occlusion that cannot be relieved (eg, a ball in the pharynx), an emergent ("slash") tracheostomy may be performed to provide the patient with an airway. Slash tracheostomies are also occasionally required in association with an upper airway examination in cats with laryngeal masses that are unable to be intubated. Ideally, a more controlled, surgical approach to tracheostomy is preferred, to minimize stress on both the patient and the surgeon.

However, it is preferable for a tracheostomy to be performed more as an elective procedure, with first oral intubation, and then subsequent surgical approach to the airway. The incision into the trachea may be transverse, longitudinal, or T-shaped, but ideally the incision should not be more than 50% of the diameter of the trachea. The tracheostomy tube should NOT be sutured to the patient, as the clinician needs to be able to remove the tube quickly in case of occlusion. Following placement of a temporary tracheostomy tube, the patient should be supervised continuously to ensure that occlusion of the tube does not occur. The high-volume, low-pressure cuff on the tracheostomy tube should not be insufflated unless the pet is undergoing mechanical ventilation or if general anesthesia is necessary (eg, for a procedure). This will minimize pressure necrosis to the trachea, and also allow limited ventilation if the lumen of the tracheostomy tube were to occlude unobserved.

Sterile technique should be observed when suctioning the tracheostomy tube. If supplemental oxygen is provided via the tracheostomy, it should be humidified, if possible. A "trach kit" should be placed near the patient, with readily available supplies for changing the tube, suction, and, if needed, sedation. When the tracheostomy tube is no longer needed, the site should be allowed to close by second intention. Closure of the skin before closure of the tracheostomy site may result in marked subcutaneous emphysema.

Intubation and PPV

For animals with severe respiratory distress that fail to respond to oxygen therapy or therapeutic intervention, intubation and intermittent PPV is an important option to consider. Ventilation removes the work of breathing from the patient, and provides humane relief for patients with respiratory distress. Ventilation may be associated with a good prognosis in animals with reversible underlying diseases; however, ventilation is labor-intensive and expensive, and important considerations must be considered (see the article "Analgesia, Anesthesia, and Chemical Restraint in the Emergent Small Animal Patient" elsewhere in this issue, for more information).

Thoracic Radiographs, Ultrasound, or Echocardiography

Thoracic radiographs are a mainstay of diagnostics for identification of intrathoracic sources of respiratory distress. Radiographs in patients with respiratory disease are beneficial, as they will help identify pulmonary infiltrates, mediastinal masses, cardiomegaly, pleural space disease, and trauma (eg, rib fractures, diaphragmatic hernias). Readers are directed to a radiology resource for additional information.

Thoracic ultrasound is also useful in characterizing the cause of respiratory distress. TFAST is a diagnostic test that is rapidly gaining popularity, relying on the use of brief ultrasound to evaluate a patient for pleural space disease.[11] This technique can be used to identify the presence of pleural effusion and pneumothorax. Advantages of TFAST include rapidity of the procedure, convenience, radiation sparing, and allowance for repeat evaluation; also this diagnostic tool can be performed with less patient stress and restraint than radiography. It can be performed in either sternal or lateral recumbency, further contributing to minimal patient stress. In a study of TFAST evaluation of dogs after trauma, it was found to have a high specificity but poor sensitivity for pneumothorax detection versus conventional thoracic radiographs. TFAST was found to have a higher sensitivity and specificity in dogs with penetrating trauma than those with blunt trauma[12] (see the article "Emergency Management and Treatment of the Poisoned Small Animal Patient" elsewhere in this issue, for more information).

Last, echocardiography is useful for assessment of chamber size and myocardial function, and can be performed in a cursory, limited fashion in the emergency setting to rapidly support a diagnosis of cardiac disease. In the emergency room, echocardiography can be used to assess the left atrial-to-aorta size ratio (LA:AO), which normally should be approximately 1:1. Increased left atrial dimensions are consistent with a cardiac cause of pulmonary infiltrates and respiratory distress (cardiogenic pulmonary edema). Short training courses for the use of echocardiography by the emergency room clinician have been shown reasonably effective to teach evaluation of left atrial enlargement.[13] In some cases, diuretic therapy may result in a decrease in the size of the left atrium, which may make the subsequent determination of cardiac disease challenging. In all cases in which cardiac disease is suspected, a complete echocardiogram and cardiac evaluation, ideally by a cardiologist, should be performed as soon as the patient is stable.

Laboratory Evaluation

Several clinicopathologic tests are important in the patient with respiratory disease. The use of arterial blood gas (ABG) or venous blood gas (VBG) analysis will allow the clinician to assess both oxygenation and ventilation. In patients, in whom primary respiratory disease cannot be definitively ruled out from cardiac disease, the use of tests such as N-terminal prohormone of brain natriuretic peptide (NT pro-BNP) or possibly troponin can be considered.

Blood Gas Analysis

ABG analysis is considered the gold standard in assessing oxygenation and ventilation. The use of blood gases may assist the clinician in confirming the severity of respiratory dysfunction; however, it is unlikely to be able to definitively provide a diagnosis.

Hypoxemia, or decreased oxygen content of the blood, is confirmed by establishing a low partial pressure of oxygen dissolved in plasma (Pao_2), typically lower than 80 mm Hg at sea level. The partial pressure of carbon dioxide ($Paco_2$) on an ABG or

VBG may be used to assess adequacy of ventilation. A $Paco_2$ greater than 40 mm Hg or partial pressure of CO_2 in mixed venous blood ($PVCO_2$) greater than 45 mm Hg is supportive of hypoventilation. In severe hypoperfusion, venous CO_2 is not an appropriate surrogate for arterial CO_2.

Historically, blood gas analysis has been available only at large referral or university hospitals, but in the past decade a variety of portable point-of care machines have become affordable and available in practices. The I-STAT (Abbott Laboratories, Abbott Park, IL) model has been widely used and is generally considered accurate and user-friendly; the IRMA (ITC, Edison, NJ) is also popular. These devices (and other similar products) are able to measure blood gas values and other blood chemistries on small volumes of blood. Disposable cartridges make each test relatively economical and the turn-around time is excellent. Larger veterinary hospitals often used the Nova Biomedical Analyzer (Nova Biomedical, Waltham, MA). Other alternatives may include local human hospitals or regional referral hospitals. Guidelines for interpretation of blood gases are shown in **Table 3**.

Collecting an ABG may be challenging to obtain technically, particularly in a dyspneic patient or small patient. For example, obtaining an ABG in a distressed, open-mouth-breathing cat is not a viable option. Therapy should not be delayed while attempting an ABG, and a patient showing respiratory distress should not be removed from supplemental oxygen for assessment of oxygen levels (pulse oximetry or ABG analysis) while breathing room air, as the treatment plan should include supplemental oxygen.

As mentioned previously, blood gas analysis is useful in evaluating oxygenation and ventilation. Oxygen levels should always be interpreted in light of the Pco_2 level and the inspired oxygen concentration (Fio_2). It is also important to remember that even though an ABG analysis may look "normal," it does not always imply normal oxygen delivery to tissues. The Pao_2 is an indicator of arterial oxygen tension and measures the dissolved oxygen in the blood (or whatever fluid is analyzed). Oxygen content of blood

Table 3
The following guidelines have been adapted from the references and serve as the recommendation for interpretation from the American College of Veterinary Emergency and Critical Care

At Sea Level	Normal Value (Arterial)	Normal Value (Venous)
pH	7.36–7.44	7.32–7.36
Pco_2	36–40 mm Hg	40–45 mm Hg
Pao_2	90–100 mm Hg	40–50 mm Hg
HCO_3-	20–24 mEq/L	24–28 mEq/L

Clinical Guidelines for Compensation	
Disturbance	
Metabolic acidosis	Each 1 mEq/L decrease in HCO_3 will decrease Pco_2 by 0.7 mm Hg
Metabolic alkalosis	Each 1 mEq/L increase in HCO_3 will increase Pco_2 by 0.7 mm Hg
Respiratory acidosis	
Acute	Each 1 mm Hg increase in Pco_2 will increase HCO_3 by 0.15 mEq/L
Chronic	Each 1 mm Hg increase in Pco_2 will increase HCO_3 by 0.35 mEq/L
Respiratory alkalosis	
Acute	Each 1 mm Hg decrease in Pco_2 will decrease HCO_3 by 0.25 mEq/L
Chronic	Each 1 mm Hg decrease in Pco_2 will decrease HCO_3 by 0.55 mEq/L

is defined as (1.34 × hemoglobin concentration × % saturation) + 0.003 Pao_2. Adequate oxygen delivery is dependent on normal cardiac function, normal hemoglobin concentrations, and the affinity that exists between oxygen and hemoglobin. Methemoglobin, and carboxyhemoglobin are 2 examples of altered hemoglobins that are markedly less effective in oxygen delivery.

Anemic animals will have lower oxygen content in the blood, and oxygen delivery in these patients is improved by transfusion of red blood cells rather than supplemental oxygen.

It is crucial that the clinician does not just look at the Pao_2 values in interpreting blood gases, but rather to look as well at the Pco_2 values. Low partial pressure of CO_2 supports that the patient is hyperventilating to maintain oxygen values, whereas high partial pressure of CO_2 supports respiratory fatigue or neuromuscular failure. The clinician should recall that providing supplemental oxygen to a patient with respiratory failure (high $Paco_2$) will improve oxygen level, but often worsen hypercarbia.

When an ABG sample is obtained, an alveolar-arterial (A-a) gradient should be calculated to assess if pulmonary dysfunction exists. For example, a dog may be able to maintain a near normal oxygen concentration (Pao_2 80 mm Hg) by hyperventilating (as detected by a low Pco_2 of 20 mm Hg), but have moderate to severe pulmonary dysfunction, A-a gradient equal to 45. Similarly, a dog with laryngeal paralysis may have severe hypoventilation (Pco_2 of 70 mm Hg) and appear to be hypoxemic (Pao_2 of 60 mm Hg), which in actuality, his A-a gradient is normal (3), indicating normal lung function. This can be detected by calculating the A-a gradient (**Box 2**) or by using the nonogram shown in **Fig. 5**.

Another useful screening tool to differentiate primary respiratory disease versus cardiac causes for respiratory distress is the NT pro-BNP. Chronic pressure or volume overload results in increased synthesis of pre-proBNP (a precursor molecule of BNP) by the ventricles, which is then processed to active BNP and inactive NT-proBNP. Multiple studies have evaluated the clinical utility of NT-proBNP and found that it can be used to detect occult cardiomyopathy in cats and to distinguish cardiac and noncardiac causes for respiratory signs in dogs.[14,15] Species-specific assays must be used for NT-proBNP evaluation, because of variation in the protein structure between species.

Last, troponin is a biomarker that is released from ischemic myocardium. Troponin elevations have been appreciated with a variety of cardiovascular diseases, including hypertrophic cardiomyopathy and pericardial effusion. However, troponin increases are unlikely to be helpful in evaluation of the patient with respiratory distress.[16]

Box 2
Calculation of the Alveolar to arterial gradient (A-a gradient)

Alveolar oxygen content is calculated using the Alveolar gas equation = (Fio_2 [Barometric pressure-water vapor pressure] − Pco_2/R), where

R = respiratory quotient, usually set at 0.8 or 0.9

Barometric pressure is in mm Hg, typically 760 at sea level

Water vapor pressure is 53 mm Hg at dog/cat body temperature, classically given at 47 for people.

Arterial content = measured using blood gas analyzer

Normal <15 mm Hg.

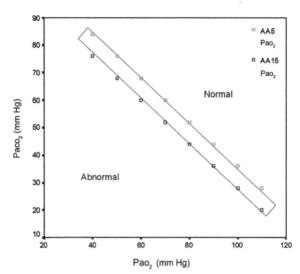

Fig. 5. Arterial oxygen to arterial carbon dioxide nonogram. Match the patient's $Paco_2$ and Pao_2 values, and determine if the value is normal or abnormal. Abnormal values support pulmonary dysfunction. Elevated Pco_2 values alone may reflect simple ventilation failure.

Troponin is well-preserved across species, so human analyzers are acceptable for dogs and cats.

SUMMARY

Respiratory distress is a common presenting complaint for animals brought to the emergency room, and it is important for clinicians to feel comfortable diagnosing and treating these animals. Prompt recognition of the localization of the source of respiratory distress based on history, pattern recognition, and physical examination findings will help to determine the underlying cause and is key to determining an appropriate therapeutic course. Careful handling, minimizing stress, and rapid and focused treatment are crucial in the management of all patients in respiratory distress.

REFERENCES

1. West JB. Respiratory physiology: the essentials. 9th edition. Philadelphia: Lippincott Williams & Wilkins; 2011.
2. Sigrist NE, Adamik KN, Doherr MG, et al. Evaluation of respiratory parameters at presentation as clinical indicators of the respiratory localization in dogs and cats with respiratory distress. J Vet Emerg Crit Care (San Antonio) 2011;21: 13–23.
3. Irizarry R, Reiss A. Beyond blood gases: making use of additional oxygenation parameters and plasma electrolytes in the emergency room. Compend Contin Educ Vet 2009;31:E1–5.
4. Manning AM. Oxygen therapy and toxicity. Vet Clin North Am Small Anim Pract 2002;32:1005–20.
5. Ponrartana S, Laberge JM, Kerlan RK, et al. Management of patients with "ex vacuo" pneumothorax after thoracocentesis. Acad Radiol 2005;12(8):980–6.

6. Felker GM, Lee KL, Bull DA, et al. Diuretic strategies in patients with acute decompensated heart failure. N Engl J Med 2011;364:797–805.
7. Schulman RL, Crochik SS, Kneller SK, et al. Investigation of pulmonary deposition of a nebulized radiopharmaceutical agent in awake cats. Am J Vet Res 2004; 65(6):806–9.
8. Cohn LA, DeClue AE, Reinero CR. Endocrine and immunologic effects of inhaled fluticasone propionate in healthy dogs. J Vet Intern Med 2008;22(1):37–43, 8.
9. Leemans J, Kirschvink N, Clercx C, et al. Effect of short-term oral and inhaled corticosteroids on airway inflammation and responsiveness in a feline acute asthma model. Vet J 2012;192(1):41–8.
10. Reinero CR, Lee-Fowler TM, Dodam JR, et al. Endotracheal nebulization of N-acetylcysteine increases airway resistance in cats with experimental asthma. J Feline Med Surg 2011;13(2):69–73.
11. Lisciandro GR. Abdominal and thoracic focused assessment with sonography for trauma, triage, and monitoring in small animals. J Vet Emerg Crit Care (San Antonio) 2011;21:104–22.
12. Lisciandro GR, Lagutchik MS, Mann KA, et al. Evaluation of a thoracic focused assessment with sonography for trauma (TFAST) protocol to detect pneumothorax and concurrent thoracic injury in 145 traumatized dogs. J Vet Emerg Crit Care (San Antonio) 2008;18:258–69.
13. Tse YC, Rush JE, Cunningham SM, et al. Evaluation of a training course in focused echocardiography for non-cardiology house officers. J Vet Emerg Crit Care, in press.
14. Fox PR, Rush JE, Reynolds CA, et al. Multicenter evaluation of plasma N-terminal probrain natriuretic peptide (NT-proBNP) as a biochemical screening test for asymptomatic (occult) cardiomyopathy in cats. J Vet Intern Med 2011;25:1010–6.
15. Ettinger SJ, Farace G, Forney SD, et al. Evaluation of plasma N-terminal pro-B-type natriuretic peptide concentrations in dogs with and without cardiac disease. J Am Vet Med Assoc 2012;240:171–80.
16. Prosek R, Sisson DD, Oyama MA, et al. Distinguishing cardiac and noncardiac dyspnea in 48 dogs using plasma atrial natriuretic factor, B-type natriuretic factor, endothelin, and cardiac troponin-I. J Vet Intern Med 2007;21(2):238–42.

Management of Cardiac Emergencies in Small Animals

Teresa C. DeFrancesco, DVM

KEYWORDS

- Heart failure • Arrhythmia • Pericardial effusion • Syncope
- Feline aortic thromboembolism • Focused echocardiography • Cardiac biomarkers

KEY POINTS

- Cardiac emergencies include a variety of different diseases, including congestive heart failure, cardiac tamponade, arrhythmogenic disease, and thromboembolic disease.
- Cardiac emergencies are life-threatening conditions that must be diagnosed quickly to avoid delays in therapy.
- A timely and accurate diagnosis leads to early relief of symptoms and improved survival.
- The increased use of thoracic ultrasound and focused echocardiography in the rapid diagnosis of HF and cardiac tamponade as well as the use of pimobendan for the treatment of HF in both dogs and cats are the most important recent advances in the management of cardiac emergencies.

Cardiac emergencies include a variety of different diseases, including congestive heart failure (HF), cardiac tamponade, arrhythmogenic disease, and thromboembolic disease. Many of these diseases are life threatening and must be diagnosed quickly and efficiently to provide relief of symptoms and to avoid delays in definitive treatment. New modalities and medications used in the diagnosis and treatment of cardiac emergencies are reviewed.

HF

The timely and accurate diagnosis of HF can be challenging. Historical and physical examination findings are not pathognomonic for HF and can be compatible with other diseases, such as primary respiratory disease. Many dogs and cats presenting with HF are in severe respiratory distress, which limits diagnostic evaluation. In acute HF, treatment consists of stabilizing the patients' clinical condition while establishing the diagnosis, the underlying cause, and any precipitating factors for the HF. In small

Disclosures: Boehringer-Ingelheim, speaker's bureau; Idexx Laboratories, speaker's bureau and research grant monies; Antech Laboratories, consultant and research grant monies.
Department of Clinical Sciences, College of Veterinary Medicine, North Carolina State University, 1052 William Moore Drive, Raleigh, NC 27607, USA
E-mail address: Teresa_defrancesco@ncsu.edu

Vet Clin Small Anim 43 (2013) 817–842
http://dx.doi.org/10.1016/j.cvsm.2013.03.012 **vetsmall.theclinics.com**
0195-5616/13/$ – see front matter © 2013 Elsevier Inc. All rights reserved.

animal veterinary medicine, the most common causes of HF are degenerative mitral valve disease (MVD) and dilated cardiomyopathy (DCM) in dogs and hypertrophic cardiomyopathy (HCM) in cats. Other less common diseases include congenital heart disease, infectious endocarditis, cardiac neoplasia, heartworm disease, or other conditions leading to pulmonary hypertension.

There is no single diagnostic test for HF. The diagnosis is based on a combination of findings, including signalment, historical interrogation of clinical signs, and results of diagnostic tests (including physical examination) and cardiac imaging (specifically, thoracic radiography and echocardiography). See **Table 1** for a summary of clinical findings that are suggestive of HF or for findings that usually refute the diagnosis of HF. The response to treatment directed at HF can also provide supportive evidence for the diagnosis of HF (ie, the furosemide-response test).

Table 1
Clinical findings in suspect HF and their reliability for diagnosis

Clinical Findings	Very Suggestive of HF	Somewhat Suggestive of HF	Usually Opposes HF Diagnosis
History	• Previous HF diagnosis • Furosemide responsive cough/dyspnea	• Family history of HF or sudden death • Previous diagnosis of heart murmur	• Coughing cat • Vomiting then dyspneic • No loss in appetite • Normal respiratory rate
Physical examination	• Dyspnea and loud murmur in small-breed dog • Gallop sound • Jugular venous distention/pulses • Positive hepatojugular reflex	• Murmur, cough, tachycardia, and dyspnea in dog • Poor pulse quality and slow capillary refill time • Soft end-inspiratory crackles	• Absence of a murmur in small-breed dog • Cough induced by tracheal palpation • Obese dog with no history of weight loss • Transient cyanosis
Imaging	• Distended pulmonary veins or caudal vena cava on radiograph • Enlarged atria on echo (LA/Ao ratio >2)	• Cardiomegaly • Perihilar to caudal dorsal interstitial-alveolar lung pattern • Pleural effusion + cardiomegaly in cats	• Bronchiolar pulmonary pattern • DOG only: large amount pleural effusion in the absence of ascites • CAT only: large amount ascites in the absence of pleural effusion
ECG	• Atrial fibrillation • Left bundle branch block	• Chamber enlargement pattern (esp cat) • Sinus tachycardia • Other tachyarrhythmia	Respiratory sinus arrhythmia
Cardiac biomarkers	DOGS NTproBNP >3000 pg/mL BNP >6 pg/mL CATS NTproBNP >1000 pg/mL Markedly elevated cTnI		DOGS NTproBNP <900 pg/mL BNP <3 pg/mL CATS Normal CTnI NTproBNP <100 pg/mL

Abbreviations: AO, aorta; BNP, B-type natriuretic peptide; cTnI, cardiac troponin I; ECG, electrocardiogram; esp, especially; LA, left atrium; NTproBNP, amine terminal pro B-type natriuretic peptide.

Rapid clinical recognition of HF includes being familiar with the common signalment with a strong predisposition for the heart disease; however, any cat or dog breed/mixed breed can develop HF.[1–9] Genetic testing for some breeds is now available, such as in Doberman pinchers with DCM, boxers with arrhythmogenic right ventricular cardiomyopathy (ARVC), and Maine coon and ragdoll cats with HCM.[10–12] See **Table 2** for the typical signalments for dogs and cats for the common causes of HF.

Patients with emergent HF will typically exhibit the following clinical signs: cough (dog), dyspnea, lethargy, syncope or episodic weakness, abdominal distention (dog), and/or partial to complete anorexia. Most cats in HF do not present for cough or abdominal distention. An antecedent event or precipitating factor is not uncommon in congestive HF, especially in cats. Corticosteroid or intravenous (IV) fluid administration, a new tachyarrhythmia, chordae tendinae rupture, left atrial rupture, concurrent systemic disease, or a stressful event can precipitate HF.[13–15]

A careful physical examination will provide further evidence supporting or refuting the diagnosis of congestive HF. **Table 3** provides a summary of typical physical examination findings in HF for canine MVD and DCM and feline HCM. Dogs with HF secondary to MVD typically have loud systolic murmurs and tachycardia.[16–18] The absence of a murmur or a soft murmur (grade II or less) or the presence of a respiratory sinus arrhythmia in a small-breed dog with respiratory signs usually refutes the diagnosis of HF. Dogs with DCM, on the other hand, typically have soft or barely audible systolic murmurs and tachyarrhythmias.[4–6] The presence of atrial fibrillation in a dog or cat with suspect HF is very suggestive of HF.[5,8,19,20] The physical examination of a cat with HF can unfortunately be somewhat nonspecific.[13] The heart rate can be fast, normal, or slow; up to 30% of cats may not have an obvious arrhythmia, murmur, or gallop on initial examination. Additionally, cats in HF are not uncommonly hypothermic.[21] In some patients with significant respiratory distress, empiric therapy to stabilize patients is started even before any further diagnostic tests are performed if the signalment, history, and physical examination are suggestive of HF. Initial empiric therapy typically includes the administration of parenteral furosemide, oxygen, and sedation (please see **Tables 4** and **5**).

Table 2
Typical signalments associated with common causes of HF

Disorder	Canine MVD	Canine Dilated Cardiomyopathy	Feline Hypertrophic Cardiomyopathy
Age	Usually older dog (>10 y), except for Cavalier King Charles spaniels, Dachshund	Usually young to middle-aged adult	Usually young to middle-aged adult
Sex	Males > females	Male > females Except in boxers whereby male = females	Males > females
Breed	Usually small breeds: Cavalier King Charles spaniels, toy/mini poodles, mini schnauzers, Pomeranians, Chihuahuas, Malteses, Bichons, Shi Tzus, Dachshunds, Cocker spaniels, Pekingeses, terriers, beagles, whippets; occasional large-breed dogs	Usually larger breeds: Dobermans, boxers, giant breeds (Newfoundlands, Irish wolfhounds, Scottish deerhounds, Saint Bernards), retrievers, Portuguese water dogs, old English sheepdogs, cocker spaniels	Usually mixed-breed cats; strong family associations in Maine coon, American and British shorthairs, Bengals, Sphinx, Himalayan, and Persian cats

Table 3
Typical physical examination findings in the common causes of HF

Cause	Heart/Rhythm and Pulse Quality	Thoracic Auscultation	Other
Canine mitral valve disease	High normal to elevated heart rate Atrial premature complexes not uncommon	Usually loud systolic murmur heard best over left apex Increased breath sounds or soft crackles on end inspiration	Cardiac cachexia or weight loss common Possible ascites and jugular venous pulsations
Canine dilated cardiomyopathy	High normal to elevated heart rate Frequent atrial or ventricular arrhythmias Atrial fibrillation very common in giant breeds	Soft systolic murmur Gallop sound Increased breath sounds or soft crackles on end inspiration	Dobermans may not have cardiac cachexia Possible ascites
Feline hypertrophic cardiomyopathy	Heart rate can be low, normal, or high with heart failure Low heart rates associated with hypothermia Poor pulse quality	Murmur or gallop Not uncommonly, heart sounds are normal Respiratory sounds can be quiet (predominant pleural effusion) or loud (predominant pulmonary edema)	With ATE, cold, painful rear legs with absent femoral pulses Noncompliant thorax with pleural effusion May not have cardiac cachexia

Abbreviation: ATE, aortic thromboembolism.

Table 4
Management recommendations of acute severe HF for dogs and cats

Dog FONS-P or FONS-D	• Furosemide: 2–4 mg/kg IM or IV bolus PRN ± CRI (max 12 mg/kg/d) • Oxygen • Nitroglycerin: 0.25–1.0 in transdermal q 8–24 h for 1–2 d or nitroprusside: 1–10 µg/kg/min IV (careful BP monitoring) • Sedation: butorphanol 0.1–0.2 mg/kg IV or IM PRN • Pimobendan: 0.25 mg/kg PO q 8 – 12 h (when able to swallow) • Dobutamine: if cardiogenic shock (hypotensive, hypothermic, low output signs) • Diltiazem/digoxin: if concurrent atrial fibrillation
Cat FONS-T or FONS-P	• Furosemide: 1–4 mg/kg IM or IV bolus PRN ± CRI (max 12 mg/kg/d) • Oxygen • Nitroglycerin: 0.25 in transdermal q 8–24 h for 1–2 d or nitroprusside: 0.5–5.0 µg/kg/min IV (careful BP monitoring) • Sedation: butorphanol 0.1–0.2 mg/kg IM *(minimize stress)* • Thoracocentesis: if pleural effusion • Pimobendan: if refractory edema, LV systolic dysfunction, or azotemia 0.25 mg/kg PO q 12 h (when able to swallow) • Puff: inhaled albuterol (2 puffs) or SQ terbutaline for peribronchiolar edema or refractory respiratory distress

Abbreviations: BP, blood pressure; CRI, continuous rate infusions; IM, intramuscularly; LV, left ventricle; max, maximum; PRN, as needed; SQ, subcutaneous.

Diagnostic imaging of the heart and lungs with thoracic radiography and echocardiography are helpful to confirm or refute a diagnosis of HF. A recent advancement in the diagnostic imaging in patients with respiratory distress is the increased use of focused echocardiography and thoracic ultrasound to improve the timely and accurate diagnosis of either left or right HF.[22,23] In the author's practice, essentially every dog or cat with respiratory distress or collapse that presents emergently will have a thoracic focused assessment with sonography for trauma (TFAST) ultrasound or an abdominal FAST (AFAST) ultrasound performed by emergency department (ED) clinicians, usually before radiography. The TFAST and AFAST ultrasound and focused echocardiogram are performed with patients in sternal recumbency while receiving oxygen supplementation typically after a low dose of sedation. The examination is brief and minimally stressful to patients and is generally less stressful than performing a thoracic radiograph. A recent joint consensus statement by the American Society of Echocardiography and the American College of Emergency Physicians supported the use of the focused cardiac ultrasound examinations to expedite the diagnosis and management of life-threatening conditions in the ED setting.[24] With some training, noncardiologist/ nonradiologist veterinarians can achieve proficiency in identifying pleural and pericardial effusions and left atrial enlargement.[25] Focused thoracic ultrasound is especially useful in cats with suspect HF because both the physical examination and radiographic findings in cats with HF are notoriously nonspecific.[13,26] Pleural effusion, a common manifestation of feline HF, obscures the cardiac silhouette, lungs, and vasculature radiographically (**Fig. 1**). With pleural effusion, the heart can be clearly visualized by ultrasound, allowing accurate assessments of chamber dimensions, specifically left atrial size (**Fig. 2**). The left atrium is most commonly indexed to the aorta in a right-sided, short-axis view at the base of the heart or a long-axis view. A left atrium/aorta ratio of 2.0 or greater is very suggestive of HF.[27,28] Normally, the left atrium/aorta ratio is less than 1.5 in cats and less than 1.3 in dogs.[29,30] The finding of pericardial effusion in cats with cardiomegaly and respiratory distress is also very suggestive of HF.[31] In addition to rapidly identifying left atrial enlargement, pleural and pericardial effusion, assessments of right and left heart enlargement, left ventricular systolic dysfunction, and mitral valve thickening can be made with echocardiography (**Fig. 3**). The emergent focused ultrasound examination has become an extension of the physical examination and has been termed by some as the *visual stethoscope*.[23] Although ultrasound is becoming more commonly available at EDs and general practices, many veterinary practitioners may not have ready access to this technology.

Thoracic radiography is still one of the highest-yield tests for the diagnosis of both suspected left and right HF. In most cases, the diagnosis of HF is based on the finding of venous distention, presence of cardiomegaly, and a consistent pulmonary pattern (**Fig. 4**). Distention of either pulmonary veins or the caudal vena cava is very suggestive of either left or right HF, respectively.[32–34] The pulmonary vein is considered distended if it is larger than its accompanying pulmonary artery. If radiographs are taken after several doses of empiric furosemide and clinical improvement, the pulmonary veins may not always appear distended with resolving pulmonary edema. Heart enlargement is usually present but may not always be a consistent finding in the diagnosis of HF. In dogs, the radiographic pulmonary pattern consistent with left HF is typically a perihilar interstitial to alveolar pattern. The pulmonary pattern is commonly asymmetric in dogs with MVD with an eccentric jet of mitral valve regurgitation or more symmetric in canine DCM.[33] The distribution of radiographic pulmonary patterns is notoriously variable in cats with cardiogenic pulmonary edema.[26] In severe HF cases, a diffuse, severe interstitial to alveolar pulmonary pattern or pleural effusion will make the cardiac silhouette and pulmonary veins impossible to visualize.

Table 5
Common drugs and dosages used in the management of cardiac emergencies

Drug	Species	Route	Dosage and Frequency
Antiarrhythmics			
Amiodarone	Dog	PO	10–25 mg/kg q 12 h × 7 d, then 5.0–7.5 mg/kg q 12 h × 14 d, then q 24 h
Diltiazem SR (Cardizem CD)	Cat	PO	10 mg/kg q 24 h (human capsules = 120 mg with sprinkles inside)
Digoxin	Dog	PO	0.003 mg/kg q 12 h
Digoxin	Dog	IV	0.0025 mg/kg q 1 h × 4 h (total 0.01 mg/kg)
Diltiazem SR (Dilacor)	Dog	PO	1–4 mg/kg q 12 h (60-mg tablets inside capsule)
Diltiazem SR (Dilacor)	Cat	PO	30 mg per cat q 12–24 h (one-half of 60-mg tablet inside a capsule)
Diltiazem	Dog	PO	0.5–1.5 mg/kg q 8 h, start low, titrate up
Diltiazem	Dog	IV	0.1 mg/kg over slow over 3–5 min, can repeat 2 times; wait 15 min in between dosing to assess response
Diltiazem	Cat	PO	7.5 mg per cat q 8 h
Esmolol	Both	IV	0.1 mg/kg can titrate up to 0.5 mg/kg, MAX effect 2–4 min
Lidocaine	Dog	IV	2-mg/kg bolus, repeat up to 8 mg/kg or adverse effect 30–80 µg/kg/min CRI
Lidocaine	Cat	IV	0.2–0.75 mg/kg slow bolus, can repeat 1–2 × MAX
Magnesium chloride	Dog	IV	0.15–0.45 meq/kg slow IV (15–20 min)
Magnesium oxide	Dog	PO	1–2 mEq/kg/d
Magnesium sulfate	Dog	IV	30 mg/kg slow IV (15–20 min), then 30 mg/kg over 12–24 h
Mexiletine	Dog	PO	5–8 mg/kg q 8 h
Procainamide	Dog	IV	2–8 mg/kg slow bolus up to MAX 16 mg/kg CRI 25–40 mcg/kg/min
Procainamide	Dog	PO	7.5–20.0 mg/kg q 6–8 h
Sotalol	Dog	PO	2 mg/kg q 12 h (lower if concurrent renal disease)
Sotalol	Cat	PO	2 mg/kg q 12 h (lower if concurrent renal disease)
ACE inhibitors			
Enalapril	Dog	PO	0.5 mg/kg q 12–24 h (start low or avoid if azotemic)
Enalapril	Cat	PO	0.5 mg/kg q 24 (start low or avoid if azotemic)
Benazepril	Dog	PO	0.5 mg/kg q 12–24 (start low or avoid if azotemic)
Benazepril	Cat	PO	0.5 mg/kg q 24 h (start low or avoid if azotemic)
Diuretics			
Furosemide	Dog	IV/SQ	2–4 mg/kg q 6–12 h PRN (MAX 12 mg/kg/d)
Furosemide	Dog	PO	1–4 mg/kg q 8–24 h PRN (MAX 12 mg/kg/d)
Furosemide	Dog	CRI	2–4 mg/kg over 2–4 h post IV bolus
Furosemide	Cat	IV/SQ	1–4 mg/kg q 8–24 h
Furosemide	Cat	PO	1–4 mg/kg q 8–12 h
Aldactazide (HTCZ + Spironolactone)	Dog	PO	0.5–1.0 mg/kg dosed based on spironolactone q 12–48 h
Torsemide	Dog	PO	One-tenth of furosemide dose

(continued on next page)

Table 5
(continued)

Drug	Species	Route	Dosage and Frequency
Vasodilators			
Nitroglycerine 2% oint	Both	Skin	0.25-in strip/5–10 kg q 8 h (for first 24 h typically)
Nitroprusside	Dog	IV	1–10 mcg/kg/min CRI (careful BP monitoring)
Nitroprusside	Cat	IV	0.5–5.0 mcg/kg/min CRI (careful BP monitoring)
Amlodipine	Cat	PO	0.625 mg q 24 h, titrate up PRN with BP monitor
Amlodipine	Dog	PO	0.1 mg/kg q 12–24 h initially, titrate up to MAX 0.25 mg/kg q 12 h monitor BP
Sildenafil	Both	PO	1–2 mg/kg q 8–12 h
Inotropes			
Digoxin	Dog	PO	0.003 mg/kg q 12 h (not to exceed 0.25 mg BID) (therapeutic levels: 0.5–0.9 ng/mL)
Digoxin	Dog	IV	0.0025 mg/kg q 1 h × 4 h (total 0.01 mg/kg)
Pimobendan	Both	PO	0.25 mg/kg q 12 h (can increase dose and frequency to q 8 h in refractory cases)
Dobutamine	Dog	IV	1–10 mcg/kg/min CRI
Dobutamine	Cat	IV	1–3 mcg/kg/min CRI
Vagolytics			
Atropine	Both	IV/SQ	0.04 mg/kg
Glycopyrrolate	Both	IV/SQ	0.005–0.02 mg/kg (generally 0.011 mg/kg)
Propantheline	Dog	PO	0.5–1.5 mg/kg q 8 h
Bronchodilator			
Terbutaline	Dog	PO	2.5–5.0 mg total dose q 8–12 h
Terbutaline	Cat	PO	1.25 mg total dose q 8–12 h
Terbutaline	Both	SQ	0.01 mg/kg q 4 h
Theophylline ER	Both	PO	10 mg/kg q 12 h
Albuterol	Both	Inhaled	2 puffs PRN (90 mcg per actuation)
Sedation/analgesia			
Butorphanol	Both	IV/SQ	0.05–0.3 mg/kg, repeat as needed
Buprenorphine	Both	IV/SQ	0.005–0.02 mg/kg q 6–8 h
Buprenorphine	Cat	Buccal	0.01–0.03 mg/kg q 8–12 h
Acepromazine	Both	IV/SQ	0.005–0.01 mg/kg once, could repeat if needed
Fentanyl	Both	IV	2–3 mcg/kg, then 1–5 mcg/kg/h CRI
Antithrombotics			
Dalteparin	Cat	SQ	100–150 IU/kg q 12 h (some advocate higher dose)
Enoxaparin	Cat	SQ	1 mg/kg q 12 h for acute treatment, 1.5 mg/kg q 24 h for prophylaxis
UF Heparin	Cat	SQ	100 U/kg IV once then 200 U/kg SQ q 8 h (APTT 1.5–2.0 ×)
UF Heparin	Cat	IV	100 U/kg once then 600 U/kg/d CRI (APTT 1.5–2.0 ×)
Aspirin	Cat	PO	81 mg per cat q 72 h OR 5 mg per cat q 24 h with food
Tissue plasminogen activator	Cat	IV	0.75 mg IV bolus, 2.5 mg IV over 30 min, 1.75 mg IV over 1 h (5 mg total)
Clopidogrel	Cat	PO	18.75 mg per cat (one-fourth of 75-mg tablet)

Abbreviations: ACE, angiotensin-converting enzyme; APTT, activated partial thromboplastin time; BP, blood pressure; CRI, continuous rate infusions; HTCZ, hydrochlorothiazide; MAX, maximum; oint, ointment; SR, sustained release; SQ, subcutaneous; UF, unfractionated.

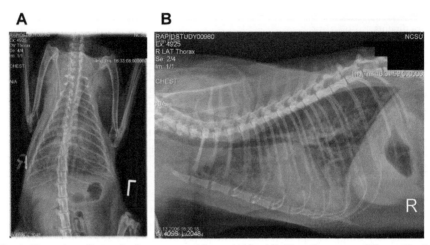

Fig. 1. Thoracic radiographs from a cat with congestive HF. Note the severe diffuse alveolar pattern and slight pleural effusion on both the dorsoventral (*A*) and lateral (*B*) projection that obscures assessment of heart size and pulmonary vessels.

Another recent advancement in the diagnosis of HF in veterinary medicine is the use of cardiac biomarkers, such as amine terminal pro B-type natriuretic peptide (NTproBNP), BNP, and cardiac troponin I (cTnI). Cardiac biomarkers are blood tests for heart disease. NTproBNP and BNP are peptide hormones released by the ventricles in response to increased stretch. Both are elevated in dogs and cats with active congestive HF.[35–38] Used in conjunction with other clinical information, the measurement of NTproBNP (Canine and Feline Cardiopet proBNP, Idexx Laboratories, Inc, Westbrook, ME) and BNP (Canine Cardio-BNP, Antech Diagnostics, Irvine, CA) are useful in establishing, increasing confidence for, or excluding the diagnosis of congestive HF in patients presenting with acute dyspnea or cough.[39] Samples need to be obtained when the animal is symptomatic for HF because the concentrations of the natriuretic peptides will decrease with treatment. Unfortunately, these assays are currently only available as send-out tests, limiting their usefulness in the emergency management of HF.

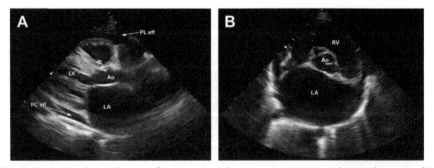

Fig. 2. Focused echocardiogram from a cat with congestive HF secondary to hypertrophic cardiomyopathy. Note easy recognition of left atrial enlargement and pleural and pericardial effusion (*arrows*) on the right-sided long-axis view (*A*). On the right-sided short-axis view, the diameter of left atrium is more than 2 times of the aortic diameter suggestive of left HF (*B*). Ao, aorta; LA, left atrium; LV, left ventricle; PC eff, pericardial effusion; PL eff, pleural effusion; RV, right ventricle.

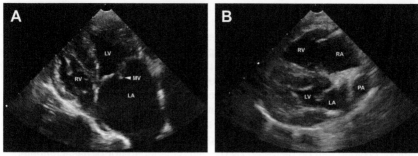

Fig. 3. Focused echocardiogram from 2 dogs, one with left HF (A) and the other with right HF (B). Note the severe left atrial and ventricular enlargement in the dog with MVD viewed from a left-sided 4-chamber view. (A) Note the severe right heart enlargement in the dog with right HF caused by severe pulmonary hypertension viewed from a right-sided long-axis view. In this view, the left heart should normally be 3 to 4 times larger than the right heart. LA, left atrium; LV, left ventricle; MV, mitral valve; PA, pulmonary artery; RA, right atrium; RV, right ventricle.

Development of point-of-care testing, more accurate reference values, and a better understanding of the influence of systemic disease on these biomarkers are in progress. Special sample handling with transfer of the EDTA plasma into a stabilizer tube is required for analysis. At the time of this writing, the only point-of-care cardiac biomarker commercially available is cTnI, a marker of myocardial injury (i-STAT Cardiac Troponin I, Abaxis, Inc, Union City, CA). cTnI may have some utility in the emergency diagnosis of HF in cats but not dogs.[40,41] Most cats with HF have a markedly elevated cTnI; however, cats with severe, primary respiratory disease may also have elevated values. Typically, the magnitude of elevation is higher in cats with HF than those with respiratory disease. In rare circumstances, the measurement of pulmonary venous and central venous pressure (CVP) can be performed when the HF diagnosis is still uncertain. A CVP greater than 15 mm Hg is suggestive of right HF.

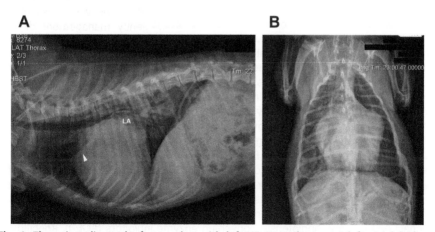

Fig. 4. Thoracic radiographs from a dog with left HF. Note the severe left atrial (LA) enlargement, pulmonary venous distention (*arrowhead*), and perihilar interstitial pulmonary pattern indicating pulmonary edema on the lateral projection (A). On the dorsoventral projection (B), the caudal pulmonary pattern is asymmetric, with the right caudal lung fields being more affected.

The immediate goal of emergency therapy is to reduce abnormal fluid accumulations and to provide adequate or improved cardiac output. Strict cage rest and minimization of stress are of the utmost importance. Initially, treatments include sedation, oxygen, furosemide, or thoracocentesis in patients with large amounts of pleural effusion. Sedation is generally administered if patients are dyspneic and anxious. Butorphanol is a very effective sedative for patients in respiratory distress, in the author's opinion. The butorphanol ranges from 0.05 to 0.3 mg/kg IV, intramuscularly (IM), or subcutaneously but is generally dosed at 0.1 mg/kg in patients with respiratory distress. Painful cats with aortic thromboembolism respond well to buprenorphine (see **Table 5**). Supplemental oxygen therapy is recommended to reduce the work of breathing. Oxygen can be delivered by oxygen cage/incubator or nasal catheter.

Furosemide (Lasix or Salix), a loop diuretic, is a mainstay in the management of congestive HF, regardless of the cause. Despite its usefulness in HF management, furosemide never improves cardiac output. The dose of furosemide is usually the most challenging issue because it needs to be tailored to the individual patient. Too high of a dose can have deleterious effects on renal perfusion and electrolytes, especially in a dog or cat with hypotension. Conversely, too low of a dose can lead to unnecessary hospitalization, expense, and potential euthanasia because of refractory or recurrent pulmonary edema. Additionally, in patients with severely decompensated HF, the best route of administration is IV because of its quicker onset of action and more predictable bioavailability.[42] The current debate about furosemide in human medicine is on the use of repeated bolus dosing versus continuous rate infusions (CRI).[43–45] The author uses a combination of repeat bolus dosing and CRIs to manage hospitalized patients with decompensated HF (see **Table 5**). The combination of a furosemide bolus followed by a CRI may have a better diuretic effect.[45] The initial emergency furosemide dose is usually higher than the discharge dose, and the best dose to administer chronically is the lowest effective dose. Generally, renal parameters and electrolytes are reevaluated with 1 to 3 days in inpatients with HF and 3 to 7 days in outpatients with HF.

Another loop diuretic of possible use in acute severe refractory canine HF is torsemide (Demadex).[46] Torsemide has a longer duration of action, decreased susceptibility to diuretic resistance, and adjunctive aldosterone antagonist properties compared with furosemide. Generally, the torsemide dosage is one-tenth of the daily furosemide dosage divided into twice-daily oral dosing.

In addition to furosemide, in patients with severely dyspneic HF, the addition of either nitroglycerin (Nitro-Bid ointment) or nitroprusside (Nitropress) is recommended because of their vasodilator actions. Nitroglycerin, a venodilator, is commonly used in a transdermal formulation in veterinary medicine. Nitroprusside, a potent IV venous and arterial vasodilator, is given by a variable dosage, starting at a low dosage of 1 or 2 ug/kg/min in dogs and even lower in cats (0.5 mcg/kg/min) and titrating upward based on blood pressure, targeting a mean blood pressure of 70 mm Hg or systolic blood pressure of 90 to 100 mm Hg.[47] Because of its potent vasodilatory effects, direct arterial blood pressure monitoring is recommended; however, if an arterial catheter cannot be placed (eg, smaller dogs and cats), continuous indirect blood pressures (eg, Doppler) should be measured.

Other vasodilators useful in the management of HF include amlodipine (Norvasc), sildenafil (Viagra), and angiotensin-converting enzyme inhibitors (ACE-I), specifically enalapril (Vasotec) or benazepril (Lotensin). Many previous studies in dogs have shown that ACE-I improve survival and quality of life in dogs with congestive HF secondary to both DCM and MVD.[48–50] Although the two ACE-I are very similar, benazepril is less dependent on renal clearance. The benefit of ACE-I seems to involve more than just their vasodilator effects. It is proposed that the inhibition of the local renin-angiotensin-aldosterone system may protect the myocardium from deleterious remodeling effects. Although enalapril has been shown to reduce pulmonary venous pressures acutely in HF,[51] ACE-I are typically withheld in the peracute management of severely decompensated HF because of the possibility of lowering intrarenal perfusion and the glomerular filtration rate. ACE-I should also be used cautiously in any patient with HF with concurrent azotemia by either dose reduction or withholding ACE-I if creatinine is greater than 2.0 g/dL. ACE-inhibition is recommended in the chronic management of all patients with HF (cats and dogs) once patients are stable and eating. After the initiation of an ACE-I, reevaluation of serum urea nitrogen, creatinine, and electrolytes is recommended in 3 to 7 days.

Sildenafil is a useful adjunctive vasodilator in the setting of symptomatic and severe pulmonary hypertension and in refractory HF associated with pulmonary hypertension.[52,53] Sildenafil is a phosphodiesterase inhibitor with greater affinity for certain vascular beds, including the pulmonary arteries. Because sildenafil is now available in a generic formulation in the United States, it can be a realistic option financially. Amlodipine, a calcium channel blocker, acts primarily as an arterial vasodilator. Amlodipine can also be used in patients with refractory or recurrent congestive HF, especially if systolic blood pressure is maintained or high (eg, >120 mm Hg systolic). Amlodipine is especially helpful in dogs with severe refractory HF caused by MVD.

The most important recent advancement in HF management is the addition of an inodilator, pimobendan (Vetmedin). Pimobendan has a dual mechanism of action; therefore, it is labeled as an inodilator. Specifically, it is a calcium-sensitizing drug that improves contractility (positive inotrope) with minimal effects on myocardial oxygen consumption. The other mechanism of action is phosphodiesterase inhibition, primarily leading to a balanced vasodilation (arterial and venous).[54] The favorable pharmacokinetic and pharmacodynamic actions of pimobendan make it essential in the management of most canine HF and possibly feline HF. Several prospective canine studies and one retrospective feline study have shown improved survival and quality of life with pimobendan either in combination or compared with ACE-I and furosemide.[55–57] In addition to its Food and Drug Administration–labeled indications for the management of HF secondary to canine DCM and MVD, it is also used to manage dogs with HF from other causes, such as heartworm disease, primary or secondary pulmonary hypertension with secondary right HF, infectious endocarditis, and some congenital heart diseases.[58] The role of pimobendan in feline HF is still evolving. Although not licensed for use in cats (or humans in the United States), pimobendan is being used more frequently in the management of feline HF. Pimobendan is typically added when a cat with HF has left ventricular systolic dysfunction identified echocardiographically, significant pleural effusion, renal insufficiency, or severe refractory pulmonary edema. There are no prospective randomized clinical trials in cats with HF evaluating pimobendan, but a recent retrospective case series suggest that it is safe at similar doses used in dogs.[59,60] A pharmacokinetic study in cats suggests that pimobendan may have a longer half-life in cats than dogs.[61] In dogs, the onset of action and peak blood levels of pimobendan and its metabolite are reached within 1 hour of administration of a single oral dose. Because of its rapid onset of action, the author has found it to be *very useful* in the management of severe acutely decompensated HF. Pimobendan is given as soon as the clinician feels that the dog or cat can take an oral medication. Dose and frequency escalation are common with recurrent or refractory HF with good clinical response.[62] Pimobendan is primarily eliminated in feces via bile (95%); only 5% of the drug and its metabolites are renally excreted, making it safe to use with concurrent renal disease and HF, which is common in older dogs with MVD.[63] The addition of pimobendan allows lower doses of furosemide and ACE-inhibitors. Adverse effects are surprisingly few. Because of the human experience, there are concerns for proarrhythmic tendencies. These concerns have, for the most part, been greatly reduced by the canine clinical trials showing no increase in arrhythmias. Since the introduction of pimobendan, the use of digoxin in the management of canine HF has decreased dramatically. The most common scenario when one may use digoxin (Digitek), usually combined with diltiazem (Cardizem), is in the management of rapid atrial fibrillation in the setting of congestive HF either caused by DCM or MVD disease, without evidence of renal insufficiency.

If patients with HF are unable to take oral medications and have signs of severe low cardiac output HF, dobutamine (Dobutrex) is recommended. Dobutamine is an IV adrenergic-positive inotrope with primarily beta-1 effects. The dosage ranges from 1 to 10 mcg/kg/min CRI, starting at a lower dose and titrating upward based on blood pressure and electrocardiogram (ECG) monitoring. Tachyarrhythmias are the main adverse effect. This drug is most useful in cardiogenic shock (eg, Doberman pincher with severe DCM, hypotension, and severe pulmonary edema). If concurrent atrial fibrillation is present, rapid IV digitalization is recommended before dobutamine to slow AV nodal conduction.

Other therapeutic considerations in the management of patients with HF include possible thoracocentesis or abdominocentesis, bronchodilators, and antiarrhythmic agents (see next section on arrhythmia management). If large-volume pleural or abdominal effusion is present and causing patient discomfort, the most effective therapeutic maneuver is the removal of the fluid by centesis. The optimal site for thoracocentesis and abdominocentesis can be guided by ultrasound. Additionally, if concurrent airway disease is suspected, empiric bronchodilator therapy may be beneficial. Many small-breed dogs with advanced valvular heart disease may also have significant airway disease that can contribute to clinical signs. Additionally, some cats with HF may develop peribronchiolar edema with associated bronchoconstriction. Inhaled albuterol (ProAir HFA) is an easy-to-administer bronchodilator with mask and spacer chamber (AeroKat). Other useful bronchodilators are terbutaline and theophylline. Bronchodilators should be used cautiously, however, because they may promote tachyarrhythmias if administered at high doses.

Treating the first episode of acutely decompensated HF is usually successful. A recent study showed an estimated 80% survival rate to discharge for dogs with acute HF that were admitted to a university ED in an urban setting.[21] Once the diagnosis and initial urgent management of HF has been performed, a plan for continued management and monitoring should be formulated. The therapeutic plan will be tailored to the individual patient based on the pathophysiology of the HF and any concurrent disease. An important and often overlooked part of the successful emergency management of congestive HF is open communication with the owner regarding the emotional, practical, and financial ability to deal with the long-term management of the animal's heart disease. Survival times for most dogs or cats in HF with treatment vary from 6 months to 1 year, depending on the underlying cause of the heart disease and comorbidities.[4,13,55,56,59,64–66]

ARRHYTHMIAS

Arrhythmias can occur with a wide range of diseases and vary greatly in their clinical signs from asymptomatic to collapse, depending on the rate, frequency, and complexity of the arrhythmia and the severity of any organic cardiac dysfunction or other noncardiac diseases.

Tachyarrhythmias are suspected on physical examination in emergently ill patients on cardiac auscultation because of either sustained or paroxysmal bursts of tachycardia, generally at heart rates of 150 to 300 beats per minute. An ECG is necessary to further characterize the tachycardia into a sinus tachycardia, a ventricular tachycardia (VT), or supraventricular tachycardia (SVT). Sinus tachycardia is a physiologic rhythm that originates in the sinus node and occurs in response to increased need for cardiac output or increased sympathetic tone. Cardiac and noncardiac diseases may result in either supraventricular or ventricular tachyarrhythmias. Noncardiac disease conditions, such as sepsis, pancreatitis, autoimmune hemolytic anemia, pheochromocytoma, gastric-dilation-volvulus, splenic disease (eg, neoplasia, torsion), and end-stage uremia, may result in supraventricular and ventricular arrhythmias in the absence of structural heart disease. Another electrical rhythm disturbance that can be seen in critically ill patients is accelerated idioventricular rhythm (AIVR). AIVR is an ectopic ventricular rhythm with a rate of 60 to 120 beats per minute. AIVR is thought to be a relatively benign arrhythmia requiring no treatment. Electrolyte disturbances, such as hypokalemia, hypocalcemia, hypomagnesium or hyperkalemia, and digoxin toxicity may cause myocardial ionic abnormalities and arrhythmias. Other cardiac causes of tachyarrhythmias include DCM, infectious endocarditis, myocarditis, severe congenital heart disease, advanced congestive HF secondary to DCM or MVD, and cardiac neoplasia. Traumatic myocarditis resulting from blunt chest trauma, possibly related to myocardial bruising or ischemia-reperfusion injury, may also result in ventricular arrhythmias.

Establishing a diagnosis of VT is made from the interpretation of the ECG. Ventricular premature beats and ventricular tachycardia have wide and bizarre QRS complexes with no associated P waves. Other findings suggestive of VT include atrioventricular (AV) dissociation and fusion beats. The QRS axis or polarity of a ventricular arrhythmia is usually negative in lead II but could be positive, particularly in VT commonly seen in boxer dogs with ARVC (**Fig. 5A**).[67]

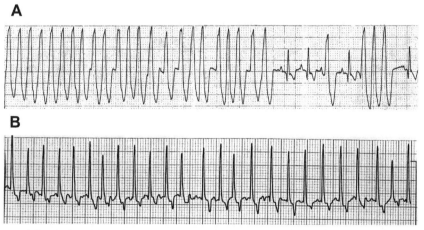

Fig. 5. (A) ECG (25 mm/s) from a syncopal Boxer dog with ARVC showing a predominant rhythm of ventricular tachycardia. Note the wide QRS tachycardia that is positive in lead II, typical for boxer ARVC. (B) ECG (25 mm/s) from a dog with congestive HF and atrial fibrillation. Note the narrow QRS irregular tachyarrhythmia with lack of P waves and varying QRS amplitude.

The need and urgency of treatment of VT depends on the hemodynamic status of patients, the severity of the arrhythmia, and underlying myocardial dysfunction. Some ventricular arrhythmias may not require specific antiarrhythmia therapy and would benefit from supportive maneuvers, such as supplemental oxygen, adequate fluid/electrolyte therapy, and treating the underlying condition, such as HF or sepsis. Ventricular arrhythmias are considered more hemodynamically significant and life threatening if they occur at a fast rate (>150/min in dogs or >250/min in cats) or in sustained runs (>30 seconds), if they are multiform, or are very premature (R-on-T phenomenon).

Acute management of ventricular arrhythmias in cats with injectable antiarrhythmic drugs is problematic because of the risk of adverse effects. The author often suppresses symptomatic feline VT with compounded oral sotalol (Betapace) (see **Table 5**). For acute management of severe and symptomatic ventricular arrhythmias in the dog, treatment recommendations include lidocaine (Xylocaine) as a 2 mg/kg IV bolus, which is often repeated to effect up to a total of 8 mg/kg or until an adverse effect is observed, such as nausea or transient neurologic tremors or seizure, waiting 3 to 5 minutes in between each bolus to evaluate efficacy. If the bolus injections are successful in controlling the VT, then a CRI of lidocaine is initiated. Because the half-life of lidocaine in dogs is approximately 60 minutes, the CRI may take 5 to 7 hours to reach a steady state; therefore, intermittent, smaller 1-mg/kg boluses may be necessary in the interim. If lidocaine is unsuccessful, ensure adequate serum potassium and magnesium concentrations, then try administering procainamide (Procan). IV procainamide boluses are given slowly over 3 to 5 minutes because of the possible development of hypotension in 2- to 8-mg/kg increments to effect, up to a total of 16 mg/kg. If the boluses are successful in controlling the arrhythmia, then a CRI of procainamide should be initiated. Alternatively, if a CRI is not feasible, IM procainamide (7–10 mg/kg) every 6 to 8 hours could be used. For oral maintenance therapy or nonurgent control of a ventricular arrhythmia, treatment recommendations in dogs include the use of sotalol (a beta-adrenergic blocker + potassium channel blocker or Vaughn Williams type II and III antiarrhythmic, respectively) or mexiletine (Mexitil) (a sodium channel blocker or Vaughn Williams type IB antiarrhythmic) or a combination of both. Sotalol is often started shortly after lidocaine if chronic oral suppression of the arrhythmia is anticipated, as in a syncopal ARVC boxer. For medically refractory, incessant VT associated with the loss of consciousness or hypotension, other antiarrhythmics, such as amiodarone (Pacerone), or electrical cardioversion may be considered.[68,69] Electrical cardioversion of VT is rarely performed in veterinary medicine but not uncommonly performed in human emergency medicine.

The management of SVT is importantly different than a ventricular arrhythmia. SVTs are usually narrow QRS complex tachycardias that include atrial fibrillation, atrial flutter, multifocal atrial tachycardia, reentrant accessory pathway, or reentrant AV nodal tachycardias. The QRS is typically positive in lead II. SVTs can be rarely aberrantly conducted resulting in a wide-complex tachycardia, which can be confused for a VT. Aside from atrial fibrillation and multifocal atrial tachycardia, most other causes of SVTs have regular QRS intervals. Atrial fibrillation is typically a sustained tachyarrhythmia, whereas regular SVTs and multifocal atrial tachycardias are typically intermittent. The ECG diagnosis of atrial fibrillation includes the lack of P waves; presence of baseline undulation waves (f waves); and a fast, irregular rhythm, sometimes with varying QRS amplitudes (see **Fig. 5**B). In the emergency setting, most dogs and cats presenting with atrial fibrillation are in congestive HF and are typically managed with a combination of digoxin and diltiazem.[70] The combination of these two drugs is superior to either drug alone at reducing the ventricular response rate of atrial fibrillation, which is the goal of therapy. In most cases, these drugs are given orally but can be given initially IV for more rapid onset of action. Treatment of other supraventricular arrhythmias depends on the frequency of the rhythm disturbance and the presence of any underlying myocardial dysfunction. If the intermittent SVT is frequent, occurring in long runs (several minutes), or is causing symptoms, treatment is recommended. It is important to emphasize that chronic, sustained SVT may result in a tachycardia-induced cardiomyopathy and congestive HF. A vagal maneuver (eg, ocular or carotid sinus massage) may be successful in transiently breaking an SVT. However, medical treatment will usually be necessary to chronically control the SVT. For peracute management of sustained, symptomatic SVT, IV diltiazem is usually successful in both dogs and cats. IV esmolol (Brevibloc), a rapid-acting beta-blocker, may also be helpful in managing SVT acutely. For oral maintenance therapy or nonurgent control of SVT, treatment recommendations include oral diltiazem, atenolol (Tenormin), or sotalol. Sotalol may be an excellent antiarrhythmic drug for a dog or cat that has both ventricular and supraventricular arrhythmias.

Bradyarrhythmias are identified with cardiac auscultation because of either a regularly slow heart rate or intermittent periods of sinus arrest. Bradycardia is generally defined as a heart rate of less than 60 beats per minute in dogs and less than 140 beats per minute in cats. An ECG is necessary to further characterize the bradycardia into sinus bradycardia, a sinus node dysfunction, atrial standstill, or high-grade AV block, and either high-grade, second-degree AV block or complete AV block. Most animals with clinically significant bradyarrhythmias present for syncope or weakness.

Sinus bradycardia is usually a result of high vagal tone caused by gastrointestinal, respiratory or central nervous system disease, or secondary to medical therapy that may cause a decreased in heart rate, such as the administration of sedative, analgesic, or negative chronotropic cardiac drugs. Overdose or an overzealous response to negative chronotropic drugs, such as a beta blockers, calcium channel blockers, or digoxin, can cause pathologic bradycardias. Sepsis and low body temperature in cats can also produce sinus bradycardia. Treatment usually is directed at the underlying cause or disease.

When sinus bradycardia occurs with excessively long pauses (several seconds), sinus node dysfunction or sick sinus syndrome (SSS) is suspected (**Fig. 6**A). SSS is an idiopathic dysfunction of the sinus node that most commonly affects miniature schnauzers and West Highland white terriers. SSS can manifest as mostly a regular sinus bradycardia with long pauses (several seconds) or as a bradycardia-tachycardia syndrome, alternating long pauses with an SVT. Dogs with bradytachycardia do not respond to medical management and will require a pacemaker to improve clinical signs. Some dogs with SSS that do not have the bradytachycardia may improve with medical management with either positive chronotropic drugs, such as a bronchodilator, or an anticholinergic agent, such as terbutaline, theophylline, or propantheline. Most dogs with significant sinus node dysfunction disease will eventually require a pacemaker to resolve their syncope. Asymptomatic dogs with SSS do not require any treatment.

Complete or third-degree and high-grade second-degree AV block is a common pathologic bradyarrhythmia identified in dogs (see **Fig. 6**B). Most dogs with high-grade AV block have no to little structural heart disease.[71,72] However, occasionally endocarditis, DCM, or neoplasia is identified echocardiographically. Many cats with complete AV block have underlying myocardial disease.[73] Most dogs present for syncope, collapse, weakness, and lethargy. Occasionally some dogs with high-grade AV block may be asymptomatic and are identified on a routine examination. Dogs with high-grade AV block have a high risk of death regardless of presence of symptoms.

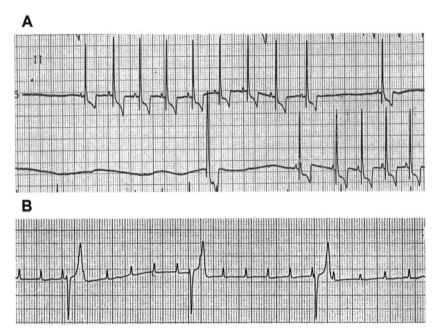

Fig. 6. (A) ECG (25 mm/s) from a syncopal miniature schnauzer with SSS. Note a predominant respiratory sinus arrhythmia with a couple of periods of sinus arrest (>2 normal R-R intervals). The markedly prolong period of sinus arrest is terminated with an escape complex. (B) ECG (25 mm/s) from a syncopal dog with complete AV block with a ventricular escape rate of approximately 40 per minute. Note complete dissociation between the P and QRS complexes.

Based on a recent study, 24% will die within 1 month of presentation and 40% within 6 months.[74] Cats with complete or third-degree AV block do not carry a similar poor prognosis. The median survival time in cats is about 1 year, with a median age of 14 years based on one study.[73] Survival in dogs, but not cats, is improved with pacemaker implantation. A pacemaker may improve symptoms for a cat or a dog with medically refractory syncope. Medical therapy is usually unrewarding in dogs with high-grade AV block. An atropine response test is always performed for high-grade second- or third-degree AV block. Most dogs with high-grade AV block will not typically respond to atropine and pacemaker implantation is recommended. Pacemakers can be implanted transvenously into the endocardium of the right ventricular or by surgically suturing an epicardial lead to the left ventricle. Pacemaker implantation improves survival time in dogs, with median survival time of 2 years with a median age of onset of approximately 11 years of age.[71] Most pacemaker implantations are successful with good client satisfaction.[75] Severe complications are not common but can be significant, ranging from a lethal arrhythmia, lead dislodgment, cardiac perforation, and infection.

Atrial standstill is a slow supraventricular rhythm in which the atria fail to contract with no discernible P waves noted on the ECG. Moderate to severe hyperkalemia, secondary to acute renal failure, urethra obstruction, uroabdomen, or Addisonian crisis, is the most common cause. Urgent management of the hyperkalemia is recommended. Another cause of atrial standstill, known as persistent atrial standstill, is an uncommon condition in dogs with cardiomyopathy that primarily affects the atria. This condition causes severe atrial enlargement and fibrosis that does not allow electrical conduction, leading to a junctional escape rhythm at about 60 beats per minute. Pacemaker implantation is recommended. Neither hyperkalemic nor persistent atrial standstill will respond to atropine.

CARDIAC TAMPONADE/PERICARDIAL EFFUSION

Cardiac tamponade refers to a physiologic state in which the pericardial effusion causes an increase in intrapericardial pressure resulting in impaired ventricular filling and low cardiac output. The most common cause of pericardial effusion in older dogs is neoplasia, most commonly right atrial hemangiosarcoma in large-breed dogs and chemodectomas (heart base tumors) in brachycephalic dogs.[76,77] Other neoplasias are possible, such as mesothelioma, lymphoma, and metastatic carcinomas. In a middle-aged large-breed dog, benign idiopathic pericardial effusion is possible; but there is always concern for occult neoplasia. Dogs with hemangiosarcoma have a poor prognosis of days to weeks.[77,78] Dogs with chemodectoma may have a better prognosis ($\sim$1–2 years) if surgical or thoracoscopically guided pericardiotomy is performed.[79] Most dogs with idiopathic pericardial effusion recur, and a pericardiotomy is recommended after the second episode of pericardial effusion. These dogs have a good prognosis.[77,78] The most common cause of pericardial effusion in cats is HF (**Box 1**).[31]

Clients usually describe clinical signs of collapse, lethargy, exercise intolerance, cough/retching, shortness of breath, abdominal distention, and inappetence. Physical examination is notable for muffled heart sounds and tachycardia with weak and variable pulses, called *pulses paradoxus*. Pulses paradoxus is recognized when an abnormally large decline in systemic arterial pressure is associated with inspiration. Pulse paradoxus is highly associated with cardiac tamponade. Other physical examination findings include slow capillary refill time, pale mucous membranes, jugular venous distention, ascites, and hepatosplenomegaly.

Echocardiography is the most sensitive and specific modality used to diagnose pericardial effusion and cardiac tamponade (**Fig. 7**). The echocardiogram will allow visualization of the following: the amount and echogenicity of the pericardial fluid, the thickness of the pericardium, and presence of a cardiac tumor. The echocardiographic criterion for cardiac tamponade is diastolic right atrial and sometimes ventricular collapse. ECG abnormalities with pericardial effusion include sinus tachycardia, low amplitude QRS (<0.5 mV), ventricular or supraventricular arrhythmias, and electrical alternans. Electrical alternans is an alternating QRS-T complex that occurs with every other beat. It is caused by the heart swinging back and forth within the pericardial space when large amounts of effusion are present. Radiographically, a classic globoid-shaped heart may be seen with a large amount pericardial effusion. However, many patients may not have the classic basketball-shaped heart if acute-onset, small-volume pericardial effusion is present, as is common with hemangiosarcoma. Other radiographic findings include a distended caudal vena cava, pleural effusion, and a mass lesion at the heart base or cranial thorax. Elevations in cTnI have been shown in dogs with pericardial effusion caused by neoplasia. cTnI is a useful additional diagnostic test in an older dog with pericardial effusion with no obvious mass identified with echocardiography. The finding of an elevated cTnI in these patients suggests a small and difficult-to-visualize neoplasia.[80,81]

Pericardiocentesis is the only effective treatment of immediate relief of cardiac tamponade. Therapy with other drugs, such as diuretics and vasodilators, may actually be harmful because they will reduce ventricular filling and cause hypotension. Placement

---

Box 1
Causes of cardiac tamponade/pericardial effusion

Hemorrhagic effusion
Idiopathic pericardial effusion
Neoplasia
  Hemangiosarcoma (most common in dogs)
  Aortic body tumor
  Mesothelioma
  Ectopic thyroid carcinoma
  Lymphosarcoma
  Metastatic carcinoma
Coagulopathy, rodenticide toxicity
Left atrial rupture (in dog with chronic mitral valve disease)
Uremia
Transudate effusions
Congestive HF (most common in cats)
Pericardioperitoneal diaphragmatic hernias
Hypoalbuminemia
Congenital pericardial cysts
Immune-mediated vasculitis
Toxemias
Uremia
Exudate effusions
Bacterial pericarditis typically caused by a penetrating wound
Fungal pericarditis
  Coccidioidomycosis
  Actinomycosis
Feline infectious peritonitis (cats only)

---

of a peripheral IV catheter and administration of IV fluids to augment cardiac output is advised while preparations are made to perform the pericardiocentesis.

Pericardiocentesis is typically performed at a referral or emergency center after an echocardiogram has confirmed the presence of pericardial fluid. Mild sedation is sometimes needed; however, some patients are so hemodynamically compromised that sedation is not necessary. Patients are placed in sternal or lateral recumbency depending on the demeanor of the patient and the preference of the veterinarian performing the procedure. ECG should be performed during the procedure to monitor for ventricular arrhythmias, which may be caused by epicardial contact with the catheter. The pericardiocentesis site is prepared aseptically. Lidocaine is infused at the puncture site on the right hemithorax between the third and sixth intercostal spaces just above the costochondral junction. Ultrasound or thoracic radiography is helpful to find the best site for the centesis. In large dogs, a large catheter (eg, 14 gauge),

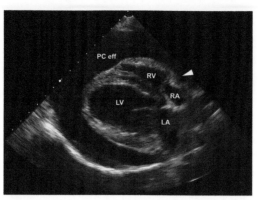

Fig. 7. Focused echocardiogram from a dog with cardiac tamponade and pericardial effusion from a right-sided long axis. Note the right atrial collapse (*arrowhead*), which is diagnostic for cardiac tamponade. LA, left atrium; LV, left ventricle; PC eff, pericardial effusion; RA, right atrium; RV, right ventricle.

often with 1 or 2 side-hole fenestrations, is inserted through a stab incision in the skin. A 3-mL syringe is attached to the end of the catheter and constant negative suction is applied. A flash of pericardial effusion into the syringe will signal entry into the pericardial space. Once in the pericardial space, the catheter is advanced over the needle stylet and extension tubing, a 3-way stopcock and 60-mL syringe are attached, and drainage of the fluid begins. Most pericardial effusions are hemorrhagic and can be similar in appearance to blood. If there is concern for possible intracardiac puncture, a sample of the fluid should be obtained and visualized for clot formation. Pericardial effusion should not clot. Complications of pericardiocentesis include death (rare) resulting from a lethal arrhythmia or coronary artery laceration, transient arrhythmias (common), pneumothorax, or intracardiac puncture. Human studies show that ultrasound-guided pericardiocentesis is associated with a reduced complication rate.[82,83] Unfortunately, analysis of the pericardial effusion is often not helpful in determining the underlying cause (see **Box 1**).[84] After the centesis, monitoring for possible re-effusion is advised, especially in a dog with presumed hemangiosarcoma.

FELINE AORTIC THROMBOEMBOLISM

Aortic thromboembolism (ATE) is one of the most devastating complications associated with feline heart disease. Most cats with ATE have severe heart disease with a severely enlarged left atrium.[13,85–87] Uncommonly, ATE has been associated with neoplasia in cats, particularly pulmonary carcinomas.[88] The most common site of embolization is the caudal aorta trifurcation (the major arterial supply to the hind limbs). The diagnosis is usually based on clinical findings of acute onset paraparesis or paralysis and pain associated with absent or diminished femoral pulses and cool temperature of the hind legs. Less commonly, a front leg may be affected. The affected footpads or nail beds may be pale or cyanotic in appearance. Vocalization and anxiety are common (**Fig. 8**). Tachypnea or respiratory distress is often present because up to two-thirds of cats will be in concurrent congestive HF.[13,85,86] Auscultation of a murmur, gallop sound, and/or arrhythmia is common; but up to 40% may not have an auscultatory abnormality.[86]

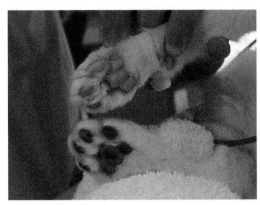

Fig. 8. A picture of a cat's foot pads with aortic thromboembolism. The front foot pads are pink, whereas the hind foot pads are cyanotic because of impaired blood flow.

Client education is an important part of the emergency management of ATE. Owners should be aware of the guarded short- and long-term prognosis. In 2 large retrospective studies, approximately 55% to 66% of cats were euthanized or died during the initial thromboembolic episode.[13,85,86] Prognosis is typically better with partial or front leg embolism. Prognosis is also associated with rectal temperature. If the initial temperature is less than 98°F, a less than 50% survival is conferred.[86] Expected course of recovery is days to weeks for a possible return of hind limb function. About 10% to 15% of cases will have some degree of permanent musculoskeletal deficiency. If a cat survives an episode of ATE, expected long-term survival varies between a few months to 1 year. Most cats with concurrent HF at the time of diagnosis have a shorter long-term prognosis than cats without initial HF. Most cats will either die of recurrence of thromboembolism or congestive HF.

No evidence exists that demonstrates any benefit of one therapy over another in the treatment of ATE. Therefore, there is variability in both the acute and chronic management of feline ATE. In general, urgent management of ATE includes analgesics, anticoagulants, antithrombotics, and treatment directed at managing HF, if present. Opiates, such as fentanyl or buprenorphine, are effective analgesics. Unfractionated heparin is the anticoagulant commonly used. In addition to heparin, an antiplatelet therapy, either aspirin or clopidogrel (Plavix), is usually initiated. Clopidogrel, an ADP receptor inhibitor that decreases platelet aggregation, is most commonly used.[89] Alternatively, aspirin could be used in lieu of clopidogrel. At some referral institutions, thrombolytic agents, such as tissue plasminogen activator, t-PA (Activase), are used infrequently in cats.[90] These drugs are expensive and carry a significant risk for bleeding complications. Ideally, one would only use t-PA within the first 3 to 6 hours following thrombus development. When using a thrombolytic agent, heparin therapy should be postponed until completion. During hospitalization, nursing care of the affected legs is of the utmost importance. No venipuncture should be performed on the affected legs. Initially, these cats may have difficulty posturing to urinate and may need to have their bladders expressed periodically to prevent overdistention of the bladder or urine scald. ECG monitoring is recommended because of possible hyperkalemic arrhythmias cause by ischemia-reperfusion injury.

For chronic anticoagulation, combination therapy or monotherapy with aspirin, clopidogrel, and/or a low molecular weight heparin (LMWH) are recommended. LMWHs, either dalteparin (Fragmin) or enoxaparin (Lovenox), are safe yet expensive injectable anticoagulants with theoretically a more predictable dose-to-response effect and more bioavailability than unfractionated heparin. The dose of LMWH is not clearly understood despite a pharmacokinetic study suggesting the need of much higher doses than what is typically used clinically with good success.[91] Even with chronic anticoagulant therapy, re-embolization is a common terminal event. Because of the guarded short-term and long-term prognosis with ATE, euthanasia is often considered an ethical and humane option.

SUMMARY

In summary, the purpose of the article is to provide updated and current management strategies for common cardiac emergencies, specifically decompensated HF, cardiac tamponade, hemodynamically significant arrhythmias, and feline ATE. These cardiac emergencies require rapid clinical assessment and treatment because these patients often have life-threatening conditions and are at risk for destabilizing quickly. Empiric stabilizing treatments are often provided before a definitive diagnosis. The increased use of thoracic ultrasound and focused echocardiography in the rapid diagnosis of HF and cardiac tamponade as well as the use of pimobendan for the treatment of HF in both dogs and cats are the most important recent advances in the management of cardiac emergencies.

REFERENCES

1. Borgarelli M, Buchanan JW. Historical review, epidemiology and natural history of degenerative mitral valve disease. J Vet Cardiol 2012;14:93–101.
2. Borgarelli M, Haggstrom J. Canine degenerative myxomatous mitral valve disease: natural history, clinical presentation and therapy. Vet Clin North Am Small Anim Pract 2010;40:651–63.
3. Pedersen HD, Lorentzen KA, Kristensen BO. Echocardiographic mitral valve prolapse in Cavalier King Charles spaniels: epidemiology and prognostic significance for regurgitation. Vet Rec 1999;144:315–20.
4. Martin MW, Stafford Johnson MJ, Celona B. Canine dilated cardiomyopathy: a retrospective study of signalment, presentation and clinical findings in 369 cases. J Small Anim Pract 2009;50:23–9.
5. Tidholm A, Jönsson L. A retrospective study of canine dilated cardiomyopathy (189 cases). J Am Anim Hosp Assoc 1997;33:544–50.
6. Meurs KM, Miller MW, Wright NA. Clinical features of dilated cardiomyopathy in Great Danes and results of a pedigree analysis: 17 cases (1990-2000). J Am Vet Med Assoc 2001;218(5):729–32.
7. Kittleson MD, Keene B, Pion PD, et al. Results of the multicenter spaniel trial (MUST): taurine- and carnitine-responsive dilated cardiomyopathy in American cocker spaniels with decreased plasma taurine concentration. J Vet Intern Med 1997;11:204–11.
8. Vollmar AC. The prevalence of cardiomyopathy in the Irish wolfhound: a clinical study of 500 dogs. J Am Anim Hosp Assoc 2000;36:125–32.
9. Trehiou-Sechi E, Tissier R, Gouni V, et al. Comparative echocardiographic and clinical features of hypertrophic cardiomyopathy in 5 breeds of cats: a retrospective analysis of 344 cases (2001-2011). J Vet Intern Med 2012;26:532–41.
10. Meurs KM, Mauceli E, Lahmers S, et al. Genome-wide association identifies a deletion in the 3'untranslated region of Striatin in a canine model of arrhythmogenic right ventricular cardiomyopathy: identification of Striatin deletion in canine ARVC. Hum Genet 2010;128:315–24.

11. Meurs KM, Lahmers S, Keene BW, et al. A splice site mutation in a gene encoding for PDK4, a mitochondrial protein, is associated with the development of dilated cardiomyopathy in the Doberman pinscher. Hum Genet 2012;131: 1319–25.

12. Meurs KM, Sanchez X, David RM, et al. A cardiac myosin binding protein C mutation in the Maine coon cat with familial hypertrophic cardiomyopathy. Hum Mol Genet 2005;14:3587–93.

13. Rush JE, Freeman LM, Fenollosa NK, et al. Population and survival characteristics of cats with hypertrophic cardiomyopathy: 260 cases (1990-1999). J Am Vet Med Assoc 2002;20:202–7.

14. Smith SA, Tobias AH, Fine DM, et al. Corticosteroid-associated congestive heart failure in 12 cats. Intern J Appl Res Vet Med 2004;2:159–70.

15. Wilson HE, Jasani S, Wagner TB, et al. Signs of left heart volume overload in severely anaemic cats. J Feline Med Surg 2010;12:904–9.

16. Häggström J, Kvart C, Hansson K. Heart sounds and murmurs: changes related to severity of chronic valvular disease in the Cavalier King Charles spaniel. J Vet Intern Med 1995;9:75–85.

17. Serfass P, Chetboul V, Sampedrano CC, et al. Retrospective study of 942 small-sized dogs: prevalence of left apical systolic heart murmur and left-sided heart failure, critical effects of breed and sex. J Vet Cardiol 2006;8:11–8.

18. Ljungvall I, Ahlstrom C, Höglund K, et al. Use of signal analysis of heart sounds and murmurs to assess severity of mitral valve regurgitation attributable to myxomatous mitral valve disease in dogs. Am J Vet Res 2009;70:604–13.

19. Menaut P, Bélanger MC, Beauchamp G, et al. Atrial fibrillation in dogs with and without structural or functional cardiac disease: a retrospective study of 109 cases. J Vet Cardiol 2005;7:75–83.

20. Côté E, Harpster NK, Laste NJ, et al. Atrial fibrillation in cats: 50 cases (1979-2002). J Am Vet Med Assoc 2004;225:256–60.

21. Goutal CM, Keir I, Kenney S, et al. Evaluation of acute congestive heart failure in dogs and cats: 145 cases (2007-2008). J Vet Emerg Crit Care 2010;20:330–7.

22. Reissig A, Copetti R, Kroegel C. Current role of emergency ultrasound of the chest. Crit Care Med 2011;39:1–8.

23. Moore CL, Copel JA. Point of care ultrasonography. N Engl J Med 2011;364: 749–57.

24. Labovitz AJ, Noble VE, Beirig M, et al. Focused cardiac ultrasound in the emergent setting: a consensus statement of the American Society of Echocardiography and American College of Emergency Physicians. J Am Soc Echocardiogr 2010;23:1225–30.

25. Tse Y, Bulmer B, Cunningham S, et al. Evaluation of a training course in focused echocardiography for the non-cardiology house officer. J Vet Emerg Crit Care 2012;22:S2–10.

26. Benigni L, Morgan N, Lamb CR. Radiographic appearance of cardiogenic pulmonary oedema in 23 cats. J Small Anim Pract 2009;50:9–14.

27. Smith S, Dukes-McEwan J. Clinical signs and left atrial size in cats with cardiovascular disease in general practice. J Small Anim Pract 2012;53:27–33.

28. Boon JA. Evaluation of size, function and hemodynamics. In: Veterinary echocardiography. 2nd edition. Ames (IA): Wiley-Blackwell; 2011. p. 184–5.

29. Abbott JA, MacLean HN. Two-dimensional echocardiographic assessment of the feline left atrium. J Vet Intern Med 2006;20:111–9.

30. Rishniw M, Erb HN. Evaluation of four 2-dimensional echocardiographic methods of assessing left atrial size in dogs. J Vet Intern Med 2000;14:429–35.

31. Hall DJ, Shofer F, Meier CK, et al. Pericardial effusion in cats: a retrospective study of clinical findings and outcome in 146 cats. J Vet Intern Med 2007;21: 1002–7.
32. Lord PF, Hansson K, Carnabuci C, et al. Radiographic heart size and its rate of increase as tests for onset of congestive heart failure in Cavalier King Charles spaniels with mitral valve regurgitation. J Vet Intern Med 2011;25:1312–9.
33. Diana A, Guglielmini C, Pivetta M, et al. Radiographic features of cardiogenic pulmonary edema in dogs with mitral regurgitation: 61 cases (1998-2007). J Am Vet Med Assoc 2009;235:1058–63.
34. Lehmkuhl LB, Bonagura JD, Biller DS, et al. Radiographic evaluation of caudal vena cava size in dogs. Vet Radiol Ultrasound 1997;38:94–100.
35. Oyama MA, Rush JE, Rozanski EA, et al. Assessment of serum N-terminal pro-B-type natriuretic peptide concentration for differentiation of congestive heart failure from primary respiratory tract disease as the cause of respiratory signs in dogs. J Am Vet Med Assoc 2009;235:1319–25.
36. DeFrancesco TC, Rush JE, Rozanski EA, et al. Prospective clinical evaluation of an ELISA B-type natriuretic peptide assay in the diagnosis of congestive heart failure in dogs presenting with cough or dyspnea. J Vet Intern Med 2007;21: 243–50.
37. Fox PR, Oyama MA, Reynolds C, et al. Utility of plasma N-terminal pro-brain natriuretic peptide (NT-proBNP) to distinguish between congestive heart failure and non-cardiac causes of acute dyspnea in cats. J Vet Cardiol 2009;11(Suppl 1): S51–61.
38. Connolly DJ, Soares Magalhaes RJ, Fuentes VL, et al. Assessment of the diagnostic accuracy of circulating natriuretic peptide concentrations to distinguish between cats with cardiac and non-cardiac causes of respiratory distress. J Vet Cardiol 2009;11(Suppl 1):S41–50.
39. Singletary GE, Rush JE, Fox PR, et al. Effect of NT-pro-BNP assay on accuracy and confidence of general practitioners in diagnosing heart failure or respiratory disease in cats with respiratory signs. J Vet Intern Med 2012;26:542–6.
40. Connoly DJ, Brodbelt DC, Copeland H, et al. Assessment of the diagnostic accuracy of circulating cardiac troponin I concentration to distinguish between cats with cardiac and non-cardiac causes of respiratory distress. J Vet Cardiol 2009; 11:71–8.
41. Herndon WE, Rishniw M, Schrope D, et al. Assessment of plasma cardiac troponin I concentration as a means to differentiate cardiac and noncardiac causes of dyspnea in cats. J Am Vet Med Assoc 2008;233:1261–4.
42. Suzuki S, Ishikawa T, Hamabe L, et al. The effect of furosemide on left atrial pressure in dogs with mitral valve regurgitation. J Vet Intern Med 2011;25:244–50.
43. Salvador DR, Rey NR, Ramos GC, et al. Continuous infusion versus bolus injection of loop diuretics in congestive heart failure. Cochrane Database Syst Rev 2005;(3):CD003178.
44. Felker GM, Lee KL, Bull DA, et al. Diuretic strategies in patients with acute decompensated heart failure. N Engl J Med 2011;364:797–805.
45. Adin DB, Taylor AW, Hill RC, et al. Intermittent bolus injection versus continuous infusion of furosemide in normal adult greyhound dogs. J Vet Intern Med 2003; 17:632–6.
46. Peddle GD, Singletary GE, Reynolds CA, et al. Effect of torsemide and furosemide on clinical, laboratory, radiographic and quality of life variables in dogs with heart failure secondary to mitral valve disease. J Vet Cardiol 2012;14: 253–9.

47. Atkins C, Bonagura J, Ettinger S, et al. Guidelines for the diagnosis and treatment of canine chronic valvular heart disease (ACVIM consensus statement). J Vet Intern Med 2009;23:1142–50.

48. Ettinger SJ, Benitz AM, Ericsson GF, et al. Effects of enalapril maleate on survival of dogs with naturally acquired heart failure. The Long-Term Investigation of Veterinary Enalapril (LIVE) Study Group. J Am Vet Med Assoc 1998;213:1573–7.

49. The COVE Study Group. Controlled clinical evaluation of enalapril in dogs with heart failure: results of the Cooperative Veterinary Enalapril Study Group. J Vet Intern Med 1995;9:243–52.

50. Pouchelon JL, Jamet N, Gouni V, et al. Effect of benazepril on survival and cardiac events in dogs with asymptomatic mitral valve disease: a retrospective study of 141 cases. J Vet Intern Med 2008;22:905–14.

51. The IMPROVE Study Group. Acute and short-term hemodynamic, echocardiographic, and clinical effects of enalapril maleate in dogs with naturally acquired heart failure: results of the Invasive Multicenter PROspective Veterinary Evaluation of Enalapril study. J Vet Intern Med 1995;9:234–42.

52. Brown AJ, Davison E, Sleeper MM. Clinical efficacy of sildenafil in treatment of pulmonary arterial hypertension in dogs. J Vet Intern Med 2010;24:850–4.

53. Bach JF, Rozanski EA, MacGregor J, et al. Retrospective evaluation of sildenafil citrate as a therapy for pulmonary hypertension in dogs. J Vet Intern Med 2006; 20:1132–5.

54. Boyle KL, Leech E. A review of the pharmacology and clinical uses of pimobendan. J Vet Emerg Crit Care 2012;22:398–408.

55. O'Grady MR, Minors SL, O'Sullivan ML, et al. Effect of pimobendan on case fatality rate in Doberman pinschers with congestive heart failure caused by dilated cardiomyopathy. J Vet Intern Med 2008;22:897–904.

56. Haggstrom J, Boswood A, O'Grady M, et al. Effect of pimobendan or benazepril hydrochloride on survival times in dogs with congestive heart failure caused by naturally occurring myxomatous mitral valve disease: the QUEST study. J Vet Intern Med 2008;22:1124–35.

57. Hambrook LE, Bennett PF. Effect of pimobendan on the clinical outcome and survival of cats with non-taurine responsive dilated cardiomyopathy. J Feline Med Surg 2012;14:233–9.

58. Atkinson KJ, Fine DM, Thombs LA, et al. Evaluation of pimobendan and N-terminal probrain natriuretic peptide in the treatment of pulmonary hypertension secondary to degenerative mitral valve disease in dogs. J Vet Intern Med 2009;23:1190–6.

59. Gordon SG, Saunders AB, Roland RM, et al. Effect of oral administration of pimobendan in cats with heart failure. J Am Vet Med Assoc 2012;241:89–94.

60. Macgregor JM, Rush JE, Laste NJ, et al. Use of pimobendan in 170 cats (2006-2010). J Vet Cardiol 2011;13:251–60.

61. Hanzlicek AS, Gehring R, KuKanich B. Pharmacokinetics of oral pimobendan in healthy cats. J Vet Cardiol 2012;14:489–96.

62. Suzuki S, Fukushima R, Ishikawa T, et al. The effect of pimobendan on left atrial pressure in dogs with mitral valve regurgitation. J Vet Intern Med 2011;25: 1328–33.

63. Nicolle AP, Chetboul V, Allerheiligen T, et al. Azotemia and glomerular filtration rate in dogs with chronic valvular disease. J Vet Intern Med 2007;21:943–9.

64. Payne J, Luis Fuentes V, Boswood A, et al. Population characteristics and survival in 127 referred cats with hypertrophic cardiomyopathy (1997 to 2005). J Small Anim Pract 2010;51:540–7.

65. Palermo V, Stafford Johnson MJ, Sala E, et al. Cardiomyopathy in Boxer dogs: a retrospective study of the clinical presentation, diagnostic findings and survival. J Vet Cardiol 2011;13:45–55.

66. Borgarelli M, Savarino P, Crosara S, et al. Survival characteristics and prognostic variables of dogs with mitral regurgitation attributable to myxomatous valve disease. J Vet Intern Med 2008;22:120–8.

67. Kraus MS, Moïse NS, Rishniw M, et al. Morphology of ventricular arrhythmias in the boxer as measured by 12-lead electrocardiography with pace-mapping comparison. J Vet Intern Med 2002;16:153–8.

68. Pedro B, López-Alvarez J, Fonfara S, et al. Retrospective evaluation of the use of amiodarone in dogs with arrhythmias (from 2003 to 2010). J Small Anim Pract 2012;53:19–26.

69. Prosek R. Electrical cardioversion of sustained ventricular tachycardia in three Boxers. J Am Vet Med Assoc 2010;236:554–7.

70. Gelzer AR, Kraus MS, Rishniw M, et al. Combination therapy with digoxin and diltiazem controls ventricular rate in chronic atrial fibrillation in dogs better than digoxin or diltiazem monotherapy: a randomized crossover study in 18 dogs. J Vet Intern Med 2009;23:499–508.

71. Wess G, Thomas WP, Berger DM, et al. Applications, complications, and outcomes of transvenous pacemaker implantation in 105 dogs (1997-2002). J Vet Intern Med 2006;20:877–84.

72. Johnson MS, Martin MW, Henley W. Results of pacemaker implantation in 104 dogs. J Small Anim Pract 2007;48:4–11.

73. Kellum HB, Stepien RL. Third-degree atrioventricular block in 21 cats (1997-2004). J Vet Intern Med 2006;20:97–103.

74. Schrope DP, Kelch WJ. Signalment, clinical signs, and prognostic indicators associated with high-grade second- or third-degree atrioventricular block in dogs: 124 cases (January 1, 1997-December 31, 1997). J Am Vet Med Assoc 2006;228(11):1710–7.

75. Oyama MA, Sisson DD, Lehmkuhl LB. Practices and outcome of artificial cardiac pacing in 154 dogs. J Vet Intern Med 2001;15:229–39.

76. MacDonald KA, Cagney O, Magne ML. Echocardiographic and clinicopathologic characterization of pericardial effusion in dogs: 107 cases (1985-2006). J Am Vet Med Assoc 2009;235:1456–61.

77. Stafford Johnson M, Martin M, Binns S, et al. A retrospective study of clinical findings, treatment and outcome in 143 dogs with pericardial effusion. J Small Anim Pract 2004;45:546–52.

78. Dunning D, Monnet E, Orton EC, et al. Analysis of prognostic indicators for dogs with pericardial effusion: 46 cases (1985-1996). J Am Vet Med Assoc 1998;212:1276–80.

79. Vicari ED, Brown DC, Holt DE, et al. Survival times of and prognostic indicators for dogs with heart base masses: 25 cases (1986-1999). J Am Vet Med Assoc 2001;219:485–7.

80. Shaw SP, Rozanski EA, Rush JE. Cardiac troponins I and T in dogs with pericardial effusion. J Vet Intern Med 2004;18:322–4.

81. Chun R, Kellihan HB, Henik RA, et al. Comparison of plasma cardiac troponin I concentrations among dogs with cardiac hemangiosarcoma, noncardiac hemangiosarcoma, other neoplasms, and pericardial effusion of nonhemangiosarcoma origin. J Am Vet Med Assoc 2010;237:806–11.

82. Ainsworth CD, Salehian O. Echo-guided pericardiocentesis: let the bubbles show the way. Circulation 2011;123(4):e210–1.

83. Tsang TS, El-Najdawi EK, Seward JB, et al. Percutaneous echocardiographically guided pericardiocentesis in pediatric patients: evaluation of safety and efficacy. J Am Soc Echocardiogr 1998;11:1072–7.
84. Sisson D, Thomas WP, Ruehl WW, et al. Diagnostic value of pericardial fluid analysis in the dog. J Am Vet Med Assoc 1984;184:51–5.
85. Laste NJ, Harpster NK. A retrospective study of 100 cases of feline distal aortic thromboembolism: 1977-1993. J Am Anim Hosp Assoc 1995;31:492–500.
86. Smith SA, Tobias AH, Jacob KA, et al. Arterial thromboembolism in cats: acute crisis in 127 cats (1992-2001) and long-term management with low-dose aspirin in 24 cases. J Vet Intern Med 2003;17:73–83.
87. Schober KE, Maerz I. Assessment of left atrial appendage flow velocity and its relation to spontaneous echocardiographic contrast in 89 cats with myocardial disease. J Vet Intern Med 2006;20:120–30.
88. Goldfinch N, Argyle DJ. Feline lung-digit syndrome: unusual metastatic patterns of primary lung tumours in cats. J Feline Med Surg 2012;14:202–8.
89. Hogan DF, Andrews DA, Green HW, et al. Antiplatelet effects and pharmacodynamics of clopidogrel in cats. J Am Vet Med Assoc 2004;225:1406–11.
90. Welch KM, Rozanski EA, Freeman LM, et al. Prospective evaluation of tissue plasminogen activator in 11 cats with arterial thromboembolism. J Feline Med Surg 2010;12:122–8.
91. Alwood AJ, Downend AB, Brooks MB, et al. Anticoagulant effects of low-molecular-weight heparins in healthy cats. J Vet Intern Med 2007;21:378–87.

Management of Urinary Tract Emergencies in Small Animals

Anusha Balakrishnan, BVSc, Kenneth J. Drobatz, DVM, MSCE*

KEYWORDS

- Urinary tract emergencies • Acute kidney injury • Feline urethral obstruction
- Uroabdomen • Ethylene glycol

KEY POINTS

- Rapid recognition and aggressive therapeutic intervention is necessary with urogenital emergencies because of the potential to become life threatening if not addressed rapidly.
- Emergencies can be divided anatomically into conditions that affect (1) the upper urinary tract, namely kidneys, renal pelvis, and ureters; and (2) the lower urinary tract, namely urinary bladder and urethra.
- Overall, the prognosis with urogenital emergencies is fair to good with appropriate medical or surgical management.

INTRODUCTION

Emergencies involving the urinary tract are commonly encountered in small animal practice, and several of these have the potential to become life threatening if not addressed rapidly. This article focuses on some of the most commonly seen urinary tract emergencies in dogs and cats, with emphasis on basic pathophysiology, diagnosis, and emergency management of these cases. These emergencies can be divided anatomically into conditions that affect:

- The upper urinary tract: kidneys, renal pelvis, ureters
- The lower urinary tract: urinary bladder, urethra

ACUTE KIDNEY INJURY

Acute kidney injury (AKI) is characterized by an abrupt, sustained decrease in renal function and loss of the kidneys' ability to excrete wastes, regulate acid-base and electrolyte balance, and concentrate urine.[1] AKI was previously referred to as acute renal failure (ARF). This recent change in nomenclature reflects a more accurate

Section of Emergency and Critical Care, Department of Clinical Studies-PHL, University of Pennsylvania School of Veterinary Medicine, 3900 Delancey Street, Philadelphia, PA 19104, USA
* Corresponding author.
E-mail address: drobatz@vet.upenn.edu

Vet Clin Small Anim 43 (2013) 843–867
http://dx.doi.org/10.1016/j.cvsm.2013.03.013   vetsmall.theclinics.com
0195-5616/13/$ – see front matter © 2013 Published by Elsevier Inc.

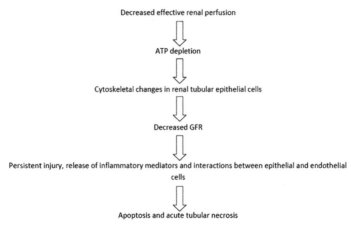

Fig. 1. Pathophysiology of intrinsic acute kidney injury (AKI). GFR, glomerular filtration rate.

understanding of the histopathologic changes that occur with an acute insult to the kidneys and encompasses a spectrum of alterations in renal function, ranging from mild to severe (**Fig. 1**). Human studies report incidence rates of AKI of 2% to 7% in all-hospital patients, and nearly 15% in critically ill patients with mortalities near 50%.[1,2] Veterinary studies have reported mortalities between 23.8% and 78.3%[3–5] in dogs and approximately 47% in cats.[6]

Acute onset of azotemia can be prerenal, renal, or postrenal in origin. AKI refers to a complex disorder that comprises multiple causative factors and occurs in a variety of settings with a range of clinical manifestations that range from a minimal but sustained increase in serum creatinine to anuric renal failure. Prerenal azotemia and other fully reversible causes of acute renal insufficiency are specifically excluded from the spectrum of AKI. Prerenal azotemia usually results from decreased renal perfusion, glomerular filtration rate (GFR), and renal blood flow. This condition can be caused by dehydration or systemic hypotension secondary to a decrease in effective circulating volume as occurs in hypovolemia or vasodilatory shock. Postrenal azotemia occurs when there is an obstruction to urine outflow as is seen with renal, ureteral, or urethral obstructions, or urine leakage caused by loss of integrity of some portion of the urinary tract. Intrinsic renal failure in dogs and cats can have a wide variety of causes and occurs when there is damage to the renal parenchyma. These causes can be classified as:

1. Toxic:
   a. Ethylene glycol (EG)
   b. Nonsteroidal antiinflammatory drugs (NSAIDs)
   c. Aminoglycoside antibiotics
   d. Lilies (cats)
   e. Grapes and raisins
   f. Heavy metals
   g. Amphotericin B
   h. Phosphate enemas
   i. Polymyxin B
   j. Sulfonamides
   k. Intravenous (IV) contrast agents
   l. Tetracyclines
   m. Mushrooms

2. Infectious:
   a. Leptospirosis
   b. Pyelonephritis
   c. Rocky Mountain spotted fever
   d. Glomerulonephritis
   e. Borreliosis
3. Others:
   a. Cardiovascular shock
   b. Systemic hypotension
   c. Burns/heatstroke
   d. Postcardiac arrest syndrome
   e. Thromboembolic disease
   f. Sepsis
   g. Anaphylaxis
   h. Prolonged general anesthesia
   i. Pigment nephropathy
   j. Transfusion reactions
   k. Snakebites
   l. Traumatic injury

PATHOPHYSIOLOGY OF AKI

AKI in humans is staged using the risk, injury, failure, loss, end-stage renal disease (RIFLE) acronym.[7,8] Serum creatinine levels and urine output (UOP) are the two most important markers used to stage AKI in people (**Table 1**). Another staging system, the Acute Kidney Injury Network (AKIN) criteria has also been recently used in human medicine (**Table 2**).[9] A recent study from 2011 evaluated a new staging system for AKI in veterinary medicine called the Veterinary Acute Kidney Injury (VAKI) scheme; this also uses increases in serum creatinine to stage patients.[5] The VAKI system stages dogs with AKI on a scale from 0 to 3, with 0 being the least severe and 3 being the most severe. **Table 3** provides more information on the VAKI classification system.

Table 1 RIFLE staging system		
	Urine Output	**Serum Creatinine**
Risk	Decrease in GFR ≥25%; <0.5 mL/kg/h for ≥6 h	≥1.5-fold increase from baseline serum creatinine
Injury	Decrease in GFR ≥50%; <0.5 mL/kg/h for ≥12 h	≥2.0-fold increase from baseline serum creatinine
Failure	Decrease in GFR ≥75%; <0.3 mL/kg/h for ≥24 h or anuria ≥12 h	≥3.0-fold increase from baseline serum creatinine; or an absolute serum creatinine ≥354 μmol/L (4.0 mg/dL) with an acute increase ≥44 μmol/L (0.5 mg/dL)
Loss	Persistent acute renal failure: complete loss of kidney function for >4 wk	
End stage	Complete loss of kidney function for >3 mo	

Data from Kellum JA, Levin N, Bouman C, et al. Developing a consensus classification system for acute renal failure. Curr Opin Crit Care 2002;8:509–14; and Bellomo R, Kellum JA, Ronco C. Defining and classifying acute renal failure: from advocacy to consensus and validation of the RIFLE criteria. Intensive Care Med 2007;11:409–13.

Table 2
AKIN staging system

	Urine Output	Serum Creatinine
Stage 1	<0.5 mL/kg/h for ≥6 h	≥26.5 μmol/L (0.3 mg/dL) or ≥150%–200% increase from baseline serum creatinine
Stage 2	<0.5 mL/kg/h for ≥12 h	>200%–299% increase from baseline serum creatinine
Stage 3	<0.3 mL/kg/h for ≥24 h or anuria ≥12 h	≥300% increase from baseline serum creatinine or absolute serum creatinine ≥354 μmol/L (4.0 mg/dL) with an acute increase of ≥44 μmol/L (0.5 mg/dL)

From Mehta RL, Kellum JA, Shah SV, et al. Acute Kidney Injury Network: report of an initiative to improve outcomes in acute kidney injury. Crit Care 2007;11:R31.

Ischemic injury is one of the most common causes of AKI, particularly in critically ill patients that are hospitalized. This condition may be caused by a reduction in effective renal perfusion caused by reduced intravascular volume (eg, hemorrhage, gastrointestinal [I] or renal losses, third spacing caused by capillary leak), reduced cardiac output (eg, cardiogenic shock, congestive heart failure [CHF], pulmonary hypertension, pulmonary thromboembolism [PTE], pericardial disease), systemic vasodilation (eg, anaphylaxis, sepsis), or renal vasoconstriction (eg, contrast nephropathy, vasopressor medications, NSAIDs).

DIAGNOSIS OF AKI

Diagnosis of AKI is usually based on history, in conjunction with physical examination (PE) findings and documentation of azotemia (which may be accompanied by oliguria or anuria in advanced cases of the disease). Various electrolyte and acid-base derangements can be seen with AKI including hyperkalemic or hypokalemia, hyperphosphatemia, and metabolic acidosis. Acutely uremic animals can also present with signs of systemic illness including lethargy, inappetence, vomiting, diarrhea, and halitosis. Uremic ulcers may be seen in these patients. Neurologic signs are also sometimes observed in these patients and may be attributed to uremic encephalopathy.

AKI can be present even if the serum creatinine is within the normal reference range, especially in hospitalized patients. A 2005 study in humans showed that even a mildly increased creatinine concentration of 0.3 mg/dL from baseline increased the risk of

Table 3
VAKI staging system

Stage 0	Creatinine increase <150% from baseline
Stage 1	Creatinine increase of 150%–199% from baseline, or: Creatinine increase of 26.5 μmol/L (0.3 mg/dL) from baseline
Stage 2	Creatinine increase of 200%–299% from baseline
Stage 3	Creatinine increase of ≥300% from baseline or an absolute creatinine value >354 μmol/L (4.0 mg/dL)

From Thoen M, Kerl M. Characterization of acute kidney injury in hospitalized dogs and evaluation of a veterinary acute kidney injury staging system. J Vet Emerg Crit Care 2011;21(6):648–57; with permission.

death by as much as 70%.[10] This is important to bear in mind because it may help identify patients with clinically significant kidney injury that may not otherwise be identified. For example, a patient whose creatinine increases from 1.5 mg/dL to 1.8 mg/dL would be in the category of stage I in the VAKI staging system. Such small increases in serum creatinine, although clinically significant, can be difficult to detect consistently because of the possibility of intermachine and intersample variability. Therefore, ideally, the same machine (one that has high precision) should be consistently used to monitor kidney values in an animal suspected of having AKI to allow detection of even the smallest changes.

GENERAL MANAGEMENT OF AKI

- The management of AKI depends largely on the underlying cause. However, the ultimate goal in all cases is to optimize hemodynamic status, restore adequate perfusion to the kidneys, and limit further injury to the renal tubules by reversal of the underlying cause.
- Aggressive IV fluid therapy to promote diuresis and reverse azotemia is the hallmark of treatment of AKI. There has been extensive research in human medicine with regard to the best type of fluid to use in cases of AKI. One of the largest studies, the Saline versus Albumin Fluid Evaluation (SAFE) study,[11] showed that albumin transfusion was safe, but not any more effective than isotonic saline in preventing death or the need for dialysis in patients in the intensive care unit (ICU). Other studies have corroborated the use of crystalloids by showing no difference between crystalloids and colloids in treating AKI. Synthetic colloids have been linked with causing or worsening AKI in several human studies in critically ill patients.[12,13]
- Because AKI is characterized by a spectrum of fluid responsiveness, close monitoring of patients is imperative to help guide therapy and detect deteriorations in renal function. Early clinical recognition of the presence of urinary casts and glucosuria may be a marker for tubular injury.
- Another upcoming area of research involves measurement of various biomarkers that are released into the blood or urine by the injured kidney at an early stage of damage. This indicator of early disease may help initiation of therapies that can stem progression or repair damage. Biomarkers ideally should be able to differentiate incipient acute tubular necrosis from other forms of acute renal dysfunction (eg, volume-responsive AKI; acute glomerular, vascular, and interstitial diseases; obstructive nephropathies), allow monitoring of the effects of treatment, and predict the need for dialysis, long-term kidney outcome, and mortality. Examples of these include interleukin 18, neutrophil gelatinase-associated lipocalin, kidney injury molecule-1, and liver fatty-acid–binding protein.[14,15] Occasional increases in the levels of these markers in the urine can occur even before serum creatinine increases.[14,15]
- Depending on the nature of injury and severity of illness, patients should be monitored closely for urine production. Placement of indwelling urinary catheters is useful in this regard, especially in patients that are tending toward oliguria or are already anuric. However, caution should be exercised before placing catheters in patients with evidence of an active urinary tract infection, in diabetic patients, in immunocompromised patients, or in patients with a coagulopathy that are at risk for bleeding. Ascending nosocomial infections are also a concern, particularly in patients already on systemic antibiotic therapy and even in otherwise healthy patients.[16]

- Careful assessment of the patient, including PE findings and monitoring tools (eg, central venous pressure, urine output monitoring, weight gain or loss) should be used. In patients showing decreased UOP, the use of diuretics and other therapy may be necessary. **Fig. 2** shows guidelines for fluid therapy for patients with AKI, and **Table 4** gives a listing of diuretics used with AKI.

MANAGEMENT OF COMMON CONDITIONS CAUSING AKI
EG Intoxication

EG is a common cause of toxicity in dogs and cats, and is found in multiple sources (eg, antifreeze, printer cartridges, paint, caulking material). In general, toxicosis is only seen after ingestion of antifreeze that is typically greater than 90% EG and concentrated (compared with other products that contain <1%–2% EG). EG toxicity can be fatal, with mortalities in cats ranging from 96% to 100% and 59% to 70% in dogs.[19–22] Cats also have a significantly lower minimum lethal dose compared with dogs (1.4 mL/kg compared with 4.4–6.6 mL/kg in dogs).[19–21]

EG by itself is nontoxic; it is the dangerous metabolites that result in severe AKI. With EG ingestion, absorption is rapid, with peak blood levels occurring about 3 hours after ingestion and clinical signs developing within 20 to 30 minutes. EG is metabolized by the enzyme alcohol dehydrogenase (ADH) into several toxic metabolites that are responsible for clinical signs. The first metabolite, glycoaldehyde, is produced after metabolism by ADH, which is the first rate-limiting step of this reaction. This metabolite is then converted to glycolic acid, which is then rapidly oxidized to glyoxylic acid (the second rate-limiting step). Glycolic acid then accumulates, resulting in metabolic

Assess patient's intravascular volume status:

Physical examination findings: Perfusion parameters (e.g., heart rate, CRT,

mucous membrane tackiness, pulse quality?), weight gain or loss

Blood work findings: Elevated lactate, elevated PCV/TS? Hypersthenuria?

Blood pressure: Increased or decreased?

Imaging: Size of the heart and vena cava on thoracic radiographs?

Central venous pressures: High, low, or normal?

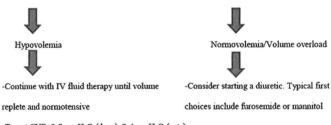

Hypovolemia   Normovolemia/Volume overload

-Continue with IV fluid therapy until volume   -Consider starting a diuretic. Typical first

replete and normotensive   choices include furosemide or mannitol

-Target CVP: 2-8 cm H_2O (dogs), 2-4 cm H_2O (cats)

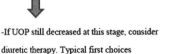

-If UOP still decreased at this stage, consider   -If UOP still inadequate and azotemia

diuretic therapy. Typical first choices   not improving, consider adding in a

include furosemide or mannitol.   second diuretic.

Fig. 2. Fluid therapy guidelines in AKI. CRT, Capillary Refill Time; CVP, Central Venous Pressure; PCV, Packed Cell Volume; TS, Total Solids.

acidosis. Glyoxylic acid is further metabolized to oxalates, formic acid, serine, glycine, and carbon dioxide. Oxalates, along with glycolic acid, are the main causes of acute tubular necrosis. Oxalates combine with calcium to form calcium oxalate monohydrate crystals within the lumen of the renal tubules, resulting in severe AKI.

Clinical signs from EG toxicity can be caused both by unmetabolized EG and its toxic metabolites. Unmetabolized EG causes signs similar to those seen with ethanol intoxication including GI (eg, nausea, hypersalivation, vomiting), renal (eg, polyuria, polydipsia), and neurologic signs (eg, ataxia and mentation changes ranging from depression to stupor). These signs occur soon after ingestion and last about 12 hours with oliguric renal failure developing within 12 to 24 hours after ingestion in cats, and 36 to 72 hours after ingestion in dogs.

Management

- Emergent treatment of EG ingestion includes decontamination via induction of emesis (if the patient is conscious and able to vomit). However, the rapid absorption of EG limits the effectiveness of this option. Emesis induction is contraindicated if the patient is already showing GI signs (such as vomiting) or neurologic signs (such as mentation changes or seizures), given the risk for causing aspiration of gastric contents. Decontamination using activated charcoal is of little use because EG is not significantly adsorbed by charcoal.
- Treatment of EG intoxication involves inhibiting metabolism of EG into its toxic metabolites and promoting excretion of unchanged EG by promoting diuresis. Treatment with the antidote (eg, either 4-methylpyrazole or ethanol) must be started within 3 hours in cats and 8 to 12 hours in dogs to ensure survival. If renal azotemia has already developed, this treatment is unlikely to be successful.[23]
  - Ethanol has traditionally been used as a competitive substrate that is capable of binding to the enzyme ADH, thereby preventing the enzyme from acting on EG and producing its toxic metabolites. Ethanol can be administered IV as a 20% solution at a dose of 5 mL/cat initially, repeated every 6 hours for 5 treatments, and then every 8 hours for 4 treatments.[23] Risks with using ethanol include possible exacerbation of neurologic signs (eg, drunkenness, obtundation), hypoglycemia (secondary to the ethanol), and worsening of serum hyperosmolality induced by EG.
  - 4-Methylpyrazole (4-MP; also called fomepizole) is another compound that is used as a direct inhibitor of ADH and can be used when hemodialysis is not available or administered while hemodialysis is being set up. 4-MP forms a complex with ADH and blocks the EG binding site, thereby preventing its metabolism. For dogs treated with 4-MP, 1 of 2 dosage regimens may be used: 20 mg/kg of body weight given IV initially, 15 mg/kg 17 hours later, and 5 mg/kg 25 and 36 hours after the initial dose, or 20 mg/kg IV initially, 15 mg/kg 12 and 24 hours later, and 5 mg/kg 36 hours after the initial dose.[24] In cats, it can be administered at a dose of 125 mg/kg IV initially, followed by intermittent doses of 31.25 mg/kg at 12, 24, and 36 hours respectively. A study published in 2010 evaluating the use of 4-MP in EG intoxication in cats showed that 4-MP was safe to use, and, when administered within 3 hours of ingestion, prevented fatal ARF induced by EG. This treatment is usually not combined with hemodialysis because 4-MP is readily dialyzed.[23,25]
- Hemodialysis is recommended for cases of ARF induced by EG to remove the circulating EG and its metabolites, as well as to filter out uremic wastes. If resources are available, hemodialysis should be considered even before there is overt evidence of ARF to ensure the best possible prognosis.

Table 4
Diuretic therapy for AKI (generally, urine output should increase within 30–60 minutes after diuretic administration)

Drug	Mechanism of Action	Adverse Effects	Dose	Comments
Furosemide	Loop diuretic; blockade of the Na-K-2Cl transporter on the luminal side of the thick ascending loop of Henle; inhibits sodium transport, reducing energy requirements of cells in the medullary thick ascending limb the loop of Henle; reduces tubular-glomerular feedback to prevent a decrease in GFR, flushes out intratubular casts, reducing tubular obstruction	Dehydration/volume contraction and prerenal azotemia; electrolyte abnormalities; hypochloremic metabolic alkalosis; ototoxicity at high doses	Wide range: 0.25–4 mg/kg IV bolus in dogs; 0.25–2 mg/kg IV bolus in cats. CRI at 0.1–2 mg/kg/h may be used thereafter, pending patient response	Typically used as a first-line diuretic in oliguric or anuric renal failure to increased UOP and tubular flow
Mannitol	Osmotic diuretic; acts at the proximal tubule and loop of Henle by extracting water from intracellular compartments; improves tubular flow; free radical scavenger; preserves mitochondrial function by reducing postischemic swelling; improves renal blood flow by inhibiting renin release, expanding intravascular volume, and reducing blood viscosity	Dehydration/volume depletion; hypernatremia; osmotic nephrosis with prolonged use (causes swelling of tubular epithelial cells caused by vacuole formation in the cytoplasm)	0.5–1.0 g/kg slow IV bolus over 20 min followed by CRI at 60–120 mg/kg/h for 24–48 h	Ineffective in anuric renal failure. Risks of volume overload. Cautious use in hyperkalemic animals or those with potential for volume overload or hypernatremia

Drug	Mechanism	Adverse effects	Dosage	Comments
Diltiazem	Calcium channel blocker; reverses renal vasoconstriction by preglomerular dilation; inhibition of tubuloglomerular feedback-induced preglomerular vasoconstriction; cytoprotective effect by preventing mitochondrial calcium accumulation; reversal of thromboxane A2–induced renal vasoconstriction	Hypotension	0.1–0.5 mg/kg slow IV, followed by 1–5 µg/kg/min CRI	Can be used in dogs with AKI secondary to leptospirosis infection[17]; monitor ECG and blood pressure during and following administration
Fenoldopam	Selective DA-1 agonist (no DA-2 or α receptor effects). Produces systemic and renal vasodilation; increases renal blood flow; direct reduction of sodium reabsorption in the proximal tubule and cortical collecting duct	—	0.8 µg/kg/min IV CRI (based on experimental studies in beagles)[18]	—
Dopamine	Increases renal blood flow; induces diuresis and natriuresis via action on DA-1 receptors	May paradoxically cause renal vasoconstriction and impair GFR because of stimulation of DA-2 and α receptors	2.5–5 µg/kg/min IV CRI	Not recommended for routine use; no evidence in the literature that suggests a benefit, particularly in cats

Abbreviation: ECG, electrocardiogram.

- Supportive care, including IV fluid therapy, antiemetic therapy, serial monitoring of blood glucose (particularly if ethanol is used as an antidote), GI support (eg, antacids, gastric acid reducing medications), and symptomatic supportive care are imperative.

Acute Pyelonephritis

Pyelonephritis is defined as inflammation of the renal pelvis and kidneys that is caused by an ascending or hematogenously acquired infection of the urinary tract. Pyelonephritis is a serious and life-threatening complication of lower urinary tract infections, and can cause severe systemic illness in animals, with potentially fatal consequences. If not treated appropriately and in a timely manner, irreversible AKI can ensue.

Depending on the severity of illness, animals with pyelonephritis can present with clinical signs of:

- Lethargy
- Inappetence or anorexia
- Vomiting
- Fever
- Renal pain
- Hematuria
- Stranguria
- Halitosis
- Polyuria/polydipsia

Pyelonephritis that progresses to cause urosepsis (defined as systemic inflammatory response to infection arising from the urinary tract) can present with more severe signs including signs of septic shock such as fever, hypotension, and cardiovascular collapse.

Acute pyelonephritis can be diagnosed based on a combination of history, clinical signs and PE findings, clinicopathologic findings, and advanced diagnostics (eg, abdominal ultrasound, pyelocentesis). Laboratory findings may reveal azotemia and other markers of AKI, leukocytosis (with possible left shift and toxic change), hemoconcentration secondary to dehydration, and hypoglycemia (secondary to urosepsis, and so forth). Urinalysis typically reveals evidence of infection (eg, increased white blood cell count with or without obvious gross bacteriuria). Abdominal imaging, such as an abdominal ultrasound, can reveal evidence of acute nephritis including enlarged kidneys with decreased corticomedullary distinction, pylectasia, and perirenal effusion (**Fig. 3**). Urine samples obtained via cystocentesis or, ideally, via pyelocentesis, should be cultured for confirmation of infection. Occult pyelonephritis may occasionally occur, wherein urine cultures may be negative, but pyelonephritis may still be present.

Management

- Animals presenting with signs of severe sepsis or septic shock should be stabilized with aggressive IV fluid therapy as indicated. Isotonic crystalloids are typically preferred for initial fluid resuscitation in these patients. Following adequate volume resuscitation, continued aggressive IV fluid therapy (eg, >2–4 mL/kg/h) should be used to promote diuresis and improve azotemia. However, caution must be exercised in using high fluid rates in animals with preexisting cardiac or pulmonary disease, or those that are oliguric or anuric, to prevent volume overload.
- Once a diagnosis of pyelonephritis is suspected, a urine sample should be collected via cystocentesis and submitted for culture and sensitivity before starting treatment with broad-spectrum antimicrobials.

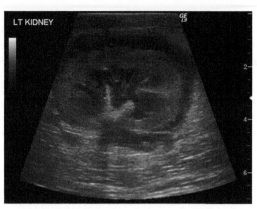

Fig. 3. Renal changes in acute pyelonephritis showing renomegaly, pylectasia and perirenal effusion.

- o Empiric antimicrobial therapy is selected based on the patient's medical history and prior antibiotic use, and clinical suspicion for the type of infection a patient is likely to have. In dogs and cats, infections with *Escherichia coli*, *Staphylococcus* spp, *Proteus* spp, and *Enterococcus* spp are commonly seen, although several other bacterial species have been documented. Pending culture results, the use of Gram staining of urine sediment can be used to help tailor appropriate antibiotic therapy.
- o Antibiotics that concentrate well in urine and the renal tissues should be selected.
  - These antibiotics include most β-lactams and trimethoprim-sulfate.
  - Fluoroquinolones are excreted in the urine predominantly in the active form, so these can be used at higher doses (10–15 mg/kg IV or by mouth, every 24 hours) in dogs but should be reserved for animals that have a prior history of more resistant organisms being cultured from their urine. Fluoroquinolones should be used cautiously in cats, because retinopathies have been documented at doses of more than 5 mg/kg/d, particularly in cats with underlying renal insufficiency.
  - After initial antimicrobial therapy is initiated, culture and sensitivity results should be evaluated to guide further therapy and alterations as necessary.
- • Appropriate analgesia is an important part of the management protocol for acute pyelonephritis because pain can contribute to increased morbidity in hospitalized patients and slow recovery times. Opioids are among the most commonly selected analgesics for this purpose, such as pure mu agonists (fentanyl at 2–5 μg/kg/h, methadone at 0.1–0.3 mg/kg IV every 6–8 hours, hydromorphone 0.005–0.1 mg/kg IV every 8 hours) and partial mu agonists (butorphanol at 0.1–0.3 mg/kg IV every 6–8 hours). Butorphanol Continuous Rate Infusions (CRIs) can also be used at 0.1 to 0.4 mg/kg/h. Buprenorphine is also widely used, particularly in cats with doses ranging from 0.01 to 0.03 mg/kg IV every 6 to 8 hours. The use of NSAIDs is generally contraindicated in patients with pyelonephritis, especially if they are hemodynamically unstable. Because of the potent renal artery vasoconstriction that can occur with NSAIDs (caused by the blocking of the locally produced prostaglandins), their use may further decrease perfusion to an already diseased kidney, thereby risking worsening renal function.

The prognosis for pyelonephritis varies with the severity of illness, presenting clinical signs and response to fluid and antibiotic therapy. In general, animals that present with severe signs of urosepsis and septic shock have a worse prognosis than animals that are only mildly azotemic. Early recognition and initiation of rational antimicrobial therapy and close monitoring are important factors that can influence outcome with this disease process. Antibiotics are typically continued for up to 2 to 4 weeks after discharge from the hospital. Repeat urine cultures should be checked between 3 and 7 days after completion of antibiotic therapy to ensure that the infection has cleared. Renal values should also be rechecked at this time to ensure that the azotemia is resolving appropriately.

Ureteral Obstruction

Ureteral obstruction is uncommon, but is still a significant cause of urinary obstruction and azotemia in dogs and cats. Ureteral calculi and ureteral strictures are among the most common causes implicated in this condition.[26–31] Based on a 2005 study evaluating 163 cats with ureteral stones, most obstructions were linked to calcium oxalate calculi.[31] In this study, 87% of the cats that had stone analysis performed had exclusively calcium oxalate stones. Other less common causes of ureteral obstruction include iatrogenic ligation (during ovariohysterectomy), neoplastic obstructions, and blood clots.

Animals with ureteral obstruction may show nonspecific clinical signs ranging from mild to severe, depending on whether 1 or both ureters are obstructed. These signs may include anorexia or inappetence, lethargy, vomiting, weight loss, inappropriate urination or thirst, halitosis, oliguria, or anuria. Animals that are bilaterally obstructed can present extremely ill with more advanced clinical signs, along with anuric renal failure.

Diagnosis of ureteral obstruction is usually difficult on PE and typically requires imaging. Plain abdominal radiographs, urinary tract ultrasonography, and contrast radiography (antegrade pyelography) have all been described,[28,31,32] with both antegrade pyelography and computed tomography (CT) being extremely sensitive and specific.[31] Ultrasonography has been shown to be effective at diagnosing hydroureter and hydronephrosis secondary to ureteral obstruction,[30] and is more commonly available.

Management

- Emergency stabilization with IV fluid therapy and correction of any electrolyte or acid-base disturbances is indicated in animals that present critically ill.
- Medical and surgical options exist for treatment of ureteral stones. Medical management options include attempting diuresis with IV fluids, whereas surgical options include ureterotomy,[33] pyelotomy, ureteral resection, and reimplantation.
- Amitriptylline, a tricyclic antidepressant, has been shown to help facilitate passage of calculi through the urinary tract by causing smooth muscle relaxation at 1 mg/kg by mouth every 24 hours in an experimental study; however, no clinical data exist supporting its use.[34]
- Mannitol, an osmotic diuretic, can also be used to help open the ureters during fluid therapy. A mannitol CRI can be used at 1 mg/kg/min for 24 hours, after a loading bolus of 0.2 to 0.5 g/kg over 20 to 30 minutes.[35]
- Ureteral stenting has recently become more widely available as a less invasive option to treat ureteral obstructions.[35]

Uroperitoneum

Uroperitoneum (or uroabdomen) is an emergency condition in which urine excavates into the peritoneal cavity, resulting in life-threatening electrolyte and acid-base derangements. Severe dehydration, hypovolemia, hyperkalemia, metabolic acidosis, profound azotemia, and severe chemical peritonitis are all consequences of uroabdomen.

Common causes of uroperitoneum in veterinary medicine include:

1. Rupture of the urinary bladder either caused by trauma or overdistension secondary to feline urethral obstruction (FUO). Iatrogenic rupture secondary to bladder palpation or cystocentesis can also occur.[36]
2. Rupture or tear of the intrapelvic portion of the urethra secondary to trauma or iatrogenic injury secondary to aggressive catheterization.
3. Ureteral rupture secondary to trauma or ureteral avulsion (along with concurrent damage to the peritoneal lining of the retroperitoneum) can cause urine leakage into the peritoneum.

Clinical signs of uroperitoneum include lethargy, anorexia, vomiting, severe abdominal pain (with secondary aggression), stranguria, hematuria, and possibly abdominal distension with a palpable fluid wave. The diagnosis of uroperitoneum should be based on PE findings and associated clinical signs mentioned earlier, clinicopathologic findings, abdominal radiographs with contrast, focused assessment of sonography in trauma (FAST) ultrasound or abdominal ultrasound, and by diagnostic abdominocentesis. The abdominocentesis can be performed either blindly or using ultrasound guidance to determine whether the free peritoneal fluid is urine. Once abdominal effusion is obtained, microscopic evaluation of the fluid should be assessed for the presence of a possible urinary tract infection, because leakage of infected urine could lead to secondary septic peritonitis. Next, abdominocentesis fluid samples should be compared for abdominal fluid blood urea nitrogen (BUN), creatinine, and potassium levels to concurrently drawn serum creatinine and potassium levels. Higher levels of BUN, creatinine, and potassium in the abdominal fluid are consistent with uroperitoneum. Fluid ratios should also be assessed for diagnostic evaluation. An abdominal fluid creatinine concentration/peripheral blood creatinine concentration ratio of greater than 2:1 is considered to predict uroabdomen in dogs, whereas an abdominal fluid potassium concentration/peripheral blood potassium concentration of greater than 1.4:1 also predicts uroabdomen in dogs.[37] In addition, contrast radiographic studies of the urinary tract, such as intravenous pyelography or cystourethrography, can help show loss of integrity of a particular part of the urinary tract and identify sites of leakage for surgical repair or medical management.

Management

- Initial cardiovascular stabilization with IV fluid therapy should be instituted as necessary, because these patients can present critically ill with signs of shock and perfusion abnormalities. Isotonic crystalloids can be used for initial stabilization with bolus doses ranging between 10 and 50 mL/kg, depending on the severity of the cardiovascular compromise.
- Electrocardiogram (ECG) monitoring and treatment of hyperkalemia should be initiated as necessary.
- Urine drainage from the abdomen is the next step after cardiovascular stabilization has been performed. Continuous passive drainage should be established to achieve stabilization and effective diuresis.
  - Placement of a percutaneous transabdominal drainage catheter such as a pigtail catheter or commercially available peritoneal dialysis catheters allows rapid removal of accumulated urine. Catheter placement should be performed by adhering to sterile technique to avoid iatrogenic introduction of infection

into the peritoneal cavity. The catheter is then attached to a sterile closed collection drainage system and the amount of fluid collected can be quantified and monitored (**Fig. 4** shows a sample pigtail transabdominal catheter).
  ○ An indwelling catheter should also be placed in the urinary bladder to keep the urinary bladder decompressed and reduce the hydrostatic pressure that may promote urine leakage into the abdominal cavity.
- Hemodialysis or peritoneal dialysis may be considered for extremely sick and uremic patients until more definitive surgical correction can be performed.
- Surgical exploration and correction is the definitive treatment of large defects; small tears in the bladder and urethra can potentially heal on their own. Patients should not undergo surgery until stable; a delay of 8 to 12 hours is appropriate if necessary to stabilize the patient's electrolytes, pain, and dehydration.

Overall, the prognosis for survival with a uroabdomen depends on the severity and location of the condition, degree of metabolic derangements caused, and rapidity of correction of these abnormalities, as well as concurrent medical problems. Various studies have reported mortalities of between 42.3% and 56.2% in dogs and 38.4% in cats.[37] The prognosis for uroabdomen remains guarded, but, with early diagnosis and aggressive, rapid management and stabilization, the prognosis can be improved.

FUO

FUO is among the most commonly seen urinary tract emergencies in cats, with several studies reporting between 2% and 13% incidence rates at veterinary teaching hospitals across North America.[38] This condition most commonly affects young male cats that seem to be predisposed because of their long, narrow urethras, although it can occur in female cats as well. Several risk factors for FUO have been proposed, including urolithiasis, lower urinary tract infections, environmental stress, and crystalluria.[38–41]

There are various causes that have been implicated; however, idiopathic cystitis progressing to FUO seems to be the most common, with an incidence of more than 50% reported in a 2008 study.[42] Urethral mucus plugs are also commonly implicated as the cause for FUO, although urinary calculi are also sometimes seen. Urethral plugs are formed when proteinaceous material leaking from an inflamed urinary bladder

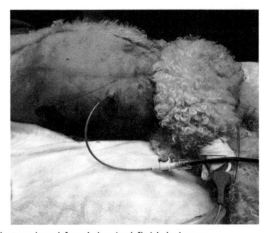

Fig. 4. Pigtail catheter placed for abdominal fluid drainage.

combines with crystals. These plugs can also comprise organic material such as tissue and red blood cells combined with aggregates of crystalline material.

Clinical signs of FUO include vomiting, stranguria, hematuria, pollakiuria, vocalization, excessive grooming or licking of the perineal area, lethargy, and more severe systemic signs (depending on the severity and duration of obstruction). PE findings may include a firm, distended, nonexpressible, and possibly painful urinary bladder. Absence of a palpable bladder in a cat presenting with these clinical signs does not necessarily rule out an FUO, because bladder rupture may have occurred; in this situation, albeit rare, cats present severely ill. Discoloration of the tip of the penis or presence of urethral mucus plugs (at the tip of the penis) may also be found on PE with FUO.

Most cats presenting with FUO are stable; however, some can present with severe cardiovascular compromise and collapse, often secondary to life-threatening electrolyte and acid-base abnormalities. Hyperkalemia, ionized hypocalcemia, and metabolic acidosis are the most commonly seen derangements. One study reported an incidence of 12% for hyperkalemia, and 6% with severe acidemia (pH <7.10).[40] Clinical signs associated with systemic electrolyte and acid-base abnormalities include dehydration or hypovolemia, bradycardia, the presence of arrhythmias, hypothermia, and weak pulses.[40,43,44]

Emergency management

- Initial cardiovascular stabilization:
  - Cardiovascular stabilization is vital in critically ill cats that are obstructed because they often present with acid-base and electrolyte derangements that can be rapidly fatal. These cats are also cardiovascularly severely compromised and can have decreased tissue perfusion secondary to both hypovolemia and cardiac dysfunction from electrolyte derangements (eg, hyperkalemia).
  - Establishing IV access: an intravenous catheter should be placed and blood drawn for an emergency database screen including a venous blood gas, Packed Cell Volume (PCV), Total Solids (TS), BUN, creatinine, glucose, serum sodium, potassium, and ionized calcium values if possible.
  - Animals presenting with signs of hypovolemia or poor tissue perfusion should be stabilized with IV fluids. A bolus of between 10 and 30 mL/kg of a balanced isotonic crystalloid is typically chosen as a starting point, followed by frequent reassessment of the patient.
  - An ECG recording should be obtained as soon as possible, especially in animals that present bradycardic or excessively tachycardic and have irregular or weak pulses. Typical arrhythmias observed in sick, hyperkalemic animals have been inconsistent with those classically observed in experimental hyperkalemia and were described in a 2008 study.[45] Some of the expected ECG changes with hyperkalemia are shown in **Table 5**.
  - Immediate management of arrhythmias secondary to hyperkalemia is needed. **Table 6** shows therapeutics for hyperkalemia.
  - Once the patient has been stabilized, therapeutic relief of the urinary obstruction should immediately follow. **Table 7** lists various sedation protocols, and **Figs. 5–8** show protocols for relief of FUO.

Relief of urinary obstruction

After cardiovascular stability is achieved, the FUO should be relieved.

- Local anesthetic agents may be used to perform epidural blocks in extremely unstable animals to avoid the risk of general anesthesia, and provide relief

Table 5
Expected ECG changes secondary to hyperkalemia

Serum Potassium (mEq/L)	Expected ECG Changes
5.5–6.49	Sinus bradycardia, sinoventricular rhythm, increased T wave amplitude
6.5–6.99	Decreased R wave amplitude, prolonged QRS complex and P-R intervals, and ST segment depression
7.0–8.5	Sinus tachycardia and tall T waves, decreased P wave amplitude, increased P wave duration and prolongation of the QT interval
8.6–10	Widening of the QRS complex, ventricular flutter, fibrillation, smooth biphasic waveform or sine wave, and asystole or ventricular tachycardia

from penile and urethral pain. A recent study described the technique for performing a coccygeal epidural block using lidocaine before catheterizing blocked cats.[46]

- Various types of urinary catheters are available for relief of the obstruction, including the standard Tom Cat, olive-tipped, polyurethane (with or without stylets for insertion), or Slippery Sam catheter.
- Antegrade urethral catheterization:
  - Fluoroscopically-guided percutaneous antegrade urethral catheterization has recently been described in blocked cats where traditional catheterization methods have been unsuccessful.[47]
  - In this procedure, an IV catheter is placed percutaneously transabdominally into the urinary bladder. Following this, iodinated contrast material is injected and a cystourethrogram performed to assess the integrity of the lower urinary tract.
  - A hydrophilic guidewire is then inserted through the catheter and, using fluoroscopy, guided down into the urethra and advanced in an antegrade fashion, exiting through the urethral tip. Through-and-through guidewire access of the lower urinary tract is thus achieved.
  - Following this, an over-the-wire urinary drainage catheter, or a 5-Fr red rubber catheter can then be passed over the wire into the urethra in a retrograde fashion into the bladder, and the guidewire can be removed through the tip of the urethra.
  - The catheter is then sutured in place routinely, and the IV catheter placed percutaneously into the bladder is removed.
- Postcatheterization care:
  - In cases in which an indwelling catheter is left in place, cats should be monitored in hospital for the next 12 to 48 hours with aggressive IV fluid therapy and analgesia (**Fig. 9**)
  - Regular monitoring of blood work (if financial limitations exist, treatments such as aggressive IV fluid therapy and pain control are of more diagnostic value, because blood work should improve with just treatment alone), especially in sick, uremic cats, may include:
    - PCV/TS
    - BUN and creatinine
    - Serum sodium, potassium, and ionized calcium
    - Acid-base parameters

Table 6
Treatment of hyperkalemia

Drug	Dose	Comments
Calcium gluconate 10%	0.5–1 mL/kg (give in mEq also) IV, slowly over 5–15 min; can be given as a faster bolus in patients that are periarrest	Treatment of choice for hyperkalemia, especially in animals that present with concurrently low ionized calcium levels. The ECG should be monitored closely throughout administration of this drug. This drug does not directly reduce potassium levels; instead it modifies the threshold potential, thereby offsetting the change in resting membrane potential caused by hyperkalemia and can be cardioprotective
Regular insulin	0.1–0.25 U/kg IV followed immediately with a 50% dextrose bolus (dose: 0.25–0.5 g/kg, IV, diluted 1:3)	Any IV fluid CRIs started subsequently are usually supplemented with between 2.5%–5% dextrose and blood glucose levels should be monitored closely over the next several hours to prevent hypoglycemia
Sodium bicarbonate	1 mEq/kg slow IV, over 10–15 min	Typically used to treat refractory hyperkalemia that has not responded to the above 2 therapies. Use of sodium bicarbonate in the face of ionized hypocalcemia can further exacerbate hypocalcemia and increase the risk of clinical signs of hypocalcemic tetany and/or seizures. Therefore, calcium levels should be monitored closely. However, it may also be beneficial with severe metabolic acidosis

○ Remove the catheter within 12 to 48 hours depending on patient stability and the gross appearance of the urine (eg, free of blood clots, isosthenuric).
○ Monitor for at least 6 to 12 hours to ensure normal urination.
○ Monitor for postobstructive diuresis:
  ■ Almost 50% of cats develop massive increases in their UOP following FUO,[48] a phenomenon called postobstructive diuresis.
  ■ Aggressive IV fluid therapy is usually necessary in these cases to keep up with the losses and prevent dehydration, and even hypovolemia.
  ■ Typical fluid rates are 40 to 60 mL/h for patients with FUO to counter this severe diuresis.

Table 7
Sedation protocols for relief of FUO

Drugs	Doses	Comments
Benzodiazepine such as midazolam or diazepam + ketamine	Midazolam/diazepam: 0.1–0.5 mg/kg IV Ketamine: 0.5–4 mg/kg IV	Should be avoided if cardiac abnormalities are present, or if underlying cardiac disease is suspected
Benzodiazepine such as midazolam or diazepam + opioids	Midazolam/diazepam: 0.1–0.8 mg/kg IV Opioids: • Butorphanol (0.1–0.8 mg/kg) • Methadone (0.1–0.4 mg/kg) • Oxymorphone (0.02–0.05 mg/kg)	Safer to use in cats with preexisting heart disease or ECG abnormalities on presentation

- As azotemia and dehydration resolve (as shown by isosthenuria and appropriate hemodilution of the patient), taper fluids to help reestablish a medullary solute gradient, because prolonged aggressive fluid therapy and diuresis often result in a medullary washout and loss of urine concentrating ability.
- Monitor ins and outs to ensure appropriate hydration and diuresis.
- Therapeutic cystocentesis:
  ○ Cystocentesis can be performed in cases in which catheterization is unsuccessful after repeated attempts. This treatment may help relieve the high hydrostatic pressure on the wall of the urinary bladder and, in some cases, may also relieve back pressure on the FUO and facilitate catheterization. Risks include bladder rupture and subsequent uroperitoneum, especially in patients that have an extremely inflamed and friable bladder wall.[34]

The prognosis for survival to discharge in most cats with FUO is good, even in critically ill cats, providing they are stabilized within the first few hours of presentation. A study from 2008 reported a guarded long-term prognosis regarding reobstruction in these cats, with more than 50% of cats in the study showing recurrence of lower urinary tract signs within a year, and more than 30% of the cats having a repeat obstruction within the next 2 years.[41] Perineal urethrostomy (PU) may need to be performed in cats that have repeated episodes of FUO, or are unable to be catheterized to relieve the obstruction. Client education is important in cases of FUO and feline lower urinary tract disease. Improved husbandry practices such as diet changes and switching to wet food, increasing water intake (eg, water fountain, grueled canned food), and environmental modifications (eg, kitty litter husbandry, including frequent, daily cleaning of litter boxes; use of favorable litter sources; and increased number of litter boxes) can all be instituted to help reduce the risk of reobstruction in these cats.

Urethral Calculi in Dogs

- Canine urethral obstruction is another commonly seen urinary emergency in small animal practice. Urethral obstruction in dogs can be caused by urethral calculi, urethral strictures, or urethral neoplasia.
- Managing an acute urethral obstruction in a dog is similar to managing a case of FUO. After initial cardiovascular stabilization and correction of life-threatening electrolyte or acid-base abnormalities (eg, hyperkalemia, metabolic acidosis), relieving the urethral obstruction is the next step.

Employ sterile technique.

Positioning: dorsal recumbency.

Clip and clean the area surrounding the penis and prepuce with a dilute antiseptic solution such as chlorhexidine.

Start catheterization using an open-ended tom cat catheter.

Lubricate the tip of the catheter with sterile lubricant gel.

Extrude the tip of the penis slightly past the prepuce.

Feed the catheter into the tip of the penis through the external urethral opening. The penis can be allowed to slip back into the prepuce once the catheter tip is well seated inside the urethra.

Hold the prepuce and retract and directit dorsally and caudally towards the tail base with the catheter still inside the tip. This:

- Straightens the urethra

- Facilitates easier dislodgement of the obstruction

- Facilitates easier passage of the catheter into the bladder.

Advance the catheter gently into the urethral passage while flushing aggressively to help alleviate the obstruction. Retract slightly if necessary and repeat flushing and advancing.

- Avoid excessive amounts of force while passing the catheter, and do not attempt to force it past an obstruction. The urethra in these cases is often extremely inflamed and friable, and can tear or rupture easily.

Fig. 5. Protocol for relief of FUO.

Use of urethral occlusion (urohydropulsion) while performing retrograde flushing to dislodge stubborn obstructions:

- Occlude the urethra around the catheter shaft using the thumb and forefinger while an assistant maintains pressure on the flush syringe to dilate the urethra by preventing reflux of the flush solution, and flush the obstructive material back into the urinary bladder.

Once the obstruction is relieved, pass the catheter further into the bladder until urine can be aspirated back.

Empty the bladder and flush several times with sterile saline until a clear solution is aspirated back. This helps remove as much grit and debris from the bladder as possible.

Leave an indwelling catheter in place, especially in cats that are uremic and critically ill, cats that have been obstructed for a long time, cats with detrusor atony, cats with possible urethral tear, or in cases in which there is significant amount of debris, grit, or blood clots in the urine that may cause a reobstruction.

- Typically, a 3.5-Fr or 5-Fr red rubber catheter is placed as an indwelling catheter and sutured in place using tape wings. This catheter is then connected to a sterileclosed collection system to facilitate monitoring of urinary output and guide fluid therapy.

Fig. 5. (*continued*)

- Passing a urinary catheter (eg, red rubber, Foley) can help dislodge smooth-surfaced stones and push them back into the bladder until more definitive treatment of the calculi, such as a cystotomy or lithotripsy, can be performed.
- Urethral calculi typically tend to lodge just behind the caudal aspect of the os penis in dogs. The use of urohydropulsion may be necessary for emergency treatment of urethral obstruction caused by urethral calculi that cannot be easily dislodged by passage of a urinary catheter.[49] Urohydropulsion is typically performed using a urinary catheter attached to a syringe filled with sterile saline (with or without a sterile lubricant mixed in equal proportions). The person performing the catheterization advances the urinary catheter into the urethral opening while an assistant maintains pressure on the flush syringe. The person performing the catheterization then occludes the urethra around the catheter shaft using the forefinger and the thumb. This technique helps dilate the urethra by preventing reflux of the flush solution, and helps flush the obstructive material back into the urinary bladder. Pulsatile pressure applied to the flush syringe may help dislodge the obstruction more quickly.

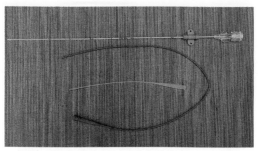

Fig. 6. Various types of urinary catheters for relief of FUO. From top to bottom: Mila™ urinary catheter, red rubber catheter, Tom Cat catheter.

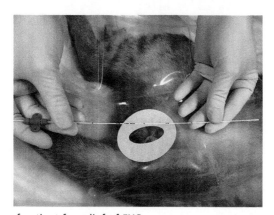

Fig. 7. Positioning of patient for relief of FUO.

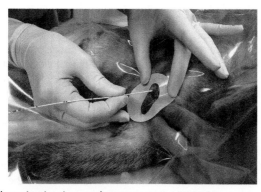

Fig. 8. Urinary catheterization in a male cat.

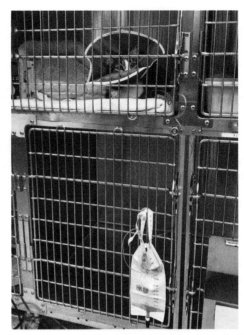

Fig. 9. Indwelling catheter in a hospitalized cat following relief of FUO.

- Clinical signs, management, and overall treatment are as discussed earlier for FUO.
- Surgical removal of the calculi is typically required to prevent reoccurrence.

SUMMARY

Rapid recognition and aggressive therapeutic intervention is necessary with urogenital emergencies because of the potential to become life threatening if not addressed rapidly. Overall, the prognosis with urogenital emergencies is fair to good with appropriate medical or surgical management.

REFERENCES

1. VA/NIH Acute Renal Failure Trial Network. Intensity of renal support in critically ill patients with acute kidney injury. N Engl J Med 2008;359(1):7–20.
2. Ali T, Khan I, Simpson W, et al. Incidence and outcomes in acute kidney injury- a comprehensive population based study. J Am Soc Nephrol 2007;18(4):1292–8.
3. Behrend EN, Grauer GF, Mani I, et al. Hospital-acquired acute renal failure in dogs: 29 cases (1983–1992). J Am Vet Med Assoc 1996;208(4):537–41.
4. Lee Y, Chang C, Chan P, et al. Prognosis of acute kidney injury in dogs using RIFLE (Risk, Injury, Failure, Loss and End-Stage renal failure)-like criteria. Vet Rec 2011;168(10):264–8.
5. Thoen M, Kerl M. Characterization of acute kidney injury in hospitalized dogs and evaluation of a veterinary acute kidney injury staging system. J Vet Emerg Crit Care 2011;21(6):648–57.
6. Worwag S, Langston C. Acute intrinsic renal failure in cats: 32 cases (1997-2004). J Am Vet Med Assoc 2008;232:728–32.

7. Kellum JA, Levin N, Bouman C, et al. Developing a consensus classification system for acute renal failure. Curr Opin Crit Care 2002;8:509–14.
8. Bellomo R, Kellum JA, Ronco C. Defining and classifying acute renal failure: from advocacy to consensus and validation of the RIFLE criteria. Intensive Care Med 2007;11:409–13.
9. Mehta RL, Kellum JA, Shah SV, et al. Acute kidney injury network: report of an initiative to improve outcomes in acute kidney injury. Crit Care 2007;11:R31.
10. Chertow GM, Burdick E, Honour M, et al. Acute kidney injury, mortality, length of stay, and costs in hospitalized patients. J Am Soc Nephrol 2005;16(11): 3365–70.
11. The SAFE Study Investigators. A comparison of albumin and saline for fluid resuscitation in the intensive care unit. N Engl J Med 2004;350:2247–56.
12. Dart AB, Mutter TC, Ruth CA, et al. Hydroxyethyl starch (HES) versus other fluid therapies: effects on kidney function. Cochrane Database Syst Rev 2010;1: CD007594.
13. Zarychanski R, Turgeon AF, Fergusson DA, et al. Renal outcomes and mortality following hydroxyethyl starch resuscitation of critically ill patients: systematic review and meta-analysis of randomized trials. Open Med 2009;3:196–209.
14. Vaidya VS, Ferguson MA, Bonventre JV. Biomarkers of acute kidney injury. Annu Rev Pharmacol Toxicol 2008;48:463–93.
15. Lameire N, Biesen WV, Vanholder R. Acute kidney injury. Lancet 2008;372:1863–5.
16. Tambyah PA, Oon J. Catheter-associated urinary tract infection. Curr Opin Infect Dis 2012;25:365–70.
17. Mathews KA, Monteith G. Evaluation of adding diltiazem therapy to standard treatment of acute renal failure caused by leptospirosis: 18 dogs (1998–2001). J Vet Emerg Crit Care 2007;17:149–58.
18. Bloom CA, Labato MA, Hazarika S, et al. Preliminary pharmacokinetics and cardiovascular effects of fenoldopam continuous rate infusion in six healthy dogs. J Vet Pharmacol Ther 2012;35:224–30.
19. Claus MA, Jandrey KE, Poppenga RH. Propylene glycol intoxication in a dog. J Vet Emerg Crit Care 2011;21(6):679–83.
20. Grauer GF, Thrall MA. Ethylene glycol (antifreeze) poisoning in the dog and cat. J Am Anim Hosp Assoc 1982;18:492–7.
21. Thrall MA, Grauer GF, Mero KN. Clinicopathologic findings in dogs and cats with ethylene glycol intoxication. J Am Vet Med Assoc 1984;184:37–41.
22. Rowland J. Incidence of ethylene glycol intoxication in dogs and cats seen at Colorado State University Veterinary Teaching Hospital. Vet Hum Toxicol 1987; 29:41–4.
23. Connally HE, Thrall MA, Hamar DW. Safety and efficacy of high dose fomepizole compared with ethanol as therapy for ethylene glycol intoxication in cats. J Vet Emerg Crit Care 2010;20(2):191–206.
24. Connally HE, Thrall MA, Forney SD, et al. Safety and efficacy of 4-methypyrazole for treatment of suspected or confirmed ethylene glycol intoxication in dogs: 107 cases (1983-1995). J Am Vet Med Assoc 1996;209:1880–3.
25. Tart KM, Powell LL. 4-Methypyrazole as a treatment in naturally occurring ethylene glycol intoxication in cats. J Vet Emerg Crit Care 2011;21(3):268–72.
26. Moon ML, Dallman MA. Calcium oxalate ureterolith in a cat. Vet Radiol 1991;32: 261–3.
27. Kyles AE, Stone EA, Gookin J, et al. Diagnosis and surgical management of obstructive ureteral calculi in cats: 11 cases (1993–1996). J Am Vet Med Assoc 1998;213:1150–6.

28. Adin CA, Herrgesell EJ, Nyland TG, et al. Antegrade pyelography for suspected ureteral obstruction in cats: 11 cases (1995–2001). J Am Vet Med Assoc 2003; 222:1576–81.
29. Dupre GP, Dee LG, Dee JF. Ureterotomies for the treatment of ureterolithiasis in two dogs. J Am Anim Hosp Assoc 1990;26:500–4.
30. Block G, Adam LG, Widmer WR, et al. Use of extracorporeal shock wave lithotripsy for treatment of nephrolithiasis and ureterolithiasis in five dogs. J Am Vet Med Assoc 1996;208:531–6.
31. Kyles AE, Hardie EM, Wooden BG, et al. Clinical, clinicopathologic, radiographic and ultrasonographic abnormalities in cats with ureteral calculi: 163 cases (1984–2002). J Am Vet Med Assoc 2005;226:932–6.
32. Kyles AE, Hardie EM, Wooden BG, et al. Management and outcome of cats with ureteral calculi: 153 cases (1984–2002). J Am Vet Med Assoc 2005; 226:937–44.
33. Roberts SF, Aronson LA, Brown DC. Postoperative mortality in cats after ureterolithotomy. Vet Surg 2011;40:438–43.
34. Achar E, Achar RA, Paiva TB, et al. Amitriptyline eliminates calculi through urinary tract smooth muscle relaxation. Kidney Int 2003;64(4):1356–64.
35. Berent AC. Ureteral obstructions in dogs and cats: a review of traditional and new interventional diagnostic and therapeutic options. J Vet Emerg Crit Care 2011;21: 86–103.
36. Aumann M, Worth LT, Drobatz KJ. Uroperitoneum in cats: 26 cases (1986–1995). J Am Anim Hosp Assoc 1998;34:315–24.
37. Schmiedt C, Tobias KM, Otto CM. Evaluation of abdominal fluid: peripheral blood creatinine and potassium ratios for diagnosis of uroperitoneum in dogs. J Vet Emerg Crit Care 2001;11(4):275–80.
38. Lekcharoensuk C, Osborne CA, Lulich JP. Epidemiologic study of risk factors for lower urinary tract diseases in cats. J Am Vet Med Assoc 2001;218:1429–35.
39. Kruger JM, Osborne CA, Goyal SM, et al. Clinical evaluation of cats with lower urinary tract disease. J Am Vet Med Assoc 1991;199:211–6.
40. Lee JA, Drobatz KJ. Characterization of the clinical characteristics, electrolytes, acid-base and renal parameters in male cats with urethral obstruction. J Vet Emerg Crit Care 2003;13:227–33.
41. Segev G, Livne H, Ranen E, et al. Urethral obstruction in cats: predisposing factors, clinical, clinicopathological characteristics and outcome. J Feline Med Surg 2011;13:101–8.
42. Gerber B, Eichenberger S, Reusch CE. Guarded long term prognosis in male cats with urethral obstruction. J Feline Med Surg 2008;10:16–23.
43. Lee JA, Drobatz KJ. Historical and physical parameters as predictors of severe hyperkalemia in male cats with urethral obstruction. J Vet Emerg Crit Care 2006;16:104–11.
44. Bass M, Howard J, Gerber B, et al. Retrospective study of indications for and outcome of perineal urethrostomy in cats. J Small Anim Pract 2005;46:227–31.
45. Tag TL, Day TK. Electrocardiographic assessment of hyperkalemia in dogs and cats. J Vet Emerg Crit Care 2008;18:61–7.
46. Hearn A, Wright BD. Coccygeal epidural with local anesthetic for catheterization and pain management in treatment of feline urethral obstruction. J Vet Emerg Crit Care 2011;21(1):50–2.
47. Holmes ES, Weisse C, Berent AC. Use of fluoroscopically guided percutaneous antegrade urethral catheterization for the treatment of urethral obstruction in male cats: 9 cases (2000-2009). J Am Vet Med Assoc 2012;241(5):603–7.

48. Francis BJ, Wells RJ, Rao S, et al. Retrospective study to characterize post-obstructive diuresis in male cats with urethral obstruction. J Feline Med Surg 2010;12:606–8.
49. Lulich JP, Osborne CA, Carlson M, et al. Nonsurgical removal of urocystoliths in dogs and cats by voiding urohydropulsion. J Am Vet Med Assoc 1993;203(5): 660–3.

Endocrine Emergencies in Dogs and Cats

Amie Koenig, DVM

KEYWORDS

- Diabetic ketoacidosis • Hyperglycemic hyperosmolar syndrome • Hypoglycemia
- Insulinoma • Hypoadrenocorticism • Pheochromocytoma • Thyroid storm
- Myxedema coma

KEY POINTS

- Diabetic ketoacidosis, hyperglycemic hyperosmolar syndrome, hypoglycemia, insulinoma, hypoadrenocorticism, pheochromocytoma, thyrotoxicosis, and myxedema coma are all examples of life-threatening complications of endocrine disease.
- Success in treatment of endocrine emergencies is contingent on early recognition and treatment.
- Many endocrine diseases presenting emergently have nonspecific signs and symptoms.
- Endocrine crises are often precipitated by concurrent disease, further making early identification difficult.

Endocrine disorders are common problems in dogs and cats. Although typically presenting with chronic, insidious, and slowly progressive signs, there are some instances when endocrine disease can present with life-threatening complications. Diabetic ketoacidosis (DKA), hyperglycemic hyperosmolar syndrome (HHS), hypoglycemia, insulinoma, hypoadrenocorticism (HA), pheochromocytoma, thyrotoxicosis, and myxedema coma are all examples of life-threatening complications of endocrine disease. Success in treatment of endocrine emergencies is contingent on early recognition and treatment. This article concentrates on clinical signs and emergency management of these endocrine crises. The reader is referred to an endocrinology textbook for further information on long-term care and treatment.

DIABETIC EMERGENCIES: DKA AND HHS

DKA and HHS are 2 diabetic crises that require emergency intervention. DKA is identified by presence of hyperglycemia, glucosuria, ketonemia, or ketonuria with a metabolic acidosis as shown by low pH, low bicarbonate, and large negative base excess

---

Disclosure: The author has received funding from Medtronic Corporation.
Department of Small Animal Medicine and Surgery, College of Veterinary Medicine, University of Georgia, Athens, GA 30602, USA
E-mail address: akoenig@uga.edu

Vet Clin Small Anim 43 (2013) 869–897
http://dx.doi.org/10.1016/j.cvsm.2013.03.004
0195-5616/13/$ – see front matter © 2013 Elsevier Inc. All rights reserved.

on arterial or venous blood gas (VBG) analysis. The criteria for HHS include severe hyperglycemia, minimal or absent serum or urine ketones, and severe hyperosmolality. (**Table 1** gives a summary of diabetic crises.)

DKA and HHS share a common yet divergent pathophysiology. In both, an absolute or relative lack of insulin renders most cells unable to use glucose for energy and promotes gluconeogenesis and glycogenolysis, thus leading to development of hyperglycemia. In addition, hormone-sensitive lipase activity is increased, thus releasing free fatty acids (FFAs) from adipocytes, which can be oxidized by many tissues to make energy. These FFAs are taken up by the liver, where they are made into triglycerides, metabolized via the tricarboxylic cycle to CO_2 and water, or formed into the ketone bodies: acetoacetate, β-hydroxybutyrate, and acetone. In the uncomplicated diabetic, triglyceride production predominates and the small amounts of ketones that are produced are completely metabolized for energy.[1]

Progression to DKA or HHS requires both a lack of insulin as well as increasing concentrations of counterregulatory (or stress) hormones, including glucagon, epinephrine, cortisol, and growth hormone. These hormones are secreted in response to a secondary stressor, although the stressor is not always identified. For example, infection, hyperadrenocorticism, pancreatitis, renal failure, neoplasia, and heart failure have all been identified in patients in diabetic crises.[2–6] The hormonal alterations contribute to development of a diabetic crisis in many ways, including stimulating hepatic glycogenolysis and gluconeogenesis, inhibiting insulin activity, potentiating the effects of glucagon and epinephrine on hepatic glycogenolysis and gluconeogenesis, and increasing protein catabolism (which subsequently impairs insulin activity in muscle and provides amino acids for hepatic gluconeogenesis). Together, these factors contribute to the hyperglycemia, osmotic diuresis, and hyperosmolality in these patients.[1]

Progression to DKA

In DKA, the counterregulatory hormones stimulate lipolysis, which increases the amount of circulating FFAs available for ketone formation. Accumulation of ketones causes ketosis. Systemic acidemia, called DKA, develops once the quantity of

Table 1
Summary of diabetic crises

	DKA	HHS
Diagnostic criteria	Hyperglycemia Glucosuria Ketonemia/ketonuria Metabolic acidosis pH <7.3, HCO_3 <15 mEq/L	Hyperglycemia (>600 mg/dL) Minimal/absent serum ketones Serum osmolality >350 mg/dL
Common clinical signs and symptoms	PU/PD Dehydration Hypovolemia Anorexia Vomiting Mental depression Weakness Ketone (acetone) breath	PU/PD Dehydration Hypovolemia Mental depression, obtundation Weakness Abnormal pupillary light reflex Seizures Stupor/coma
Common concurrent conditions	Pancreatitis Urinary tract infection Hyperadrenocorticism Corticosteroid administration Hepatomegaly	Renal failure CHF

ketoacids overwhelms metabolic pathways and buffering systems. Ketoacids cause osmotic diuresis and, coupled with lack of water intake and ongoing losses (eg, vomiting, diarrhea), contribute to the development of dehydration. Prerenal azotemia results as intravascular volume is reduced and this decline in glomerular filtration rate (GFR) causes glucose and ketones to accumulate at an accelerated rate, exacerbating the clinical state. To maintain serum electroneutrality, negatively charged ketoacids are excreted with positively charged ions such as sodium, potassium, magnesium, and calcium, leading to electrolyte deficiencies.[1]

Progression to HHS

The pathogenesis of HHS is similar to that of DKA, except that in HHS, it is thought that the presence of small amounts of insulin and hepatic glucagon resistance inhibit lipolysis, thereby preventing ketosis.[7,8] Lower concentrations of growth hormone have also been documented in patients with HHS.[8,9] In HHS, the primary result of hormonal alterations is hyperglycemia, which promotes osmotic diuresis, thus leading to a vicious circle of progressive dehydration and hyperosmolality. To achieve the magnitude of hyperglycemia that is seen in HHS, a reduction in GFR is required, because otherwise there is no maximum rate of glucose loss via the kidney.[10,11] (All glucose that enters the kidney in excess of the renal threshold is excreted in the urine in a normal animal). An inverse correlation exists between GFR and serum glucose in diabetics.[10] Renal failure and congestive heart failure (CHF) are common in cats with HHS and they can also exacerbate the hyperglycemia as a result of their reduction of GFR.[3] Human HHS survivors have also shown a reduced thirst response, despite increasing vasopressin levels, which may also contribute to dehydration and decreased GFR.[12]

Clinical Signs and Symptoms

Both DKA and HHS may be identified in new or previously diagnosed and treated diabetics. Polyuria (PU), polydipsia (PD), polyphagia, and weight loss are consistent with a diagnosis of diabetes mellitus (DM). PU and PD develop when the magnitude of hyperglycemia exceeds renal threshold, and an osmotic diuresis ensues. Decreased glucose transport into the satiety center is perceived as starvation, and the patient often develops a ravenous appetite. Weight loss occurs as adipose tissue is broken down to provide energy for cells, because their normal energy source, glucose, is unavailable.

The onset of DKA is typically accompanied by lethargy, mental depression, anorexia, vomiting, diarrhea, weakness, and other signs consistent with comorbid disease. Onset of HHS is often associated with hyporexia, lethargy, vomiting, and weakness. In addition, some owners report a history of heart or renal disease or recent-onset neurologic signs, such as circling, pacing, mentation changes, or seizures.[2-6]

Physical examination

Physical examination findings in DKA and HHS can vary with the severity and chronicity of the syndrome and any concurrent diseases. Either condition can present as hypovolemic shock, with or without hypotension. In the typical patient with DKA, dehydration, thin body condition, mental depression, weakness, vomiting, and ketone (acetone) breath are common findings.[2-6] In HHS, dehydration is typically severe, and neurologic abnormalities, including depression (most common), obtundation, stupor, or coma, may be present. Weakness, ataxia, abnormal pupillary light reflexes, or seizure activity may also be noted.[3] Neurologic signs are believed to develop secondary to cerebral dehydration induced by severe hyperosmolality.

Diagnosis

Clinically ill diabetic animals warrant a full diagnostic evaluation, including a complete blood count (CBC), chemistry, VBG, urinalysis (including ketone measurement), urine culture, and imaging. Clinicopathologic abnormalities vary with underlying disease process and are not specific for DKA or HHS. Anemia, hemoconcentration, and stress or inflammatory leukograms may be seen. Likewise, azotemia, hyperphosphatemia, increased liver enzyme activities, and electrolyte deficiencies may be seen with both diabetic crises. Hyperbilirubinemia, hypercholesterolemia, and hypertriglyceridemia are more common in cats with DKA than those with HHS.[3] Although it is not possible to differentiate HHS from DKA based on the severity of metabolic acidosis, VBG quantifies the degree of acidemia resulting from ketoacids, lactate, and uremic acids.[3] The presence of ketones should be identified by measuring urine or serum ketones using a urine dipstick or point-of-care blood ketone meter.[13–15]

Profound electrolyte abnormalities may be seen with both DKA and HHS. Although the total body content of potassium is reduced, patients with DKA and HHS may initially have normal or increased blood concentrations as a result of acidosis, severe hyperosmolality,[16] insulin deficiency, or poor renal perfusion. Potassium levels decline with therapy as acidosis improves and as insulin drives glucose and potassium into cells. Serum sodium level may also be misleading, because severe hyperglycemia pulls water into the vasculature and dilutes the serum sodium level, causing a pseudohyponatremia.[17] As the glucose level decreases, the sodium level increases. The true corrected sodium level can be estimated by the following equation: $Na^+_{(corr)} = 1.6 \times$ ([measured glucose – normal glucose]/100) + $Na^+_{(measured)}$.

Additional diagnostics such as thoracic and abdominal radiographs, abdominal ultrasonography, thyroid levels, and other endocrine testing, feline leukemia virus/feline immunodeficiency virus, heartworm testing, and echocardiogram may be indicated based on clinical findings and suspected underlying disease processes.

Emergency Management of Diabetic Crises

Goals of therapy for patients with HHS and DKA are to (1) replace dehydration deficit and vascular volume, (2) manage electrolyte abnormalities, (3) initiate insulin therapy to help reduce glucose levels and reverse ketone production in DKA, and (4) treat underlying diseases.

Fluid therapy

In hypovolemic patients, intravenous (IV) shock fluid therapy should be initiated using a replacement crystalloid. Once the patient is volume resuscitated, the fluid plan should account for the dehydration deficit, ongoing losses, and maintenance needs. A buffered isotonic replacement crystalloid (eg, lactated Ringer's solution [LRS, Baxter Healthcare Corp, Deerflied IL], Normosol-R, Hospira, Lake Forest, IL LRS, Braun Medical Inc, Irvine CA) is a good initial choice for most patients. The use of fluid therapy alone aids in reduction of blood glucose concentration via dilution and by increasing GFR, which enhances urinary glucose excretion.[18]

Treating a patient with HHS and concurrent CHF presents a dilemma, because IV fluids may exacerbate heart failure. Rehydration must be performed more slowly and cautiously. Nasoesophageal tubes offer an effective means of rehydration, with less risk of volume overload. Specific cardiac therapy is dependent on the type of underlying cardiac dysfunction. A positive inotrope (eg, dobutamine, medium-dose dopamine) or inodilator (ie, pimobendan) may also be indicated to improve cardiac output and perfusion of the kidneys.

Managing electrolytes

Potassium, magnesium, and phosphorus deficiencies should be treated before initiating insulin therapy, because insulin causes rapid decline in these electrolytes as they are driven into cells or are consumed to make energy via glycolysis. Severe electrolyte deficiencies may precipitate life-threatening complications or death. Once these 3 electrolytes are within reference range, insulin therapy may begin (see later discussion). Again, electrolyte levels may decline rapidly with insulin therapy, and deficiencies commonly develop, even if these electrolyte levels are normal or elevated at the time insulin is begun. This finding is particularly true in patients with DKA. Therefore, electrolytes should be monitored frequently (every 6–8 hours initially) and fluids and electrolyte content should be altered appropriately. Hypernatremia should be corrected slowly, with a decrease of no more than 0.5 to 1 mEq/L per hour.[19] **Table 2** presents more information on electrolyte supplementation.

Bicarbonate therapy is rarely needed to treat diabetic crises. Bicarbonate therapy administered before potassium replenishment may be detrimental and potentially life-threatening, because it further exacerbates hypokalemia as hydrogen ions moving out of cells to buffer the bicarbonate are exchanged for potassium. Sodium bicarbonate administration can also cause hypernatremia, hyperosmolality, or paradoxic central nervous system (CNS) acidosis, leading to depression, stupor, coma, or death. Bicarbonate therapy is generally reserved for those patients with severe acidemia

Table 2
Electrolyte supplementation guide for diabetic crises

Electrolyte	Form	Dose for Supplementation	Consequence of Severe Deficiency
Potassium	Potassium chloride	20–80 mEq K$^+$/L of fluids (dependent on serum potassium concentration) up to a maximum rate of 0.5 mEq/k$^+$g/h	Hypotension, arrhythmias, weakness, cervical ventroflexion, hypoventilation
Phosphorus	Potassium phosphates (sodium phosphate also available)	0.01–0.2 mmol/kg/h or give 25% of potassium supplementation (see KCl, above) as K-Phos and 75% as KCl	Hemolysis, weakness, obtundation
Magnesium	Magnesium sulfate	0.75–1 mEq/kg given as CRI over 24 h	Refractory hypokalemia, hypotension, obtundation, seizures, weakness, arrhythmias
Bicarbonate	Sodium bicarbonate	Rarely needed as the acidemia corrects with fluid therapy and reversal of ketosis. Slowly give one-quarter to one-third of the following: mEq of bicarbonate required = 0.3 × body weight in kg × (desired plasma bicarbonate mEq/L − measured plasma bicarbonate mEq/L)	Severe acidemia can cause hypotension, arrhythmias, neurologic manifestations

(pH <7.1, bicarbonate <8 mmol/L) and signs consistent with severe metabolic acidosis such as refractory hypotension, arrhythmias, and presence of stupor or coma.

Insulin therapy
Insulin therapy should not begin until the patient's hypovolemia is corrected and the dehydration and electrolytes are improved, typically after at least 4 to 6 hours. In addition, serum potassium levels should be at least 3.5 mmol/L before initiation of insulin. The goals of insulin therapy for the patient with DKA are to slowly decrease blood glucose levels and to inhibit further lipolysis and ketogenesis. The use of long-acting insulin is not recommended in the emergent or critically ill patient with DKA or HHS. Instead, regular insulin (Humulin R, Eli Lilly and Co, Indianapolis IN) should be administered using either an intermittent intramuscular (IM) or IV continuous rate infusion (CRI) protocol (**Table 3**). Use of lispro insulin (Humalog, Eli Lilly and Co, Indianapolis IN) has also been described for treating 6 dogs with DKA.[20] Subcutaneous injections of insulin should not be given, because absorption may be poor or unpredictable in a dehydrated or hypotensive patient. Insulin is less critical for reversal of HHS, because much of the syndrome can be improved just by addressing fluid deficit and GFR. Insulin doses should be reduced by 50% when treating HHS; this facilitates a slow decline in blood glucose and prevents cerebral edema, which could occur because of rapid decline in blood glucose concentration. With both DKA and HHS protocols, the goal is to decrease the glucose levels by no more than 50 to 75 mg/dL/h.[21] Blood glucose should be measured every 2 to 4 hours and the insulin dose adjusted to achieve the

Table 3		
Insulin protocols for DKA and HHS		
Insulin Protocol Type	**Initial Dose for DKA**	**Initial Dose for HHS**	**Subsequent Management**
---	---	---	---
Intermittent IM	0.2–0.25 U/kg of regular insulin, then 0.1 U/kg every 2–4 h	0.1 U/kg of regular insulin, then 0.05 U/kg every 2–4 h	Check blood glucose every 4 h. Goal is to reduce blood glucose by 50–70 mg/dL/h. Subsequent insulin doses are increased or decreased by ~25% to meet this goal. Add dextrose to fluids when glucose <250 mg/dL
IV regular insulin CRI	Dilute 1.1 U/kg (cat) to 2.2 U/kg (dog) of regular insulin in 250 mL 0.9% NaCl. Start this solution at 10 mL/h	Dilute 0.5 U/kg (cat) to 1.0 U/kg (dog) of regular insulin in 250 mL 0.9% NaCl. Start this solution at 10 mL/h	Check blood glucose every 2 h and adjust CRI rate as necessary (see **Table 4**)
IV lispro insulin CRI	Dilute 2.2 U/kg lispro insulin in 250 mL 0.9% NaCl. Start the solution at 10 mL/h	Use of lispro has not been described for treating HHS	Use of lispro insulin has been reported in only 6 dogs with DKA. Check blood glucose every 2 h and adjust CRI rate as necessary (see **Table 4**)

Abbreviation: IV, intravenous.

desired rate of decline (**Table 4** outlines blood glucose monitoring and insulin dose adjustments).

Postcrisis Therapy for DM

Regular insulin protocols should be continued until the animal is eating, at which time the patient is moved to a long-acting insulin such as NPH (neutral protamine Hagedorn [Humulin NPH, Eli Lilly and Co, Indianapolis IN]), protamine zinc (ProZinc, Boehringer Ingelheim Vetmedica Inc, St Joseph MO), or glargine (Lantus, Sanofi-aventis, Bridgewater, NJ). Additional long-term DM therapy should include dietary management and routine patient monitoring. Attentive monitoring, diligent treatment of DM, and diagnosis and treatment of any concurrent diseases are imperative to prevent DKA recurrence.

Prognosis

The prognosis for DKA depends on the severity of the acidemia, the type and severity of underlying disease, and the financial limitations of the pet owner, as well as their long-term commitment to treating a diabetic pet. The death and euthanasia rate for veterinary patients with DKA has been reported to be 7% to 30%.[2,4,22] In 1 study, azotemia, metabolic acidosis, and hyperosmolality were more severe in cats that died.[4] In dogs, nonsurvivors had lower ionized calcium concentration, hematocrit, and venous pH. Base deficit was associated with outcome, such that each 1 mEq/L increase in base deficit yielded a 9% increase in likelihood of discharge from the hospital.[2] Recurrence rates for DKA in dogs and cats are reportedly as high as 42%.[4]

HHS tends to have a higher mortality, because of the severity of the metabolic derangement and underlying diseases. No clear prognostic indicators have been identified in dogs and cats. Cats with HHS reportedly have a survival to discharge of 35.3% but a long-term survival (>2 months) of only 12%.[3]

HYPOGLYCEMIA CAUSED BY EXOGENOUS OR ENDOGENOUS INSULIN EXCESS

Blood glucose concentration is maintained by a balance between insulin and glucagon, cortisol, epinephrine, and growth hormone. When glucose use exceeds glucose production, hypoglycemia ensues. Causes of hypoglycemia can be broadly divided into (1) excess insulin or insulinlike substances, (2) excess glucose use, and (3) decreased glucose production (**Box 1**). Artifactual or spurious measures caused by improper sample handling or glucometer inaccuracy should also be ruled out.

Exogenous Insulin Overdose

Overdoses of exogenous insulin are commonly administered to diabetic pets. These overdoses can occur when insulin is administered in quantities greater than prescribed,

Table 4
Example of an insulin CRI adjustment chart

Blood Glucose (mg/dL)	Insulin CRI Rate (mL/hr)	Maintenance/Replacement Fluid Composition
>250	10	As is
200–250	7	plus 2.5% dextrose
150–199	5	plus 2.5% dextrose
100–149	5	plus 5% dextrose
<100	0	plus 5% dextrose

Box 1
Differentials for hypoglycemia

Excess insulin or Insulin-like Factors

Exogenous insulin overdose

Insulinoma and other neoplasia

Toxins (eg, xylitol, ethanol) and medications (eg, sulfonylureas, β-blockers)

Excess Glucose Utilization

Infection (eg, sepsis, *Babesia*)

Pregnancy

Paraneoplastic syndrome

Extreme exercise (hunting dog) or seizures

Reduced Glucose Production

Neonates

Hepatic dysfunction (eg, portosystemic shunt, hepatitis, lipidosis, cirrhosis, storage diseases)

HA

β-Blockers

Deficiencies of glucose regulating hormones or enzymes

Spurious

Polycythemia or leukocytosis

Collection or storage problems

---

when the prescribed dose is higher than the animal needs, or when the patient is hyporexic and the insulin dose is not reduced. Exogenous insulin overdose should be suspected in any hypoglycemic diabetic patient receiving insulin.

Insulinoma

Insulinoma is a functional insulin-secreting tumor of pancreatic β cells. Most commonly, the tumor is an adenocarcinoma. Insulinomas are most common in middle-aged to older larger breed dogs, although many breeds are affected. There is no apparent gender predilection. Insulinomas have also been reported in cats, albeit rarely.[23–26]

Clinical Signs and Symptoms

Glucose is the obligate energy source for the brain and enters the brain by a concentration gradient-dependent facilitated diffusion. Clinical signs are both neurologic, caused by neuroglycopenia (cerebral hypoglycemia), and systemic, caused by catecholamines released in response to the hypoglycemia. Chronic hypoglycemia can cause hypoglycemic unawareness (lack of clinical signs) as a result of upregulated cerebral glucose uptake. Clinical signs are typically episodic and may be precipitated by fasting, excitement, or exercise.

Diagnosis

The diagnosis of an insulinoma, although rare, should be suspected when hypoglycemia is the only or the major finding in an animal with consistent clinical signs (eg, lethargy, malaise, collapse, weakness, vomiting, tremors, seizures). Blood work is typically normal aside from hypoglycemia. Nonspecific increases in liver enzyme activities and hypokalemia caused by insulin driving potassium into cells may also be seen.[23–26]

Insulinoma is confirmed by identifying a normal or increased insulin concentration on a blood sample taken during a hypoglycemic episode (glucose <60 mg/dL). For patients with episodic hypoglycemia, a supervised fast or multiple blood glucose checks may be necessary to identify hypoglycemia. If insulin levels are equivocal, a calculated amended insulin/glucose ratio (AIGR) <30 mg/dL suggests insulinoma: AIGR = (insulin × 100) ÷ (plasma glucose – 30). Use of the ratio has fallen out of favor, because patients with other causes of hypoglycemia can also have an abnormal ratio.[24,25] Performing the test on at least 4 samples may improve the sensitivity of the test.[27] In addition, low fructosamine concentrations, which reflect the blood glucose concentration over the previous 1 to 2 weeks, have also been identified in dogs with insulinoma.[28–30] Provocative testing such as the glucagon tolerance test, oral glucose tolerance test, tolbutamide tolerance test, and epinephrine stimulation test have been tried but are no more sensitive than other tests and may precipitate hypoglycemia.[26]

Thoracic radiographs and abdominal ultrasonography are used to look for evidence of metastatic disease. Abdominal ultrasonography is also used to try to identify a mass in the pancreas, although it is not a particularly sensitive method and failure to identify a mass does not rule out the presence of insulinoma.[31] Computed tomography, magnetic resonance imaging, and scintigraphy can also be considered as diagnostic aids.[31] Surgical exploration may be used in an attempt to identify the insulinoma.

Emergency Management of a Hypoglycemic Crisis

For symptomatic hypoglycemic patients, the most rapid and effective treatment is dextrose (0.5–1 mL/kg of 50% dextrose, diluted, IV). However, in animals with suspected or confirmed insulinomas, boluses of dextrose should be used with caution, because they may stimulate release of more insulin from the tumor, leading to a vicious cycle of dextrose bolus followed by rebound hypoglycemia. An infusion of dextrose may be tried in lieu of or after a bolus to maintain blood glucose concentration. Dextrose infusions are formulated by adding 50% dextrose to a maintenance or replacement crystalloid solution, typically to make a final dextrose concentration of 2.5% to 5% (add 50–100 mL of 50% dextrose to a 1-L bag of crystalloids). Dextrose infusion may need to be continued for hours to days after exogenous insulin overdose, depending on the type of insulin and magnitude of the overdose. Once the patient is able to eat, small frequent meals that are low in simple carbohydrates and high in protein, fat and complex carbohydrates help maintain euglycemia. Blood glucose should be monitored every 2 to 4 hours to ensure adequate and not excessive supplementation and determine when it is possible to taper off the dextrose infusion.

Glucocorticoids, such as prednisone or dexamethasone, antagonize insulin effects and stimulate gluconeogenesis, and this may help stabilize the blood glucose concentration in the patient with an insulinoma. An infusion of glucagon is also an effective method for treating animals with refractory hypoglycemia caused by insulinoma or exogenous insulin overdose.[32] **Table 5** presents information about dosing.

The goal of emergent therapy is to eliminate clinical signs of hypoglycemia; it may not be necessary or even possible to return the glucose to reference range. Neuroglycopenic symptoms should resolve or markedly improve within a few minutes of resolution of the hypoglycemia; although prolonged, severe neuroglycopenia can cause irreparable neuronal damage.

Table 5
Drugs for use in endocrine emergencies

Drug	Dose/Route	Indication/Mechanism of Action	Comments
Amlodipine	Dog: 0.1–0.4 mg/kg by mouth every 12–24 h Cat: 0.625–1.25 mg per cat by mouth every 24 h	For chronic management of hypertension Calcium channel blocker, arterial vasodilator	Start low and titrate upwards, if needed In dogs, often used in conjunction with angiotensin-converting enzyme inhibitor for managing chronic hypertension
Atenolol	Dog: 0.25–1 mg/kg by mouth every 12 h Cat: 6.25–12.5 mg per cat by mouth every 12–24 h	For control of arrhythmias in hyperthyroid storm, possibly in pheochromocytoma Selective β_1-blocker	In pheochromocytoma, use only after complete α receptor blockade or could precipitate hypertensive crisis
Dexamethasone	0.1–0.5 mg/kg IV as initial dose, then 0.05–0.1 mg/kg IV every 12 h	Antagonizes insulin, increases blood glucose in hypoglycemia Glucocorticoid supplementation for HA	Does not interfere with cortisol assay Doses up to 2.0 mg/kg have been reported; this is likely excessive because it is equivalent to ~14 mg/kg prednisone
Dextrose	Bolus: 0.5–1 mL/kg of 50% dextrose (diluted), followed by CRI of 2.5%–5% dextrose (or more) as needed in fluids	Provides source of glucose to treat hypoglycemia Stimulates insulin secretion in hyperkalemia	Avoid dextrose bolus in patients with suspected insulinoma Solutions >5% are ideally administered via central line
Diazoxide	Start with 5 mg/kg by mouth twice daily; increase as needed to a maximum of 30 mg/kg by mouth twice daily to control clinical signs	Inhibits pancreatic insulin secretion For chronic medical management of insulinoma	
Desoxycorticosterone pivalate (DOCP)	Start with 2.2 mg/kg IM or subcutaneously every 25 d. Titrate subsequent dose and interval based on electrolyte monitoring	Mineralocorticoid replacement for HA	For chronic therapy. Give with prednisone because has no glucocorticoid activity Must not be given IV
Esmolol	CRI of 10–200 µg/kg/min Can be preceded by loading dose of 0.25–0.5 mg/kg IV over 2 min	Selective β_1-blocker For control of arrhythmias in thyroid storm, possibly in pheochromocytoma	In pheochromocytoma, use only after complete α receptor blockade or could precipitate hypertensive crisis

Drug	Dosage	Indication	Comments
Fludrocortisone (Florinef)	Start at 0.01 mg/kg by mouth every 12 h, titrate upwards every 1–2 wk as needed (based on electrolytes) until stable	For HA: provides both mineralocorticoids and glucocorticoid	Patient may or may not also require routine daily prednisone
Furosemide	1–4 mg/kg IV every 1–2 h during crisis or 0.66 mg/kg/h as CRI	Loop diuretic for treating pulmonary edema in heart failure, may be needed to treat patients with thyroid storm with secondary CHF	Chronic therapy: start 2 mg/kg by mouth every 12 h (dogs) or 6.25 mg/cat by mouth every 12–24 h (cats) adjusted as needed to control edema
Glucagon	Bolus 50 ng/kg IV followed by CRI of 5–10 ng/kg/min (up to 40 ng/kg/min) to effect	For acute management of hypoglycemic crisis caused by insulinoma or insulin overdose. Stimulates glycogenolysis and gluconeogenesis	Reconstitute based on manufacturer's instructions to a 1000-ng/mL solution
Hydrocortisone	0.3–0.5 mg/kg/h as IV infusion for a few hours or give 2–4 mg/kg IV every 8 h	Glucocorticoid with mild mineralocorticoid effects, for use in acute hypoadrenal crisis	Use only after ACTH stimulation test has been completed
Ipodate sodium or calcium	50 mg by mouth every 12 h or 100–200 mg per cat by mouth every 24 h	For reduction of thyroid hormone secretion in hyperthyroid storm Blocks conversion of T_4 to T_3 Blocks T_3 receptors	May be available only from compounding pharmacy
Methimazole (Tapazole)	Start with 2.5 mg by mouth or to the inner pinna (using transdermal product) every 12–24 h	For treatment of hyperthyroidism, inhibits thyroid hormone synthesis	Treatment of hyperthyroidism decreases GFR, monitor for azotemia
Nitroprusside	Start 0.5 μg/kg/min, titrate upwards to desired blood pressure (typically <200 mm Hg, reducing systolic blood pressure by ~25% over 4 h)	For acute hypertensive crisis in thyroid storm or pheochromocytoma Nitrates cause vasodilation independent of catecholamines	Continuous direct or frequent indirect blood pressure monitoring is essential
Phenoxybenzamine	Start with 0.25 mg/kg by mouth twice a day; increase dose gradually every few days until signs of hypotension or adverse drug reaction occur up to a maximum dosage of 2.5 mg/kg by mouth every 12 h	For acute hypertensive crisis in thyroid storm or pheochromocytoma α-Blocker	Takes multiple days to reach maximum receptor blockade. Allow 2 wk of therapy before surgery

(continued on next page)

Table 5
(continued)

Drug	Dose/Route	Indication/Mechanism of Action	Comments
Prednisone Prednisolone	1. For HA: 0.1–0.22 mg/kg, then taper to lowest dose needed to control clinical signs 2. For insulinoma: 0.25–0.5 mg/kg by mouth every 12 h	1. Glucocorticoid supplementation for HA 2. Antagonize insulin, increases blood glucose in insulinoma	1. Use only after ACTH stimulation test has been completed Prednisolone is preferred for cats
Propranolol	For susceptible arrhythmias: 0.02 mg/kg IV slowly Dog: 0.1–0.2 mg/kg by mouth every 8 h Cat: 2.5 mg by mouth (up to 10 mg) per cat every 8–12 h	Nonselective β-blocker Used to treat arrhythmias in hyperthyroid storm, possibly in pheochromocytoma	In pheochromocytoma, use only after complete α-receptor blockade or could precipitate hypertensive crisis
Thyroid hormone (levothyroxine)	For myxedema coma: 5 μg/kg (0.005 mg/kg) IV every 12 h during crisis For long-term management: 0.02 mg/kg by mouth every 12 h	For thyroid supplementation in dogs with hypothyroidism	Preferentially use IV for hypothyroid crisis/myxedema coma. If IV is unavailable, give orally or via a nasogastric tube

Data from Plumb DC. Plumb's veterinary drug handbook. 7th edition. Stockholm (WI): PharmaVet; 2011.

Postcrisis Management of Insulinoma

Surgical excision is the treatment of choice for insulinomas, because it results in the longest survival times. However, metastatic disease is evident at surgery in up to 50% of cases, and occult metastasis is present in most dogs. Thus, surgery is considered a palliative procedure for all animals, even when a single lesion is initially identified.[23,24,26] The primary tumor is not always identifiable at surgery. When found, the primary tumor and suspected metastatic lesions should be removed, if possible, and submitted for histopathology.

Medical management for patients not undergoing surgery or those with metastatic disease may include dietary management, glucocorticoids, and chemotherapy. Small, frequent meals that are low in simple carbohydrates and high in protein, fat and complex carbohydrates help maintain euglycemia. Glucocorticoids such as prednisone, hydrocortisone, or dexamethasone (see **Table 5**) antagonize insulin effects and stimulate gluconeogenesis and are indicated for long-term management of the insulinoma patient. Diazoxide (10–60 mg/kg by mouth divided every 12 hours to effect) inhibits pancreatic secretion, stimulates gluconeogenesis and glycogenolysis, and inhibits cellular uptake of glucose. Chemotherapy with streptozocin (which destroys pancreatic β-cells), octreotide (which suppresses insulin synthesis and release), and alloxan (a β-cell cytotoxin) are also management options.

Prognosis

The prognosis for insulinoma is dependent on extent of disease or metastasis and on management choices. Survival is from 74 days up to a median of more than 3.5 years for dogs undergoing surgery followed by medical management after recurrence.[33,34]

HYPOADRENOCORTICISM

Hypoadrenocorticism (HA), also called Addison's disease, is classically a deficiency of cortisol and mineralocorticoids, although isolated cortisol deficiency can also occur. Primary HA occurs secondary to destruction of the adrenal cortex either because of immune-mediated destruction (most common in dogs), neoplasia, infection, hemorrhage, iatrogenic causes (eg, mitotane, trilostane), or hemorrhage. Most patients with HA have deficiencies in both cortisol and mineralocorticoids. Secondary HA is the absence of cortisol, which occurs when the pituitary fails to produce adrenocorticotropin hormone (ACTH), which stimulates adrenal cortisol production. These patients are deficient only in cortisol. Secondary HA is typically caused by destruction or damage to the pituitary such as by neoplasia, trauma, or infection or inflammation. Both tertiary HA, which is lack of corticotrophin-releasing hormone secretion, and isolated mineralocorticoid deficiency are rare.[1]

Cortisol and mineralocorticoids have varied and important functions in the body. The mineralocorticoid aldosterone is part of the renin, angiotensin, aldosterone system, which is activated by hypovolemia, hypotension, and low blood sodium concentration. Aldosterone is vital to maintaining electrolyte concentrations by stimulating sodium and chloride reabsorption and potassium excretion in the cortical collecting duct of the renal tubule. Water follows the sodium and results in expansion of vascular volume. Cortisol is also important for maintaining water balance and vascular volume. Cortisol has multiple effects on the vasculature, including maintaining endothelial integrity, vascular permeability, and sensitivity to catecholamines, thus helping maintain blood pressure. In addition, cortisol helps maintain blood glucose concentration by stimulating gluconeogenesis and lipolysis and antagonizing insulin. Cortisol suppresses inflammation and is trophic for the bone marrow, stimulating erythropoiesis.[1,35]

HA is most common in young to middle-aged dogs and is rare in cats. Females are affected more often than males, except in certain breeds, in which they are affected with equal frequency. Although dogs of any breed can be affected, certain breeds seem to have an increased risk or genetic predisposition, including Nova Scotia duck tolling retrievers, poodles, Portuguese water dogs, West Highland white terriers, and English springer spaniels.[36–38]

Clinical Signs and Symptoms

HA is often called the Great Pretender because the spectrum of clinical signs is nonspecific and can be consistent with multiple other disease processes. Clinical signs can be intermittent or waxing and waning in nearly half of the reported cases. Although most dogs have chronic clinical signs, an acute exacerbation may be precipitated by a stressful event, such as a trip to the groomer or veterinarian, a stay at a boarding facility, or changes in the household.

Clinical signs primarily include lethargy, weakness, PU/PD, and gastrointestinal (GI) signs, including anorexia, vomiting, diarrhea, or abdominal pain. Tremors/shaking, collapse, melena, hematochezia, and hematemesis may also be seen.[39,40]

Physical examination findings are dependent on the stage of disease and range from simple dehydration to signs of hypovolemic and vasodilatory shock, including muffled heart sounds, weak pulses, prolonged capillary refill time, hypotension, hypothermia, and severe dehydration. These findings are a product of fluid losses from the GI tract, renal water losses that accompany renal sodium wasting, and reduced vascular sensitivity to catecholamines. Dogs with mineralocorticoid deficiency may be bradycardic because of hyperkalemia, and an electrocardiogram may show evidence of this hyperkalemia (eg, blunted or absent P waves, tented T waves, and widened QRS complexes).

Diagnosis

Attaining a definitive diagnosis of HA requires adrenal testing, although history and routine blood work may provide a high degree of suspicion (**Table 6**). Electrolyte abnormalities associated with HA include hyperkalemia, hyponatremia, and hypochloremia, although they are not unique to this disorder.[40] These abnormalities occur because the aldosterone deficiency prevents normal sodium reabsorption and potassium excretion in the cortical collecting duct. Chloride changes typically accompany and parallel sodium abnormalities.

Testing for HA

The electrolyte abnormalities give rise to the popular Na/K ratio as a screening test for HA. An Na/K ratio less than 27:1 has a sensitivity of 70% to 89% and specificity of 94% to 97% for HA, whereas lower ratios are more specific for the diagnosis.[41,42] A recent study reported that combining Na/K ratio and lymphocyte count was consistently more sensitive and specific when compared with either variable alone, suggesting that this combination may be a good screening test.[41] Although most dogs in the study had normal lymphocyte counts, dogs with HA had significantly higher counts (median 2.38 [range 0.80–8.20] $\times$ 10^3 cells/μL) than those without HA (median 1.07 [range 0–6.00] $\times$ 10^3 cells/μL).[41]

The gold standard for diagnosis of HA remains the ACTH stimulation test. To perform an ACTH stimulation test, a baseline blood sample is obtained, 5 μg/kg (maximum of 250 μg/dog) of synthetic ACTH (cosyntropin) is given IM or IV, and a second sample is taken an hour later; cortisol concentrations are measured on both samples. Dogs with HA have either a severely blunted or absent response to ACTH.

Table 6
Common clinicopathologic abnormalities in dogs with HA

Clinicopathologic Abnormality	Reasons for Abnormalities
Anemia, normochromic, normocytic, nonregenerative	Loss of red blood cells via GI hemorrhage; lack of steroids contributes (cortisol stimulates erythroid production)
Lack of stress leukogram (ie, neutrophil count not increased, may have eosinophilia or lymphocytosis)	Lack of steroids. A stress leukogram is expected in an animal as sick as an Addisonian
High alanine aminotransferase level	Poor perfusion of liver (shock)
Hypoalbuminemia	Probably multifactorial: GI losses, decreased synthesis, decreased nutrient intake and absorption
Hypoglycemia	Cortisol is needed to stimulate gluconeogenesis and glycogen storage. Patients are not typically symptomatic for hypoglycemia
Hypercalcemia (total), with or without ionized hypercalcemia	Exact mechanism unknown, may be caused by hemoconcentration, decreased GFR, and decreased renal calcium excretion. Resolves with supportive care, no specific therapy required
Increased blood urea nitrogen (BUN) and creatinine	Dehydration and hypovolemia; increased BUN can also result from GI bleeding
Hyperphosphatemia	Decreased renal excretion as a result of dehydration and hypovolemia
Dilute urine (specific gravity <1.030 in face of azotemia)	Renal sodium wasting

Basal cortisol levels can also be used as a diagnostic tool for HA. In 1 study, basal cortisol lower than 1 μg/dL was 100% sensitive and 98% specific for HA; basal cortisol lower than 2 μg/dL was 100% sensitive but only 78% specific.[43] Ratios of endogenous cortisol/ACTH and aldosterone/renin have been found to provide specific diagnosis of primary hypocortisolism and hypoaldosteronism. Whereas plasma concentrations of these individual hormones overlapped between healthy dogs and dogs with HA, the ratios of endogenous cortisol/ACTH and aldosterone/renin identified each group without overlap.[44]

Imaging
There are no specific radiographic abnormalities in animals with HA. If thoracic radiographs are taken before completing resuscitation, they may show signs of hypovolemia, including microcardia, reduced pulmonary vasculature size, or small caudal vena cava size.[40] Megaesophagus has also been reported in dogs with HA.

Abdominal ultrasonography may identify the presence of small adrenal glands. Dogs with HA have significantly thinner adrenal glands than healthy dogs and dogs with non-HA illness. A left adrenal gland that measured less than 3.2 mm thick was highly suggestive of HA in 28 of 29 dogs.[45]

Emergency Management of HA
Therapy for HA is aimed at reversing the hypovolemia, shock, hyperkalemia, and hypoglycemia and then providing replacement hormones.

The cause of death for patients with HA is typically the result of hypovolemic shock, so aggressive fluid resuscitation is imperative. A shock bolus (20–30 mL/kg, IV) of a replacement crystalloid such as Normosol-R, LRS, 0.9% NaCl, or Plasmalyte-A, is indicated. Many sources advocate use of 0.9% NaCl (with 154 mEq Na/L) as the preferred resuscitation solution; however, multiple cases of myelinolysis have occurred in dogs with HA that had rapid correction of their hyponatremia.[46–48] Several days after the rapid increase in sodium, myelinolysis manifests as neurologic signs, including lethargy, weakness, ataxia, hypermetria, and trouble swallowing, which may take weeks to months to resolve, if at all. A lower sodium resuscitation fluid, such as LRS (with 130 mEq Na/L) may be indicated to prevent this complication. Regardless of fluid chosen, serum sodium should not increase by more than 0.5 mEq/L/h in a patient with chronic hyponatremia, particularly when the initial sodium is 120 mEq/L or lower.

Hyperkalemia associated with HA typically improves with fluid resuscitation alone. However, in patients with life-threatening hyperkalemia (manifesting bradycardia or arrhythmias), more specific, rapidly acting therapy such as calcium gluconate (as a cardioprotective agent) or insulin, dextrose, bicarbonate, or a β-agonist (to lower potassium levels) are indicated. **Table 7** presents more information regarding these therapies.

In conjunction with fluid therapy, supplementation with glucocorticoids is indicated for any animal suspected of having an HA crisis. Glucocorticoids help reduce GI signs and, more importantly, stabilize the vascular volume and blood pressure. Dexamethasone is typically used until the ACTH stimulation is completed, because dexamethasone is not measured in the cortisol assay. Hydrocortisone or prednisone/prednisolone can also be considered once adrenal testing is completed (see **Table 5** for more information).

Additional supportive and symptomatic therapy for GI complications such as gastric acid reducers (eg, histamine 2 blockers, proton pump inhibitors), sucralfate, and antiemetics is indicated. For animals with GI hemorrhage, antibiotic coverage (eg, ampicillin, 22 mg/kg IV every 8 hours) may reduce risk of bacterial translocation across the compromised mucosal surface.

Postcrisis Management of HA

Once the patient has been stabilized and the results of the ACTH stimulation have returned, long-term therapy can begin. Glucocorticoid deficiency is typically managed with oral prednisone and titrated to the lowest dose needed; the physiologic glucocorticoid dose needed to control HA is lower than traditional antiinflammatory doses. (See **Table 5** for dosing.) Patients usually also need extra supplementation at times of stress, such as during periods of illness, hospitalization, travel, or changes in living conditions.

Mineralocorticoid-deficient patients also require mineralocorticoid replacement; however, the need for supplementation in the midst of the HA crisis is debated. Most patients can be stabilized with intensive fluid resuscitation and glucocorticoids alone; some clinicians prefer to initiate mineralocorticoid therapy during the crisis. Fludrocortisone (Florinef) is a short-acting synthetic glucocorticoid that also has mineralocorticoid activity; it can be given orally or rectally. Desoxycorticosterone pivalate (DOCP, Percorten-V) is a long-acting parenteral mineralocorticoid given IM once per month. (See **Table 5** for dosing.) Complications are unlikely if DOCP is administered to a suspected Addisonian that is later determined to have a normal ACTH stimulation test.[49] Dogs receiving DOCP usually require concurrent prednisone therapy, whereas those receiving fludrocortisone often do not require daily glucocorticoid supplementation.

Table 7
Treatments for hyperkalemia

Treatment	Dose	Mechanism	Comments
IV replacement crystalloid fluids	Many	Dilution of potassium, diuresis	Low concentration of K^+ in balanced replacement crystalloids should not worsen hyperkalemia
Calcium gluconate, 10% solution	0.5–1.5 mL/kg over 10–20 min	Rapidly cardioprotective by increasing the threshold potential	Does not lower potassium, protects heart, whereas other methods are used to reduce potassium; monitor electrocardiograph and slow or discontinue infusion if arrhythmias occur
Regular insulin	0.25–0.5 U/kg IV or IM given with dextrose bolus (4 mL of 50% dextrose IV per unit insulin given)	Insulin stimulates obligate cotransport of glucose and potassium into cells	Rapid onset. Must also supplement dextrose in fluids until insulin effect wears off
Dextrose	0.5–1 mL/kg bolus followed by CRI of 2.5%–5% dextrose solution	Stimulate endogenous insulin production, also maintains blood glucose after exogenous insulin administration	Also addresses hypoglycemia common with HA
Albuterol (β-agonist)	Cat: 2 puffs (90 μg/puff) Dog weighing 30 kg (60 lb): 0.5 mL of 0.5% solution nebulized in 4 mL of saline	Cat: Using mask and spacer device, breathe 7–10 s	Best dose for hyperkalemia unknown, this dose is based on asthmatic therapy Dose can be repeated every half an hour for 2–4 h in crisis
Sodium Bicarbonate	1–3 mEq/kg over 30 min	Potassium moves into the cell in exchange for hydrogen as pH increases	Slow onset of action

Subsequent doses of DOCP are determined by serum sodium and potassium levels 12 days after the first dose; if hyponatremia or hyperkalemia is present, the next dose is increased by 5% to 10%, and vice versa. Electrolytes should be measured again at 25 days; if hyponatremia or hyperkalemia is present, the interval until the next dose is decreased to 24 days. If hypernatremia or hypokalemia is present, the interval until the next dose can be extended to 26 days. These rechecks are continued in this way until the optimal dose is identified, after which rechecks can be extended to 2 to 4 times yearly in otherwise normal, well-controlled animals. For fludrocortisone therapy, electrolytes should be monitored every 1 to 2 weeks initially and therapy should be tailored based on results. It is not uncommon for dogs to require steady increases in fludrocortisone dose over the first year or so.

Prognosis

With intensive fluid resuscitation followed by committed and attentive follow-up care and hormonal supplementation, most patients with HA live normal lives.[40]

PHEOCHROMOCYTOMA

Pheochromocytoma is an uncommon tumor of the catecholamine-secreting chromaffin cells of the adrenal medulla reported in dogs, cats, and other species. Pheochromocytoma can be malignant or locally invasive and has been reported in a multitude of metastatic sites.[50–53] Pheochromocytoma has also been reported in dogs with concurrent hyperadrenocorticism.[54]

Clinical Signs and Symptoms

Clinical signs and physical examination findings associated with pheochromocytoma are often intermittent, because they occur during surges of catecholamine secretion, and include weakness, collapse, tachypnea, tachyarrhythmias, hypertension, and seizures.[50–53] Retinal or retroperitoneal hemorrhage and epistaxis have also been reported.[55–57] Acute presentation of pheochromocytoma is usually associated with severe hypertension, hemorrhage, or arrhythmias, which require emergent intervention.

Presumptive diagnosis is based on history, clinical signs, and presence of an adrenal mass identified on ultrasonography. Invasion into the caudal vena cava is also frequently reported.[51,52,56,58] Plasma and urine catecholamines, metanephrines, and ratios of these (particularly the urine normetadrenaline/creatinine ratio) show promise for diagnosis of pheochromocytoma but are not readily available.[59–61] Most often, definitive diagnosis is via histopathology of surgically excised tumors.

Emergency Management of Pheochromocytoma

α-Blockade using the α_1-antagonist phenoxybenzamine reduces hypertension that is the result of catecholamine-mediated vasoconstriction. Because it takes several days for maximal α -blockade, severe hypertension manifesting with neurologic signs, retinal detachment, or hemorrhage requires more rapid intervention. Fast-acting vasodilator drugs such as nitroprusside or hydralazine can be used; both drugs have a rapid onset of action, and nitroprusside can also be rapidly titrated to effect. Other blood pressure-lowering drugs such as amlodipine and benazepril/enalapril do not lower the blood pressure rapidly enough in a crisis but may be useful long-term. In human medicine, magnesium sulfate has been advocated as a treatment of hypertension for patients with pheochromocytoma under anesthesia or in crisis.[62,63] Magnesium blocks catecholamine receptors and also inhibits the release of catecholamines from the adrenal medulla and peripheral nerve terminals. Magnesium also causes vasodilation and has some antiarrhythmic properties. There are no data on the efficacy of magnesium for treating pheochromocytoma in veterinary medicine. (See **Table 5** for dosing.)

Arrhythmias seen with pheochromocytoma may include atrial tachycardia, ventricular premature contractions, ventricular tachycardia, and atrioventricular block. Use of β-blockers to treat arrhythmias should be avoided until α-blockade is in full effect. Early β-blockade prevents β_2-mediated vasodilation, thus leaving α-mediated vasoconstriction unopposed and possibly precipitating a hypertensive crisis. Magnesium may be useful in treating pheochromocytoma-induced arrhythmias.[62] Depending on the type of arrhythmia, lidocaine, procainamide, and diltiazem can be tried if arrhythmias are ongoing and life-threatening. Severe retroperitoneal hemorrhage or epistaxis may require shock fluid therapy to restore circulating volume and red blood cell transfusions to improve blood oxygen content.

Postcrisis Management of Pheochromocytoma

Surgical excision of the tumor is the treatment of choice, although perioperative morbidity and mortality can be high.[50–52] Hypertension, hypotension, extreme tachycardia, and arrhythmias have all been documented during surgery and anesthesia for pheochromocytoma excision. Dogs treated with phenyoxybenzamine for 2 weeks before surgery had decreased mortality compared with dogs that were not pretreated with phenoxybenzamine (13% vs 48%, respectively).[50] Other factors associated with increased mortality in 1 or more studies include longer surgical time, intraoperative arrhythmias,[50] large tumors, and acute adrenal hemorrhage.[64]

HYPERTHYROIDISM: THYROTOXICOSIS AND THYROID STORM

Hyperthyroidism in the cat is typically the result of a functional thyroxine (T_4)-secreting thyroid adenoma. Less commonly, cats and dogs present with functional thyroid adenocarcinomas. Thyroid storm (TS) is a rare, acute exacerbation of thyrotoxicosis marked by fever and CNS, cardiovascular, and GI or hepatic signs. This constellation of clinical signs is well recognized in human medicine as TS. TS is a less well-described entity in veterinary medicine, although feline hyperthyroid crises often include 1 or more of these abnormalities.

What causes an animal to progress from being hyperthyroid to TS is not clear. As in other endocrinopathies, there is believed to be a catalyst, although it is not always recognized. Infections, other endocrinopathies, concurrent diseases, and antithyroid treatments, including radioiodine therapy, methimazole, or surgery, may contribute to development of TS. In 1 human study, TS was most common in newly diagnosed hyperthyroid patients, with most cases occurring in the first year of treatment. In addition, TS seemed to be more common in patients who took their antithyroid medications irregularly or stopped taking them altogether.[65]

The levels of total and free thyroid hormones in patients with TS are not different from those in patients with hyperthyroidism without crisis.[66,67] It is hypothesized that a rapid change in thyroid level, an alteration in thyroid-binding hormone number or affinity, or an increased sensitivity to catecholamines may contribute to development of TS.[68]

Clinical Signs and Symptoms

Thyroid hormone is instrumental in function of most tissues in the body and increases metabolic rate and oxygen consumption by most tissues. Clinical signs of thyrotoxicosis in the cat involve the respiratory, cardiovascular, and neurologic systems.

Thyroid hormone increases the number and sensitivity of β-receptors in the heart and acts as a positive inotrope and chronotrope, which may account for some of the cardiovascular signs associated with thyroid excess and TS. Tachycardia, arrhythmias, gallop rhythm, and murmurs may all be identified in thyrotoxic cats. Thyroid hormone also sensitizes the vasculature to catecholamines, contributing to hypertension. Tachypnea, respiratory distress, and abnormal auscultation may be seen as a consequence of heart failure. Hypertension can lead to neurologic signs, including acute blindness from retinal hemorrhage or retinal detachment, seizures, depressed mentation or stupor, and sudden death.[69,70] Weakness and cervical ventroflexion can be seen secondary to severe hypokalemia,[71] and loss of limb function as a result of thromboembolism has also been reported.[72] Other clinical findings associated with hyperthyroidism include weight loss, polyphagia, increased activity, and enlargement of the thyroid gland.

The definition of TS in human medicine includes presence of GI or hepatic signs. In 1 human study, presence of nausea, vomiting, or diarrhea was not frequent in patients with non-TS thyrotoxicosis. The significance of this finding is unclear in veterinary medicine, because many cats with hyperthyroidism have GI signs as a presenting complaint.[73]

Diagnosis

Presumptive diagnosis of TS is made by identifying compatible clinical signs in an animal with known or suspected hyperthyroidism. Some presenting with TS may already be undergoing therapy for hyperthyroidism, so the index of suspicion should be heightened for those patients. Hyperthyroidism can be confirmed by identifying an increased total T_4, increased free T_4 with a high normal total T_4, or failure to suppress with triiodothyronine (T_3) suppression test. Technetium scan of the thyroid is also an accurate way of diagnosing hyperthyroidism and identifying ectopic tissue.[74,75]

To rule out other causes of crisis and identify any underlying catalysts for TS, a complete patient evaluation is warranted, including a CBC, chemistry, urinalysis, urine culture, retroviral testing, and thoracic and abdominal imaging. Clinicopathologic abnormalities are as expected for any case of hyperthyroidism, and may include mild erythrocytosis, macrocytosis, a stress leukogram, increased liver enzyme activities, hypokalemia, and mild hyperglycemia. Thoracic radiographs may reveal cardiomegaly or biatrial enlargement, with or without evidence of CHF, pulmonary edema, or pleural effusion. Echocardiogram may show left ventricular and interventricular hypertrophy and atrial enlargement.[76,77]

Emergency Management of Thyrotoxicosis/TS

Treatment of thyrotoxic crisis or TS must address the systemic manifestations of thyrotoxicosis as well as reduce the hormone excess. In the midst of a thyroid crisis, eliminating clinical signs is accomplished most rapidly by reducing tachycardia, tachyarrhythmias, and hypertension. Arrhythmias in TS can typically be treated via β-blockade using esmolol, atenolol, or propranolol. Esmolol is a short-acting selective $β_1$-blocker that must be administered as CRI. Atenolol is also a selective $β_1$-blocker, but only available orally. Propranolol is a nonselective β-blocker that can be given both injectably and orally. β-Blockers should be used with caution in patients with CHF, because β-blockade can reduce cardiac contractility and exacerbate CHF. A hypertensive crisis may require a rapidly acting vasodilatory drug such as nitroprusside or hydralazine. Both can be given injectably; nitroprusside is give as a CRI and is titrated to effect. Amlodipine takes several days to reach maximal effect, so it is effective for treating hypertension only in the noncrisis state. See **Table 5** for drug doses.

Reducing thyroid levels is crucial for effective treatment of TS. Methimazole prevents synthesis of new thyroid hormone and can be given orally, rectally, and transdermally.[78,79] Plasmapheresis or plasma exchange could also be used to reduce blood thyroid hormone levels, but these are not readily available.[80] Because large quantities of hormone can be stored in the thyroid, additional treatment is aimed at reducing hormone release from the thyroid gland. Iodine, in the form of sodium or potassium iodide or potassium iodate, reduces thyroid hormone concentrations by inhibiting oxidation of iodide in the thyroid gland, formation of thyroid hormone within follicles, and secretion of hormone from the gland.[81,82] These drugs must be given at least 1 hour after methimazole to prevent increased iodine uptake and subsequent hormone production by the thyroid. However, when given in conjunction with antithyroid medications, the thyroid levels decrease dramatically. Iopanoic acid (50–100 mg, twice a day, by mouth) decreases conversion of T_4 to T_3 and decreased mean serum T_3 concentrations by more than 50% in 1 study.[83] Ipodate (sodium or calcium) also decreases conversion of T_4 to T_3 and may also block T_3 receptors and effects of thyroid-stimulating hormone (TSH).[82] It is not available commercially, but may be available via compounding pharmacies. See **Table 5** for dosing.

Symptomatic and supportive care is the final phase of treatment of TS and may continue after the crisis is past. Concurrent cardiac failure may require oxygen therapy, furosemide diuresis, and venodilation with nitroglycerin paste. Additional cardiac medications such as pimobendan, an angiotensin-converting enzyme inhibitor (eg, benazepril, enalapril) and a calcium channel blocker (eg, diltiazem) may also be indicated based on echocardiographic evaluation. β-Blockade is continued at least until the hyperthyroidism is definitively treated. Cats that remain hypertensive after the TS crisis should be treated with an antihypertensive drug such as amlodipine, because β-blockade alone is not sufficient to treat ongoing hypertension.[84]

Miscellaneous therapies that may be indicated for TS include antithrombotic therapy and electrolyte or dextrose supplementation. Anticoagulants, such as heparin or warfarin, or antiplatelet drugs, such as aspirin or clopidogrel, may be indicated for cats with evidence of thrombosis or spontaneous contrast in the atria on echocardiogram. Potassium supplementation (IV or by mouth) may be required to treat hypokalemia. IV fluids containing dextrose may help replenish hepatic glycogen levels.[68] Any concurrent disease processes should also be addressed, because they may have contributed to development of TS.

Postcrisis Management of Hyperthyroidism

Once the thyrotoxic crisis has passed, hyperthyroidism must be managed long-term. Chronic methimazole therapy, radioactive iodine (I^{131}), surgical thyroidectomy, and dietary management are all possible strategies.[79] There are no data in veterinary medicine regarding which of these may be the best or least ideal therapy in regards to preventing recurrence of TS. In human medicine, definitive therapy with radioactive iodine or surgery is preferred.[68] Hypertension may also require chronic management. Thyrotoxic cardiac changes are largely reversible with appropriate treatment of the hyperthyroidism, and patients with historical thyrotoxicity-induced CHF may be amenable to withdrawal of cardiac medications.

Prognosis

Prognosis for a true TS is unknown for veterinary patients. Mortality in humans is reportedly 10% to 75%.[65,67,68] Early recognition and appropriate, timely interventions are likely imperative for a positive outcome.

HYPOTHYROIDISM: MYXEDEMA COMA

As reviewed earlier, thyroid hormone plays pivotal roles in the body. It governs the metabolic rate and is essential to normal function of most tissues, including the neurologic and cardiovascular systems. Severe hypothyroidism rarely manifests as myxedema coma, a life-threatening condition marked by altered mental status, hypothermia, and mucinous skin edema.[68,85–87] Hypotension, hypoventilation, and other signs of hypothyroidism may also be present (**Box 2**).[88] As with many endocrine crises, myxedema coma is often precipitated by another condition, such as an infection,

Box 2
Clinical signs associated with hypothyroidism

Reduced Metabolism

Weight gain[a]

Weakness, lethargy[a]

Exercise intolerance

Cold intolerance

Neurologic/Muscular

Peripheral neuropathy

Paraparesis/tetraparesis

Lameness (unilateral, forelimb)

Variable cranial nerve dysfunction

Central vestibular signs

Megaesophagus

Laryngeal paralysis

Cognitive dysfunction

Ophthalmic

Corneal lipid

Corneal ulceration

Lipid aqueous

Lipemia retinalis

Retinal detachment

Cardiovascular

Sinus bradycardia

Reduced cardiac contractility

Reduced electrocardiograph voltages, inverted T waves

Atherosclerosis

Vascular events

Dermatologic

Bilateral, symmetric alopecia[a]

Hyperpigmentation

Scaly skin

Seborrhea sicca

Seborrhea oleosa

Pyoderma

Reproductive (Possibly)

Unpredictable cycling in females

Spontaneous abortions

Weak or stillborn pups

Low libido

Testicular atrophy

Low sperm count

[a] The most common clinical findings.

nonthyroidal illness, certain drugs, diet, or even cold weather, that overwhelms the normal compensatory mechanisms of the body.[68]

The term myxedema coma is a misnomer, because coma is rare. Both central and peripheral neurologic deficits may be seen in hypothyroidism, although peripheral deficits are more common. CNS deficits can occur in hypothyroidism as a result of myxedema coma, atherosclerosis, hyperlipidemia, or presence of a pituitary tumor causing secondary hypothyroidism. The most common central neurologic manifestations include weakness and dull mentation or stupor caused by cerebral edema. Concurrent dilutional hyponatremia may also contribute to neurologic signs. Profound weakness and cerebral edema can also contribute to hypoventilation and hypoxemia.[89]

Hypothermia occurs because the metabolic rate decreases in the absence of thyroid hormone, and this subsequently reduces the amount of heat generated as a by-product of cellular respiration. Cerebral edema or presence of a pituitary tumor can interfere with the hypothalamic thermoregulatory set point, and shivering is also decreased as a result of lack of thyroid stimulation of muscular activity.[89] Bradycardia and hypotension may also occur, because thyroid hormone normally indirectly stimulates cardiac rate and contractility by increasing the number of β-adrenergic receptors and sensitizing the cardiovascular system to catecholamines.

Myxedema, also known as cutaneous mucinosis, is a nonpitting edema of the skin that occurs in severe hypothyroidism when glycosaminoglycans and water accumulate within the interstitium of the dermis. The myxedema tends to be most prominent over the head and face and can be a clue to the presence of this hypothyroid crisis.

Diagnosis

Presumptive diagnosis of myxedema coma is via history, physical examination and supportive findings on diagnostic evaluation. Given the severity of clinical signs, a complete diagnostic workup, including CBC, chemistry, urinalysis, urine culture, and thoracic and abdominal imaging, is indicated. General clinicopathologic abnormalities include mild nonregenerative anemia (because T_4 stimulates erythropoiesis), hyperlipidemia, hypercholesterolemia (because T_4 governs cholesterol synthesis and degradation), hypoglycemia, a dilutional hyponatremia, and increased alkaline phosphatase levels.[85,87,90]

Thyroid testing

Confirmation of hypothyroidism requires specific thyroid testing. Dogs with myxedema coma should have thyroid function tests that are consistent with hypothyroidism, including a low free T_4 by equilibrium dialysis, low total T_4, and an increased TSH.[87,90] Secondary hypothyroidism (TSH deficiency) is rare, and tertiary hypothyroidism (thyrotropin-releasing hormone deficiency) has not been documented in dogs.

Emergency Management of Myxedema Coma

Successful treatment of a hypothyroid crisis must include stabilization of the cardiovascular and respiratory systems and supplementation of thyroid hormone. The first step is to ensure a patent airway and adequate ventilation based on blood gas analysis. Oxygen should be supplemented if the animal is hypoxic; the patient should be intubated and ventilated if hypercapnic.[85] Hypotension should be managed with judicious fluid therapy, because cardiac dysfunction and retention of free water may predispose the patient to fluid overload. An initial bolus of 20 to 30 mL/kg of replacement crystalloids (such as LRS or Normosol-R) is often indicated, with repeat boluses and development of a postresuscitation fluid therapy plan based on response to therapy.

Slow rewarming of the patient is also indicated; rapid rewarming causes vasodilation, which can exacerbate hypotension.

True myxedema coma is life-threatening and requires empirical thyroid hormone supplementation before the return of thyroid function tests. IV levothyroxine (5 μg/kg [0.005 mg/kg] every 12 hours) is recommended. To prevent overtaxing a weak heart, a lower dose may be indicated if significant underlying heart disease or heart failure is present. Once the patient is stable and able to swallow oral medications, oral levothyroxine therapy should be started (see **Table 5**). If injectable levothyroxine is unavailable from a local pharmacy or hospital, enteral supplementation can be attempted via a nasoesophageal or orogastric tube in those unable to swallow.

Postcrisis Management of Hypothyroidism

After stabilization, lifelong supplementation with oral T_4 is required. Therapy is titrated using routine measurement of T_4, initially monthly until clinical signs resolve and the T4 is within or just above reference range 4 to 6 hours after dosing, then 1 to 2 times yearly in an otherwise asymptomatic and clinically well patient.[91]

Prognosis

Prognosis for myxedema coma hinges on timely recognition and institution of appropriate therapy. Successful treatment has been reported in dogs with severe hypothyroidism.[87,90] In humans, mortality has historically been up to 70% but has improved to 20% to 25% with intensive care and hormonal therapy.[68]

SUMMARY

Endocrine emergencies present with a wide spectrum of nonspecific signs and symptoms.

Familiarity with the clinical presentations of these endocrine crises facilitates early recognition, appropriate treatment, and improved outcomes for patients.

REFERENCES

DIABETIC EMERGENCIES

1. Hall JE. Guyton and hall textbook of medical physiology. 12th edition. Philadelphia PA: Saunders; 2011.
2. Hume DZ, Drobatz KJ, Hess RS. Outcome of dogs with diabetic ketoacidosis: 127 dogs (1993–2003). J Vet Intern Med 2006;20(3):547–55.
3. Koenig A, Drobatz KJ, Beale AB, et al. Hypergylcemic, hyperosmolar syndrome in feline diabetics: 17 cases (1995–2001). J Vet Emerg Crit Care 2004;14(1): 30–40.
4. Bruskiewicz KA, Nelson RW, Feldman EC, et al. Diabetic ketosis and ketoacidosis in cats: 42 cases (1980–1995). J Am Vet Med Assoc 1997;211(2):188–92.
5. Nichols R, Crenshaw KL. Complications and concurrent disease associated with diabetic ketoacidosis and other severe forms of diabetes mellitus. Vet Clin North Am Small Anim Pract 1995;25(3):617–24.
6. Macintire DK. Treatment of diabetic ketoacidosis in dogs by continuous low-dose intravenous infusion of insulin. J Am Vet Med Assoc 1993;202(8):1266–72.
7. McGarry JD, Woeltje KF, Kuwajima M, et al. Regulation of ketogenesis and the renaissance of carnitine palmitoyltransferase. Diabetes Metab Rev 1989;5(3): 271–84.

8. Chupin M, Charbonnel B, Chupin F. C-peptide blood levels in keto-acidosis and in hyperosmolar non-ketotic diabetic coma. Acta Diabetol Lat 1981;18(2):123–8.
9. Gerich JE, Martin MM, Recant L. Clinical and metabolic characteristics of hyperosmolar nonketotic coma. Diabetes 1971;20(4):228–38.
10. Kandel G, Aberman A. Selected developments in understanding of diabetic ketoacidosis. Can Med Assoc J 1983;128(4):392–7.
11. Owen OE, Licht JH, Sapir DG. Renal function and effects of partial rehydration during diabetic ketoacidosis. Diabetes 1981;30(6):510–8.
12. McKenna K, Morris AD, Azam H, et al. Exaggerated vasopressin secretion and attenuated osmoregulated thirst in human survivors of hyperosmolar coma. Diabetologia 1999;42(5):534–8.
13. Hoenig M, Dorfman M, Koenig A. Use of a hand-held meter for the measurement of blood beta-hydroxybutyrate in dogs and cats. J Vet Emerg Crit Care 2008;18:86–7.
14. Zeugswetter F, Pagitz M. Ketone measurements using dipstick methodology in cats with diabetes mellitus. J Small Anim Pract 2009;50(1):4–8.
15. Tommaso M, Aste G, Rocconi F, et al. Evaluation of a portable meter to measure ketonemia and comparison with ketonuria for the diagnosis of canine diabetic ketoacidosis. J Vet Intern Med 2009;23(3):466–71.
16. Montolieu J, Revert L. Lethal hyperkalemia associated with severe hyperglycemia in diabetic patients with renal failure. Am J Kidney Dis 1985;5:47–8.
17. Katz MA. Hyperglycemia-induced hyponatremia: calculation of expected serum sodium depression. N Engl J Med 1973;289(16):843–4.
18. West ML, Marsden PA, Singer GG, et al. Quantitative analysis of glucose loss during acute therapy for hyperglycemic, hyperosmolar syndrome. Diabetes Care 1986;9(5):465–71.
19. Kahn A, Brachet E, Blum D. Controlled fall in natremia and risk of seizures in hypertonic dehydration. Intensive Care Med 1979;5(1):27–31.
20. Sears KW, Drobatz K, Hess R. Use of lispro insulin for treatment of diabetic ketoacidosis in dogs. J Vet Emerg Crit Care 2012;22(2):211–8.
21. American Diabetes Association (Position Statement). Hyperglycemic crises in patients with diabetes mellitus. Diabetes Care 2001;24(1):154–61.
22. Claus MA, Silverstein D, Shofer FS, et al. Comparison of regular insulin infusion doses in critically ill diabetic cats: 29 cases (1999-2007). J Vet Emerg Crit Care 2010;20(5):509–17.

HYPOGLYCEMIA: EXOGENOUS AND ENDOGENOUS INSULIN OVERDOSE (INSULINOMA)

23. Dunn JK, Bostock DE, Herrtage ME, et al. Insulin-secreting tumors of the canine pancreas: clinical and pathological features of 11 cases. J Small Anim Pract 1993;34:325–31.
24. Caywood DD, Klausner JS, O'Leary TP, et al. Pancreatic insulin secreting neoplasms: clinical, diagnostic and prognostic features in 73 dogs. J Am Anim Hosp Assoc 1988;24:577–84.
25. Leifer CE, Peterson ME, Matus RE. Insulin-secreting tumor: diagnosis and medical and surgical management in 55 dogs. J Am Vet Med Assoc 1986;188(1):60–4.
26. Kruth SA, Feldman EC, Kennedy PC. Insulin-secreting islet cell tumors: establishing a diagnosis and the clinical course for 25 dogs. J Am Vet Med Assoc 1982;181(1):54–8.

27. Siliart B, Stambouli F. Laboratory diagnosis of insulinoma in the dog: a retrospective study and a new diagnostic procedure. J Small Anim Pract 1996;37(8): 367–70.
28. Mellanby RJ, Herrtage ME. Insulinoma in a normoglycaemic dog with low serum fructosamine. J Small Anim Pract 2002;43(11):506–8.
29. Loste A, Marca MC, Pérez M, et al. Clinical value of fructosamine measurements in non-healthy dogs. Vet Res Commun 2001;25(2):109–15.
30. Thoresen SI, Aleksandersen M, Lønaas L, et al. Pancreatic insulin secreting carcinoma in a dog: fructosamine for determining persistent hypoglycaemia. J Small Anim Pract 1995;36(6):282–6.
31. Robben JH, Pollak YW, Kirpensteijn J, et al. Comparison of ultrasonography, computed tomography, and single-photon emission computed tomography for the detection and localization of canine insulinoma. J Vet Intern Med 2005;19(1): 15–22.
32. Fischer JR, Smith SA, Harkin KR. Glucagon constant-rate infusion: a novel strategy for the management of hyperinsulinemic-hypoglycemic crisis in the dog. J Am Anim Hosp Assoc 2000;36:27–32.
33. Polton GA, White RN, Brearley MJ, et al. Improved survival in a retrospective cohort of 28 dogs with insulinoma. J Small Anim Pract 2007;48(3):151–6.
34. Tobin RL, Nelson RW, Lucroy MD, et al. Outcome of surgical versus medical treatment of dogs with beta cell neoplasia: 39 cases (1990–1997). J Am Vet Med Assoc 1999;215(2):226–30.

HYPOADRENOCORTICISM

35. Kemppainen RJ, Behrend E. Adrenal physiology. Vet Clin North Am 1997;27: 173–86.
36. Hughes AM, Nelson RW, Faula TR, et al. Clinical features and heritability of hypoadrenocorticism in Nova Scotia duck tolling retrievers: 25 cases (1994–2006). J Am Vet Med Assoc 2007;231:407–12.
37. Oberbauer AM, Bell JS, Belanger JM, et al. Genetic evaluation of Addison's disease in the Portuguese water dog. BMC Vet Res 2006;2:15.
38. Famula TR, Belanger JM, Oberbauer AM. Heritability and complex segregation analysis of hypoadrenocorticism in the standard poodle. J Small Anim Pract 2003;44:8–12.
39. Thompson AL, Scott-Moncrieff JC, Anderson JD. Comparison of classic hypoadrenocorticism with glucocorticoid-deficient hypoadrenocorticism in dogs: 46 cases (1985–2005). J Am Vet Med Assoc 2007;230:1190–4.
40. Peterson ME, Kintzer PP, Kass PH. Pretreatment clinical and laboratory findings in 225 dogs with hypoadrenocorticism. J Am Vet Med Assoc 1996;208:85–91.
41. Seth M, Drobatz K, Church D, et al. White blood cell count and the sodium to potassium ratio to screen for hypoadrenocorticism in dogs. J Vet Intern Med 2011; 25(6):1351–6.
42. Adler JA. Abnormalities of serum electrolyte concentrations in dogs with hypoadrenocorticism. J Vet Intern Med 2007;21:1168–73.
43. Lennon EM, Boyle TW, Hutchins RG, et al. Use of basal serum or plasma cortisol concentrations to rule out a diagnosis of hypoadrenocorticism in dogs: 123 cases (2000–2005). J Am Vet Med Assoc 2007;231:413–6.
44. Javadi S, Galac S, Boer P, et al. Aldosterone-to-renin and cortisol-to-adrenocorticotropic hormone ratios in healthy dogs and dogs with primary hypoadrenocorticism. J Vet Intern Med 2006;20:556–61.

45. Wenger M, Mueller C, Kook PH, et al. Ultrasonographic evaluation of adrenal glands in dogs with primary hypoadrenocorticism or mimicking diseases. Vet Rec 2010;167:207–10.
46. Macmillan KL. Neurological complications following treatment of canine hypoadrenocorticism. Can Vet J 2003;44:490–2.
47. Brady CA, Vite CH, Drobatz KJ. Severe neurological sequelae in a dog after treatment of hypoadrenal crisis. J Am Vet Med Assoc 1999;215:222.
48. O'Brien DP, Kroll RA, Johnson GC, et al. Myelinolysis after correction of hyponatremia in two dogs. J Vet Intern Med 1994;8:40–8.
49. Chow E, Campbell WR, Turnier JC, et al. Toxicity of desoxycorticosterone pivalate given at high dosages to clinically normal beagles for six months. Am J Vet Res 1993;54:1954–61.

PHEOCHROMOCYTOMA

50. Herrera MA, Mehl ML, Kass PH, et al. Predictive factors and the effect of phenoxybenzamine on outcome in dogs undergoing adrenalectomy for pheochromocytoma. J Vet Intern Med 2008;22(6):1333–9.
51. Barthez PY, Marks SL, Woo J, et al. Pheochromocytoma in dogs: 61 cases (1984–1995). J Vet Intern Med 1997;11(5):272–8.
52. Gilson SD, Withrow SJ, Wheeler SL, et al. Pheochromocytoma in 50 dogs. J Vet Intern Med 1994;8(3):228–32.
53. Out G. Pheochromocytoma in dogs: a retrospective study of nine cases [1981–1987]. Can Vet J 1989;30(6):526–7.
54. von Dehn J, Nelson RW, Feldman EC, et al. Pheochromocytoma and hyperadrenocorticism in dogs: six cases (1982-1992). J Am Vet Med Assoc 1995;207(3):322–4.
55. Leblanc NL, Stepien RL, Ellison Bentley E. Ocular lesions associated with systemic hypertension in dogs: 65 cases (2005-2007). J Am Vet Med Assoc 2011;238(7):915–21.
56. Santamarina G, Espino L, Vila M, et al. Aortic thromboembolism and retroperitoneal hemorrhage associated with a pheochromocytoma in a dog. J Vet Intern Med 2003;17(6):917–22.
57. Williams JE, Hackner SG. Pheochromocytoma presenting as acute retroperitoneal hemorrhage in a dog. J Vet Emerg Crit Care 2001;11(3):221–7.
58. Schoeman JP, Stidwort MF. Budd-Chiari-like syndrome associated with an adrenal phaeochromocytoma in a dog. J Small Anim Pract 2001;42(4):191–4.
59. Kook PH, Grest P, Quante S, et al. Urinary catecholamine and metadrenaline to creatinine ratios in dogs with a phaeochromocytoma. Vet Rec 2010;166(6):169–74.
60. Wimpole JA, Adagra CF, Billson MF, et al. Plasma free metanephrines in healthy cats, cats with non-adrenal disease and a cat with suspected phaeochromocytoma. J Feline Med Surg 2010;12(6):435–40.
61. Kook PH, Boretti FS, Hersberger M, et al. Urinary catecholamine and metanephrine to creatinine ratios in healthy dogs at home and in a hospital environment and in 2 dogs with pheochromocytoma. J Vet Intern Med 2007;21(3):388–93.
62. Lord MS, Augoustides JG. Perioperative management of pheochromocytoma: focus on magnesium, clevidipine, and vasopressin. J Cardiothorac Vasc Anesth 2012;26(3):526–31.
63. James MF. Use of magnesium sulphate in the anaesthetic management of pheochromocytoma: a review of 17 anaesthetists. Br J Anaesth 1989;62:616–23.

64. Lang JM, Schertel E, Kennedy S, et al. Elective and emergency surgical management of adrenal gland tumors: 60 cases (1999-2006). J Am Anim Hosp Assoc 2011;47(6):428–35.

THYROTOXICOSIS/THYROID STORM

65. Akamizu T, Satoh T, Isozaki O, et al. Diagnostic criteria, clinical features, and incidence of thyroid storm based on nationwide surveys. Thyroid 2012;22(7): 661–79.
66. Jacobs HS, Mackie DB, Eastman CJ, et al. Total and free triiodothyronine and thyroxine levels in thyroid storm and recurrent hyperthyroidism. Lancet 1973; 2(7823):236–8.
67. Tietgens ST, Leinung MC. Thyroid storm. Med Clin North Am 1995;79(1):169–84.
68. Klubo-Gwiezdzinska J, Wartofsky L. Thyroid emergencies. Med Clin North Am 2012;96(2):385–403.
69. Maggio F, DeFrancesco TC, Atkins CE, et al. Ocular lesions associated with systemic hypertension in cats: 69 cases (1985–1998). J Am Vet Med Assoc 2000; 217(5):695–702.
70. Joseph RJ, Peterson ME. Review and comparison of neuromuscular and central nervous system manifestations of hyperthyroidism in cats and humans. Progr Vet Neurol 1992;3(4):114–8.
71. Nemzek JA, Kruger JM, Walshaw R, et al. Acute onset of hypokalemia and muscular weakness in four hyperthyroid cats. J Am Vet Med Assoc 1994; 205(1):65–8, 24.
72. Smith SA, Tobias AH, Jacob KA, et al. Arterial thromboembolism in cats: acute crisis in 127 cases (1992–2001) and long-term management with low-dose aspirin in 24 cases. J Vet Intern Med 2003;17(1):73–83.
73. Meric S. Recognizing the clinical features of feline hyperthyroidism. Vet Med 1989;84(10):956–63.
74. Shiel RE, Mooney CT. Testing for hyperthyroidism in cats. Vet Clin North Am Small Anim Pract 2007;37(4):672–91.
75. Harvey AM, Hibbert A, Barrett EL. Scintigraphic findings in 120 hyperthyroid cats. J Feline Med Surg 2009;11:96–106.
76. Chastain CB, Panciera D. Echocardiographic variables before and after radioiodine treatment. Small Anim Clin Endo 2006;16(1):5.
77. Bond BR, Fox PR, Peterson ME, et al. Echocardiographic findings in 103 cats with hyperthyroidism. J Am Vet Med Assoc 1988;192(11):1546–9.
78. Sartor LL, Trepanier LA, Kroll MM, et al. Efficacy and safety of transdermal methimazole in the treatment of cats with hyperthyroidism. J Vet Intern Med 2004;18(5): 651–5.
79. Trepanier LA. Pharmacologic management of feline hyperthyroidism. Vet Clin North Am Small Anim Pract 2007;37:775–88.
80. Carhill A, Gutierrez A, Lakhia R, et al. Surviving the storm: two cases of thyroid storm successfully treated with plasmapheresis. BMJ Case Rep 2012;2012. pii: bcr2012006696.
81. Foster DJ, Thoday KL. Use of propranolol and potassium iodate in the presurgical management of hyperthyroid cats. J Small Anim Pract 1999;40:307–15.
82. Murray LA, Peterson ME. Ipodate treatment of hyperthyroidism in cats. J Am Vet Med Assoc 1997;211(1):63–7.
83. Gallagher AE, Panciera DL. Efficacy of iopanoic acid for treatment of spontaneous hyperthyroidism in cats. J Feline Med Surg 2011;13:441–7.

84. Henik R, Stepien R, Wenholz L, et al. Efficacy of atenolol as a single antihypertensive agent in hyperthyroid cats. J Feline Med Surg 2008;10(6):577–82.

MYXEDEMA COMA

85. Atkinson K, Aubert I. Myxedema coma leading to respiratory depression in a dog. Can Vet J 2004;45(4):318–20.
86. Panciera DL. Conditions associated with canine hypothyroidism. Vet Clin North Am Small Anim Pract 2001;31(5):935–50.
87. Henik RA, Dixon RM. Intravenous administration of levothyroxine for treatment of suspected myxedema coma complicated by severe hypothermia in a dog. J Am Vet Med Assoc 2000;216(5):713–7.
88. Dixon RM, Reid SW, Mooney CT. Epidemiological, clinical, haematological and biochemical characteristics of canine hypothyroidism. Vet Rec 1999;145(17): 481–7.
89. Fliers E, Wiersinga WM. Myxedema coma. Rev Endocr Metab Disord 2003;4(2): 137–41.
90. Pullen WH, Hess RS. Hypothyroid dogs treated with intravenous levothyroxine. J Vet Intern Med 2006;20(1):32–7.
91. Dixon RM, Reid SW, Mooney CT. Treatment and therapeutic monitoring of canine hypothyroidism. J Small Anim Pract 2002;43(8):334–40.

[illegible] H, [illegible] ... dogs. J [illegible] Med [illegible] Surg 2008;10(5):[illegible]

MYXEDEMA COMA

[illegible] K, [illegible] Myxedema coma [illegible] dog. [illegible]

[illegible] conditions associated with canine hypothyroidism. [illegible]

[illegible] [illegible] hypothyroidism [illegible] ... complicated by [illegible]

[illegible]

Surgical Considerations in the Emergent Small Animal Patient

Jennifer J. Devey, DVM

KEYWORDS

- Damage control • Veterinary surgery • Emergency surgery • Hemostasis • Surgery
- Wounds

KEY POINTS

- To ensure a successful outcome when performing emergency surgery, the clinician must have the knowledge to be able to assess the patient to determine that surgical intervention is necessary, and to determine the urgency of the procedure.
- The emergency clinician should be prepared to perform potentially life-saving surgical procedures, including surgical cutdowns for airway and vascular access, procedures for control of severe hemorrhage, and emergency thoracotomy to control hemorrhage or perform open chest cardiac massage.
- Constant evaluation and assessment of patients and attention to detail are essential to ensuring a positive outcome.
- Records of patients that experience morbidity or those that die or are euthanized should be regularly reviewed to assess team performance and to make improvements where necessary.

In veterinary medicine, many critically ill, emergency patients will present with injuries or diseases that require surgery as part of resuscitation and/or definitive care. Although some surgical diseases or injuries require advanced training and a board-certified surgeon to perform the surgery (eg, hemilaminectomy for a herniated disc), some of these patients will require surgery urgently. The emergency clinician should be prepared to perform potentially life-saving surgical procedures, including surgical cutdowns for airway and vascular access, procedures for control of severe hemorrhage, and emergency thoracotomy to control hemorrhage or perform open chest cardiac massage. Emergency celiotomy may be required to control hemorrhage from trauma (necessitating liver, splenic, or renal surgery), gastric derotation and gastropexy for correction of gastric volvulus, gastrotomy or enterotomy for removal of foreign bodies, gastric or intestinal resections, urinary bladder repair, Cesarean section, and ovariohysterectomy for pyometra. The veterinarian must also know how to debride, drain (if indicated), and suture wounds. Many seriously ill or injured patients

6675 Welch Road, Saanichton, British Columbia V8M 1W6, Canada
E-mail address: jendevey@aol.com

Vet Clin Small Anim 43 (2013) 899–914
http://dx.doi.org/10.1016/j.cvsm.2013.03.001
0195-5616/13/$ – see front matter © 2013 Elsevier Inc. All rights reserved.
vetsmall.theclinics.com

may require enteral nutritional support and the clinician should be competent at placing esophagostomy, gastrostomy, and enterostomy feeding tubes. The reader is referred to a surgical reference for more detail on the specifics of each surgical procedure.

"Time, trash, and trauma" must be minimized. Prolonged operative times have been associated with higher morbidity, making speed essential, especially in more critically ill or injured patients.[1–3] In extremely critical patients it may be appropriate to have the surgeon gowned and packs open even before induction of anesthesia to minimize the amount of time the patient spends anesthetized. Indwelling implants or foreign material, such as drains and suture material ("trash"), should be minimized. The surgeon must have a thorough knowledge of anatomy, as surgery for the critically ill or injured can be complicated and challenging. Necrotic tissue should be removed. Surgical technique should be as precise as possible and tissues must be handled gently.

TIMING OF EMERGENCY SURGERY

In the case of a *truly* emergency life-saving surgical procedure where death is imminent, the surgery should not be delayed for any reason. An emergency primary survey evaluating the airway, breathing, circulation, and level of consciousness (dysfunction) (ABCDs) should be completed rapidly, but a secondary survey or complete physical examination may not have been performed, the patient may not have had a diagnostic workup, and the surgical site may not have been clipped and prepared. In the patient that is close to, or has experienced a cardiopulmonary arrest, the surgical procedure should be performed with little regard for asepsis; however, a clean surgery should be attempted.

In situations in which imminent life-saving surgery is not necessary, appropriate resuscitation and stabilization of the patient are essential before induction of anesthesia. If the patient is not responding to volume resuscitation and supportive care it should be kept in mind that the surgical procedure may be an integral part of the resuscitation and stabilization.

A team of a minimum of 3 people, surgeon, assistant surgeon, and anesthetist/circulating nurse, is very important in the management of more critical emergency surgical patients. If this team is not available, if the hospital does not have all the necessary equipment or instruments, or if the clinician does not have the necessary skills or knowledge, consideration should be given to referring the patient. Good judgment must be exercised, because the risks of performing the surgery must be weighed against the risks of transport and delayed surgery.

READINESS

Readiness includes a well-organized, prepared operating room in the event emergency surgery is indicated. The anesthetic machine should be set up appropriately with sufficient inhalant in the vaporizer and an attached breathing circuit. All electronic equipment should be set up and plugged in. Essential equipment in the operating room should include patient cardiorespiratory monitors, an anesthetic ventilator, fluid pumps, fluid warmers, forced air warming devices, suction, and electrocautery. The surgery table should be prepared (eg, heating blanket, cautery). Intravenous (IV) fluids (isotonic crystalloid and synthetic colloid) should be available, along with drip sets, extension sets, and a pressure infuser bag. Blood products should be accessible, and materials for autotransfusion should be available.

All vital sterile supplies should be set up and ready. This includes instrument packs, electrocautery handle, suction tubing, light handle covers, and scalpel blades. Ideally, a headlight and magnification loupes should be available. A sterile suction canister should be available for collection of blood for possible autotransfusion.

Because of the limited availability of blood and blood products in most veterinary hospitals, autotransfusion may be required in the severely hemorrhaging patient. If a trauma patient is bleeding into a cavity, such as the thorax or abdomen, an attempt should be made to collect the blood aseptically for possible reinfusion.[4] Blood should be collected into sterile containers and administered IV using a filter. Anticoagulant is not necessary unless the bleeding is very active, as blood within body cavities rapidly undergoes fibrinolysis, and is generally devoid of platelets and fibrinogen.[5] For this reason, patients receiving massive blood transfusions of autotransfused blood will often need fresh frozen plasma transfusions to provide coagulation factors. Ideally, blood from the abdomen is not recommended for use for autotransfusion until it has been determined that there is no gross contamination from a ruptured bowel or neoplasia (eg, hemangiosarcoma). In dire situations, the blood may have to be auto-transfused without aseptic collection, possibly contaminated with infectious organisms or cells from a neoplastic source, and delivered without a filter.[4,6–8] Patients have survived under these conditions.[4,6,8,9]

Readiness not only refers to the physical facility, but also to personnel. All personnel must possess the knowledge to rapidly recognize potentially life-threatening problems; they must also know how to find, set up, and use all equipment that might be necessary for emergency surgery. Staff training is vital and cannot be overemphasized. Training should take the form of didactic sessions in addition to mock emergency situations. Written and/or posted protocols are highly recommended, because during the panic of true emergencies, it is easy to forget important components of treatment and stabilization. Protocols should be easy to understand and follow, and should be regularly reviewed and revised as needed.

PREOPERATIVE PATIENT ASSESSMENT

In the stable patient, a complete physical examination should be performed before induction of anesthesia. This includes an objective assessment of the 5 vital signs: temperature, pulse, respiration, blood pressure, and pain.[10,11] The respiratory pattern (eg, rate, effort), airway sounds in all quadrants of the thorax, and the presence of cough should be evaluated in all patients, as patients with abdominal disease or trauma many have concurrent pneumothorax, secondary aspiration pneumonia, or metastatic disease. The cardiovascular system should be assessed based on heart rate, pulse quality, capillary refill time, and blood pressure. In addition to blood pressure, an attempt should be made to evaluate venous volume as approximately 70% of the blood volume is in the venous side of the circulation. Although no studies have been performed, observation of jugular vein filling likely provides an estimation of central venous pressure (assuming no intrathoracic pathology).[12] The jugular vein should be clipped and evaluated for distention when the vessel is held off at the thoracic inlet. A patient with a flat jugular vein is likely hypovolemic. Perfusion can be further assessed in some patients by measuring toe web temperature.[13] A difference of greater than 4°C indicates altered peripheral perfusion either secondary to global hypoperfusion or limb injury.

The abdomen should be palpated, auscultated, and percussed with the goal of localizing pain, and detecting the presence of a fluid wave, gas-distended organs, or solid masses. Auscultation of the abdomen should precede palpation, as palpation can cause gut sounds to diminish. A rectal examination should be performed, and evidence of blood, melena, pelvic fractures, or other pathology should be noted. Periumbilical hemorrhage (Cullen's sign) may be seen with a hemoabdomen. Distended superficial epigastric veins are consistent with increased intra-abdominal pressure, which can be associated with decreased preload and, consequently, reduced cardiac output.

A neurologic assessment should be performed of both central and peripheral nerves, and any abnormalities should be noted. A neurovascular assessment of the paws should be performed whenever limb injuries are present or spinal injury is suspected. The skin and mucous membranes should be evaluated for petechiation or ecchymoses.

In the emergent surgical patient, diagnostic tests are indicated to determine the extent of the illness or injury and to help confirm a diagnosis and the need for surgical intervention. The choice of tests will vary based on the presenting disease or injury. A previously healthy patient with a minor wound that can be sutured under sedation and local anesthesia may not require any tests, whereas a patient with a septic peritonitis will ideally have a complete diagnostic workup, including a complete blood count (CBC) with microscopic evaluation of a blood smear for the cell differential, cell morphology, and platelet estimate; electrolytes; blood gas (venous or arterial); coagulation profile; complete biochemical profile; and urinalysis. Cultures of wounds and abdominal fluid may also be indicated. Unstable patients ideally should have immediate diagnostics performed, including a packed cell volume (PCV) and total solids (TS), blood glucose (BG), blood urea nitrogen or creatinine, electrolytes, and a blood gas.

Thoracic radiographs should be evaluated in every trauma patient, and in any patient in which respiratory pathology is suspected. Abdominal radiographs are indicated in every patient with an abdominal injury or disease. Contrast studies, including a barium series, IV urography, cystography, or angiography may be required. When performing a barium series, water-soluble contrast material should be used instead of barium if there is any concern for gastrointestinal perforation or pulmonary aspiration. Abdominal ultrasound is useful for determining the presence of free fluid and for diagnosing many causes of acute abdomen, unless there is a significant amount of air within the peritoneal cavity.[14,15] (Please see the article "The Use of Ultrasound for Dogs and Cats in the Emergency Room [AFAST and TFAST]" elsewhere in this issue for more information.)

Paracentesis should be performed in any patient with either pleural or abdominal effusion. For abdominocentesis a 4-quadrant centesis (unless ultrasound-guided centesis is available) should be performed in patients with suspected ascites, abdominal trauma, or peritonitis. Abdominocentesis may be falsely negative, and ultrasound-guided paracentesis or diagnostic peritoneal lavage may improve diagnostic yield.[16] A PCV, TS, white blood cell count, and microscopic examination of the fluid should be performed to evaluate white blood cell morphology and to assess for the presence of bacteria. In the dog, an abdominal fluid glucose level that is at least 20 mg/dL less than the glucose level in the blood is strongly supportive of septic peritonitis.[17] A fluid lactate greater than 2.5 mg/dL is also suggestive of septic peritonitis in the dog.[18] Evidence of septic peritonitis is an indication for emergency surgery.

Other biochemical tests comparing blood versus abdominal fluid concentrations include alkaline phosphatase, total bilirubin, potassium, and creatinine. Alkaline phosphatase concentrations that are higher in the abdominal fluid compared with the serum suggest intestinal leakage.[19] Bilirubin concentrations that are higher in the abdominal fluid than serum indicate a disruption of the biliary tract (eg, bile peritonitis) and the need for emergency surgery.[20] Potassium and creatinine concentrations that are higher in the abdominal fluid than in the serum are consistent with urinary tract rupture and the need for urgent exploratory surgery, although temporary peritoneal drainage may be an appropriate course of action if the patient is too unstable for emergency surgery.[21]

INSTRUMENTS

Wound packs should be available and sterilized (**Box 1**). A major surgical pack must contain all the instruments for performing almost any major surgery (**Box 2**). Both should contain good-quality instruments. A hemostat that falls off a blood vessel at an inopportune moment may contribute to significant patient morbidity. Scissors should be sharp and should be checked regularly to ensure that sharpening or replacement is not indicated. Curved instruments are preferred over straight because they allow for better visualization of tissues to be cut and are more maneuverable.

The surgical instruments should be packed with the emergency surgery in mind and the instruments that the surgeon may require first should be placed on top. A separate peel pack (sterilized, but not sealed) should contain the necessary instruments for gaining rapid entry to an abdomen or thorax, as well as instruments needed for providing rapid hemostasis.

Stapling equipment is invaluable in saving time and preventing patient morbidity when used appropriately. Stapling equipment can be used to perform rapid lung lobectomy, liver lobectomy, gastric resection, intestinal anastomosis, vascular ligation, and fascia and skin closure. The tissues must be able to be compressed to 2-mm thickness for use of the 4.8-mm staples, 1.5-mm thickness for the 3.5-mm staples, and 1.0-mm thickness for the 2.5-mm staples.[22] Staple lines may need to be oversewn with suture. Vascular clips provide rapid, safe vascular ligation, provided the vessels are between one-third and two-thirds the diameter of the clip. A tissue bumper of 2 to 3 mm should be left to prevent the clip from slipping off of the blood vessel.

PATIENT PREPARATION

Wide surgical skin preparation is always indicated in the emergent patient, as the skin may need to be mobilized and tubes or drains may need to be placed outside of the direct surgical field. The dimensions of the prepared field will vary with the individual surgery but, ideally, should include a minimum of 6 to 8 in (15–20 cm) from the farthest extent of the anticipated surgical incision or incisions. When preparing for abdominal surgery, the thorax should be included, as access to the caudal thorax may be needed when performing cranial abdominal procedures. If catheterization of the femoral artery or vein might be indicated intraoperatively for large-bore vascular access, the inguinal region should be prepared.[23]

Box 1
Wound pack
Scalpel handle
Mayo-Hegar needle holder
Brown-Adson tissue forceps
Curved Metzenbaum scissors
Curved Halstead mosquito forceps (minimum 3)
Curved Kelly or Crile forceps (minimum 3)
Small bowl
4 × 4 sponges (minimum 10)
Skin drape

Box 2
Major pack

Saline bowls (small and large)

2 scalpel handles (#3)

Backhaus towel clamps: small (minimum 8)

Backhaus towel clamps: large (minimum 4)

Curved Mayo scissors (small and large)

Curved Metzenbaum scissors (small and large)

Curved Halstead mosquito forceps (minimum 6)

Curved Kelly or Crile forceps (minimum 6)

Curved Rochester-Carmalt hemostatic forceps (minimum 4)

Curved Foerster sponge forceps

Doyen forceps (2)

Allis tissue forceps (minimum 4)

Right-angle forceps (small and large)

DeBakey tissue forceps (fine-tipped)

Russian thumb forceps

Brown-Adson tissue forceps

Mayo-Hegar needle holders (small and large)

Poole suction tip

Yankauer suction tip

Silastic tubing for suction

5-Fr red rubber tubing

Bulb syringe

Laparotomy pads (5)

Cotton towels (4 small)

Gauze sponges 4 × 4 (20)

Skin drapes

Appropriate skin antiseptics should be applied before the surgical procedure. Chlorhexidine and povidone iodine are the 2 most common surgical antiseptics used in veterinary medicine. Chlorhexidine, which acts by disrupting the cell wall and precipitating cell proteins, has a spectrum of activity against most gram-positive and some gram-negative bacteria (including *Escherichia coli* and *Pseudomonas aeruginosa*).[24,25] Chlorhexidine is effective against yeast but it is ineffective against bacterial spores and mycobacteria.[24,25] It is not inactivated by the presence of organic material and it binds to keratin, thus it has residual antibacterial activity.[24,25] There is an approximately 90% bactericidal effect within 30 seconds of contact time.[26,27] Although a 5-minute to 7-minute preparation time is recommended, it is possible that two 30-second scrubs are sufficient.[26,27]

Povidone iodine solutions act by penetrating the cell wall where they oxidize the intracellular contents, replacing the microbial contents with iodine. Povidone iodine has a broad spectrum of activity against gram-positive and gram-negative bacteria, fungi, yeast, and mycobacteria, but it is considered ineffective against bacterial spores.[25] An approximately 90% bactericidal effect is expected within 30 seconds, although a minimum of 2 minutes of contact time is advised, and a 5-minute to 7-minute scrub time is recommended.[25] Alternating the surgical solution with alcohol wipes may reduce efficacy because contact time of the iodine with the skin will be decreased. It is inactivated by the presence of blood, plasma, and organic material, so the presence of any of these rapidly diminishes the residual bactericidal activity.[25]

Pseudomonas and Serratia marcescens can rapidly develop resistance to chlorhexidine by forming a biofilm.[27–30] A similar problem has been noted with povidone iodine; therefore, keeping gauze squares soaking in either of these antiseptic solutions in containers for any long period of time should be avoided.[27–30]

PATIENT POSITIONING

Appropriate patient positioning is essential to ensuring good surgical exposure; however, the position of the patient may have negative consequences on ventilation and hemodynamic status. Abdominal masses, a large spleen, or a gravid uterus can effectively occlude the abdominal vena cava when the patient is placed in dorsal recumbency, thus significantly decreasing preload and, therefore, cardiac output. Placing the patient at a slight angle may avoid this complication.

Patients placed in dorsal recumbency with the limbs held in a fully extended position cannot ventilate well. Bending the thoracic limbs at the elbows to a 90° angle and then securing the patient to the table will help prevent ventilatory compromise (spontaneous or mechanical). Larger dogs placed in lateral recumbency rapidly develop atelectasis of the dependent lung and should be ventilated as soon as anesthesia is induced. Patients placed in sternal recumbency and held in position with sandbags or molded trays also may not be able to adequately ventilate. Patients placed in a tilted position with the head down may have difficulty moving their diaphragm on inspiration. These positions should be avoided whenever possible.

HEMOSTASIS

Accurate hemostasis is important in all patients, but is even more so in critically ill or injured patients. Coagulopathies are not uncommon in these patients, and even minor oozing of blood can lead to significant blood loss. Blood loss from subcutaneous vessels, omental vessels, and mesenteric vessels can be significant in patients that are hypocoagulable. Blood clots and hematomas should be avoided because both can lead to delayed healing and an increased likelihood of infection. To estimate losses for fluid replacement purposes, an estimate of the volume of blood loss should be made. A gross estimate is that a "fistful" of blood represents approximately 200 to 500 mL depending on the size of the fist. Likewise, a 4 × 4 sponge, when soaked, holds approximately 5 to 18 mL of blood, and a laparotomy sponge holds approximately 50 to 100 mL.[31,32]

Temporary control of hemorrhage into parenchymal organs can be achieved by placing atraumatic vascular clamps (eg, Satinsky clamp, bulldog clamp) or a Rumel tourniquet. A modified Rumel tourniquet can be formed by passing a small-bore red rubber tube around the vascular pedicle and then bringing the tube ends together. A pair of hemostatic forceps are slid down both tube ends until the vessel is approximated, at which point they are clamped. Many of the major abdominal vessels can be safely occluded for short periods of time (**Table 1**). The safety margin is likely less in the face of significant preexisting hypoperfusion, and these time limits should be

Table 1
Time limits for vascular occlusion

Blood Vessel	Occlusion Time Limit
Ascending aorta (proximal to the left subclavian)	2–3 min
Descending thoracic aorta	5–10 min
Portal triad	10–15 min
Hepatic artery	30 min
Splenic artery and vein	15–20 min
Renal artery and vein	30 min
Abdominal aorta	30 min
Caudal vena cava (distal to liver)	Can ligate

Data from Refs.[31,65,68]

used as a guideline only. In patients with severe liver hemorrhage, temporary control may be achieved by performing a modified Pringle maneuver, which occludes the portal triad of the portal vein, hepatic artery, and common bile duct (**Fig. 1**). This will control approximately 70% of the blood flow to the liver, and provide a short period of time to clearly identify the injury and definitively control the hemorrhage.

Topical hemostatic agents can also be used to control hemorrhage in certain situations. Fibrin glues, collagen, gelatin sponges, and oxidized cellulose are available products.[33,34] Newer kaolin-based products developed for use by the military appear to be extremely effective at controlling life-threatening hemorrhage.[35]

Definitive hemostasis can be achieved by use of direct pressure, suturing of wounds (compression of vessels), electrosurgery, ligation of blood vessels, vascular clips, omental packing, cyanoacrylate, hemostatic agents, or removal of the hemorrhaging tissue.[36]

Electrosurgery is indispensable for rapid and efficient control of hemorrhage. It causes heat-induced protein denaturation and tissue coagulation, and can be used to control hemorrhage from arteries up to 1 mm and veins up to 2 mm in diameter. Monopolar electrosurgery passes a current from the electrode through the patient to a ground plate, and requires a dry field.[37] In contrast, bipolar electrosurgery passes

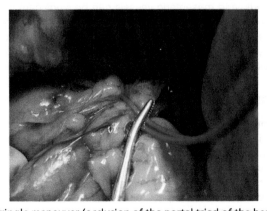

Fig. 1. Modified Pringle maneuver (occlusion of the portal triad of the hepatic artery, portal vein, and common bile duct) using a modified Rumel tourniquet.

a current between 2 electrodes. When used inappropriately, thermal damage can result, leading to ischemia and delayed healing.

FEEDING TUBES AND NASOGASTRIC DECOMPRESSION

A conscious decision should be made with regard to placement of a feeding tube in each patient undergoing major surgery. Ideally, a nasogastric tube should be placed in all dogs for postoperative decompression and early enteral feeding, and in cats with evidence of gastroparesis.[38] Gastric decompression helps decrease the chance for bloat, decreases interference with diaphragmatic excursions, and has been proven to significantly decrease the time for normal gastric motility to return.[38,39] A gastrojejunostomy or jejunostomy feeding tube should be placed in all patients with upper gastrointestinal surgery (including hepatobiliary and pancreatic surgery), if there are any concerns that enteral nutrition will not be tolerated within 24 to 36 hours.

PERITONEAL LAVAGE

Before closing the abdomen, the abdominal cavity should be flushed with warm isotonic fluids, with the number of liters of saline used depending on the degree of contamination. It has been recommended that approximately 200 to 300 mL/kg minimum, or until the lavage effluent is clear, be used to lavage a contaminated or infected abdomen. The use of intraperitoneal antibiotics is not indicated, as they have not been shown to have any beneficial effects.[40,41] No benefit has been demonstrated with the use of antiseptics in the lavage fluid and negative effects can include chemical peritonitis, increased adhesion formation, and delayed healing of intestinal anastomoses.[42,43]

PERITONEAL DRAINAGE

In cases of peritonitis, peritoneal drainage is indicated if the source of the contamination has not been completely controlled, if an anaerobic infection is likely, if a second laparotomy is planned, or if significant peritonitis exists. The 2 main options for peritoneal drainage include open peritoneal drainage and closed suction drainage.

Open abdominal drainage has many disadvantages, including protein loss, electrolyte abnormalities, fluid loss, potential for ascending infection, and risk of evisceration. Closed suction drainage is an effective alternative to open abdominal drainage in many situations. After irrigation, closed suction drains are placed in the cranial abdomen and the abdomen is closed. The drains are left in place until the amount of fluid being produced is within physiologic limits (1–2 mL/kg per day) and the fluid cytology shows no signs of active inflammation or infection.[44] This method of drainage is effective in many patients and minimizes morbidity.

TRAUMA TRIAD OF DEATH

The trauma triad of death is defined in human medicine as hypothermia, acidosis, and coagulopathy.[45] Hypothermia can develop secondary to evaporative or conductive losses, cold air in the anesthetic circuits, use of room-temperature fluids (especially boluses of cold fluid to patients that develop hypotension intraoperatively), and the presence of open body cavities or extensive tissue exposure.[46,47] To counteract this, warming circuits should be used on anesthetic machines, fluids should be warmed, surgery tables should be heated, and patients should be kept warm with warm water circulating blankets, forced warm air circuits, and warm lavage fluids.

Acidosis may develop secondary to poor tissue perfusion.[46,47] Concurrent respiratory acidosis may develop secondary to hypoventilation.[46,47] Because almost all anesthetic drugs have a negative impact on respiration, all anesthetized patients should be ventilated (ideally mechanically) and the carbon dioxide tension should be monitored using capnography or frequent blood gas assessment. Euvolemia and normal blood pressure should be maintained using synthetic colloid fluids and blood products, as indicated. Infusion of large volumes of crystalloid fluids should be avoided to minimize dilution of hemoglobin, blood proteins, and clotting factors. Blood pressure ideally should be measured directly via an arterial catheter; however, if this is not possible, then blood pressure should be measured indirectly using a Doppler ultrasonic flow detector. Doppler is preferred over oscillometric devices, because it is more accurate in smaller and hypotensive patients and allows the surgeon and anesthetist to assess flow in addition to blood pressure.[48] Red blood cell transfusions may be indicated when there has been an acute blood loss of more than 20% of the patient's blood volume, or if perfusion parameters are not improving with fluid resuscitation with non–hemoglobin-containing fluids.[49,50] Patients with acute blood loss should have a hemoglobin concentration of at least 7 g/dL before undergoing major surgery.[49,50]

Coagulopathy may develop secondary to ongoing blood loss and hemodilution with crystalloid fluids and synthetic colloid fluids.[46,47] In addition, acidosis and hypothermia alter the efficiency of the coagulation cascade, which is a series of enzyme reactions. A high index of suspicion must be maintained in patients at risk for bleeding disorders and fresh frozen plasma should be administered before evidence of a clinical coagulopathy whenever possible. Close attention should be paid to accurate hemostasis and active measures should be taken to avoid acidosis and hypothermia.

DAMAGE CONTROL

In cases of severe trauma that require surgery to control life-threatening hemorrhage, current human recommendations are to keep the operative time to 90 minutes or less to avoid the trauma triad of death.[51] The goal of damage control is to control major hemorrhage, control leakage from hollow organs, provide diversions for the bowel or urinary tract as needed, pack the abdomen, and recover the patient as soon as possible.[45,52] Deviating from these principles has been shown to worsen mortality.[53] Packing of the abdomen is performed using towels, which provide direct pressure to oozing wounds. Once packing is complete, the abdomen may not be able to be closed primarily without causing excessive intra-abdominal pressure. This increase in intra-abdominal pressure can lead to abdominal compartment syndrome, which may lead to decreased organ perfusion and secondary renal and gut failure.[47] To avoid excessive pressure during closure of the linea alba, a vacuum-assisted dressing should be placed.[54] Alternatively, a sterile sheet of plastic (eg, large IV fluid bag cut open into a sheet) may need to be sutured to the edges of the linea alba. Both provide a waterproof dressing, which helps to prevent heat loss and protein loss, while simultaneously minimizing the likelihood that abdominal compartment syndrome will develop. The patient is rewarmed, the acidosis is treated, and coagulation is normalized. Once the patient is more stable, the abdomen is reexplored (usually within 24 hours), and more definitive surgery is performed as indicated.[46,47]

WOUNDS

Trauma-induced wounds are a common presenting complaint in emergency patients. Initial wound handling can significantly affect the long-term outcome. Secondary problems with wound healing and patient morbidity often relate to inappropriate wound handling during the initial stages. Generally, tissues heal the fastest when there is good blood supply, no tension, and no movement. Problems with sepsis secondary to wounds come from inadequate debridement of necrotic tissue, insufficient irrigation, inappropriate choice of antibiotics, and inadequate resuscitation. Attention should always be paid to ensure the patient is receiving appropriate systemic treatment and proper nutrition during the healing process.

Gloves should be worn during initial wound handling and the wound should be protected immediately from desiccation and contamination. Initially, a sterile water-soluble gel followed by a sterile dressing or sterile saline-soaked gauze sponges should be placed on the wound.

The wound should be cleaned and irrigated and nonviable tissue should be debrided as soon as possible. Many wounds will require the use of general anesthesia; however, superficial wounds that do not require extensive debridement can be managed under sedation and local anesthesia.

Animals may present with fairly extensive wounds that can be severely contaminated with ground-in road dirt. These wounds require extensive irrigation using sterile isotonic fluids delivered under pressure. Although the exact volume of irrigation is unknown, 50 to 100 mL per centimeter of laceration has been suggested.[55] The ideal pressure generated by the irrigator is unknown, but a pressure of 8 to 12 psi will reduce infection without causing damage to the tissues.[42,55] This can be performed using an 18-gauge needle and a 35-mL syringe, which typically generates 11 to 13 psi, or by using mechanical lavage systems.[42,55] Irrigation should not be done blindly as this may force infection or foreign material farther into the wound and potentially into healthy tissues. Tap water can be used for irrigation of extremely large wounds. Although it is not ideal, it has not be associated with a worse outcome in humans when compared with the use of saline.[56,57]

The goal of surgical management of wounds should be to explore and remove any foreign material, control hemorrhage, and remove necrotic tissue. Tissue viability is assessed by evaluating the blood flow: edges should bleed and the color should be pink, and the tissue should be warm. Muscle should contract when incised. Floating fat is nonviable and should be removed. Bone fragments with no periosteum or muscle attachment are likely nonviable and should be removed or used for a cortical bone graft, if needed.

The debridement technique varies depending on the tissue. Gentle tissue handling is very important because traumatic tissue handling can lead to vascular compromise, direct tissue damage, poor healing, and increased likelihood of infection. Skin should be cut back to clean, bleeding (ideally) edges using sharp dissection with a scalpel blade. Staged debridement may be required if there is limited skin present. Fat and fascia should be liberally excised to clean, healthy tissue. Mayo scissors are used for cutting heavy tissue, such as fascia. Metzenbaum scissors are finer and used for cutting thin tissue. Muscle should be debrided if it does not bleed or contract in response to being incised. Tendons should be removed if there is no peritenon or if it is contaminated; however, if it is vital to the area, it should be saved, and anastomosed if possible. Embedded debris should be removed from exposed bone using the edge of a scalpel blade. Manipulation of bone fragments should be minimized so as to avoid disrupting blood supply from the periosteum and surrounding soft tissues.

Drains are often used in the management of wounds. Indications include a need for dead space obliteration, elimination of fluid accumulation, and prevention of air or fluid accumulation. Drains are classified as either active or passive. An active drain (eg, Jackson Pratt) has a suction system attached, whereas a passive drain (eg, penrose) does not. Active drains are preferred over passive drains because they decrease the likelihood of infection, keep the skin dry, provide continuous drainage, and allow the effluent to be monitored.

Closing a wound inappropriately will lead to complications. Wounds that should not be closed include nondissecting puncture wounds, wounds that could not be debrided or irrigated adequately, wounds that are more than 6 hours old and could not be converted to fresh wounds, and infected wounds. Wounds that are closed under significant tension will likely dehisce, and these wounds also should not be closed.

Extensive degloving injuries and large open wounds may benefit from the use of vacuum-assisted closure, which places the wound under negative pressure, thus promoting removal of fluid, improving circulation, and encouraging the development of granulation tissue.[54] This technique should be used with caution in wounds that have not been adequately debrided because premature placement may lead to complications, including infection and delayed healing.[54]

Wounds should be bandaged in such a way as to promote healing. A sterile dressing should be placed over every incision until a fibrin seal has formed (minimum 24 hours) to prevent contamination of the wound from external sources.[58,59]

POSTOPERATIVE CARE

Following major surgery, patients will require close monitoring and treatment with fluid therapy, analgesics, and antibiotics. Pain should be managed aggressively. Analgesics should be given on a scheduled basis, and the analgesic plan reassessed as needed, because every patient's injury and tolerance to pain is different. Good intraoperative pain control will help with postoperative pain control. Constant rate infusions are very effective at keeping patients comfortable and pain-free. Supplemental oxygen and/or ventilatory support may also be required. More critical patients and those that have had an intestinal resection and anastomosis performed may benefit from being provided with supplemental oxygen for at least 2 hours postoperatively, as this has been shown to improve tissue healing and reduce the risk of infection.[60] Urinary catheters should be placed in patients with difficulties with either ambulation or urination. Other treatment, such as chest tube aspiration and care, care of suction drains, and bandage changes will vary depending on the type of injury and the surgery performed. Monitoring will be dictated by the underlying trauma and status of the patient; however, a minimum of temperature, heart rate, respiratory rate and effort, and blood pressure should be assessed hourly until the patient is normothermic and stable. Critical patients will usually require blood work postoperatively; the tests will vary with the patient, but typically include PCV/TS/BG, albumin, electrolyte, blood gas, CBC and coagulation profile monitoring. In hemodynamically stable patients, an attempt should be made to start enteral nutritional support as soon as 6 to 12 hours postoperatively, and certainly within 24 to 48 hours.[61–64]

SUMMARY

Every hospital, whether a general practice, referral hospital, or emergency clinic, admits emergency patients. Some have minor illnesses and injuries, and some are extremely critical. Some of these patients will require surgery within a matter of minutes to hours of arrival. Ensuring the hospital is always prepared to deal with these patients, if and when they arrive, is paramount to ensuring a successful outcome. This preparation includes ensuring the hospital is appropriately equipped, and ensuring the veterinary team has the necessary knowledge and skills. Constant evaluation and assessment of patients and attention to detail is also essential to ensuring a positive outcome. Records of patients that experience morbidity or those that die or are eutha-nized should be regularly reviewed to assess team performance and to make improve-ments where necessary.

REFERENCES

1. Cruse PJ, Foord R. A five-year prospective study of 23 649 surgical wounds. Arch Surg 1973;107:206–10.
2. Pessaux P, Msika S, Atalla D, et al. Risk factors for postoperative infectious complications in noncolorectal abdominal surgery: a multivariate analysis based on a prospective multicenter study of 4718 patients. Arch Surg 2003; 138:314–24.
3. Proctor LD, Davenport DL, Bernard AC, et al. General surgical operative dura-tion is associated with increased risk adjusted infectious complication rates and length of hospital stay. J Am Coll Surg 2010;210:60–5.
4. Crowe DT. Autotransfusion in the critically injured patient: a historic review and current recommendations. J Vet Emerg Crit Care 1981;4:14–39.
5. Broadie TA, Glover JL, Bang N, et al. Clotting competence of intracavitary blood in trauma victims. Ann Emerg Med 1981;10:121–30.
6. Bowley DM, Barker P, Boffard KD. Intraoperative blood salvage in penetrating abdominal trauma: a randomised, controlled trial. World J Surg 2006;30: 1074–80.
7. Griswold RA, Ortner AB. The use of autotransfusion in surgery of the serous cavities. Surg Gynecol Obstet 1943;77:167–77.
8. Smith RN, Yaw PB, Glover JL. Autotransfusion of contaminated intraperitoneal blood: an experimental study. J Trauma 1978;18:341–4.
9. Desmond MJ, Thomas MJ, Gillon J, et al. Perioperative red cell salvage. Trans-fusion 1996;36:644–51.
10. Joint Commission on Accreditation of Health Care Organizations. Pain manage-ment and assessment: an organizational approach. JCAHO publication PAM-100. Oakbrook Terrace (IL): Joint Commission on Accreditation of Healthcare Organizations; 2000.
11. Lynch M. Pain as the fifth vital sign. J Intraven Nurs 2001;2:85–94.
12. Crowe DT. Assessment and management of the severely polytraumatized small animal patient. J Vet Emerg Crit Care 2006;16:264–75.
13. Vincent JL, Moraine JJ, van der Linden P. Toe temperature versus transcuta-neous oxygen tension monitoring during acute circulatory failure. Intensive Care Med 1988;14:64–8.
14. Boysen SR, Rozanski EA, Tidwell AS, et al. Evaluation of focused assessment with sonography for trauma protocol to detect free abdominal fluid in dogs involved in motor vehicle accidents. J Am Vet Med Assoc 2004;225: 1198–204.
15. Von Kuenssberg Jehle D, Stiller G, Wagner D. Sensitivity in detecting free intra-peritoneal fluid with the pelvic views of the FAST exam. Am J Emerg Med 2003; 21:476–8.
16. Crowe DT, Crane SW. Diagnostic abdominal paracentesis and lavage in evalu-ations of abdominal injuries in dogs and cats: clinical and experimental investi-gations. J Am Vet Med Assoc 1986;168:700–5.
17. Bonczynski JJ, Ludwig LL, Barton LJ, et al. Comparison of peritoneal fluid and peripheral blood pH, bicarbonate, glucose, and lactate concentration as a diag-nostic tool for septic peritonitis in dogs and cats. Vet Surg 2003;32:161–6.

18. Levin GM, Bonczynski JJ, Ludwig LL, et al. Lactate as a diagnostic test for septic peritoneal effusions in dogs and cats. J Am Anim Hosp Assoc 2004;40: 364–71.
19. Jaffin JH, Ochsner MG, Cole FJ, et al. Alkaline phosphatase levels in diagnostic peritoneal lavage fluid as a predictor of hollow visceral injury. J Trauma 1993;34: 829–33.
20. Ludwig LL, McLoughlin MA, Graves TK, et al. Surgical treatment of bile peritonitis in 24 dogs and 2 cats: a retrospective study (1987–1994). Vet Surg 1997; 26:90–8.
21. Schmeidt C, Tobias KM, Otto CM. Evaluation of abdominal fluid: peripheral blood creatinine and potassium ratios for diagnosis of uroperitoneum in dogs. J Vet Emerg Crit Care 2001;11:275–80.
22. Tobias KM. Surgical stapling devices in veterinary medicine: a review. Vet Surg 2007;36:341–9.
23. Crowe DT. Dealing with visceral injuries of the cranial abdomen. Vet Med 1988; 83:20–35.
24. Boyce JM, Pittett D. Guideline for hand hygiene in health-care settings; recommendations of the healthcare infection practices advisory committee and the HIPCAC/SHEA/APIC/IDSA hand hygiene task force. MMWR Recomm Rep 2002;51(RR16):1–44.
25. Rutala WA, Weber DJ, Healthcare Infection Control Practices Advisory Committee, CDC Guideline for disinfection and sterilization of healthcare facilities, 2008.
26. Magram AJ, Horan TC, Pearson ML, et al. Guideline for prevention of surgical site infection. Infect Control Hosp Epidemiol 1999;20:247–78.
27. Reichman DE, Greenberg JA. Reducing surgical site infections: a review. Rev Obstet Gynecol 2009;2:212–41.
28. Marrie TJ, Costerton W. Prolonged survival of Serratia marcescens in chlorhexidine. Appl Environ Microbiol 1981;42:1093–102.
29. Sheldon AT. Antiseptic "resistance": real or perceived threat? Clin Infect Dis 2005;40:1650–6.
30. Vali L, Davies SE, Lai LL, et al. Frequency of biocide resistance genes, antibiotic resistance and the effect of chlorhexidine exposure on clinical methicillin-resistant Staphylococcus aureus isolates. J Antimicrob Chemother 2008;61:524–32.
31. Crowe DT, Devey JJ. Assessment and management of the hemorrhaging patient. Vet Clin North Am Small Anim Pract 1994;24:434–61.
32. Zeltzman P, Downs MO. Surgical sponges in small animal surgery. Compend Contin Educ Pract Vet 2011;33:E1–7.
33. Erne JB, Mann FA. Surgical hemostasis. Compend Contin Educ Pract 2003;25: 732–40.
34. Silver IA. Tissue adhesives. Vet Rec 1976;98:405–9.
35. Kheirabadi B. Evaluation of topical hemostatic agents for combat wound treatment. US Army Med Dep J 2011;2:25–37.
36. Herold L, Devey J, Kirby R, et al. Clinical evaluation and management of hemoperitoneum in dogs. J Vet Emerg Crit Care 2008;18:40–53.
37. Fucci V, Elkins AD. Electrosurgery: principles and guidelines in veterinary medicine. Compend Contin Educ Pract Vet 1991;13:407–15.
38. Crowe DT. Use of a nasogastric tube for gastric and esophageal decompression in the dog and cat. J Am Vet Med Assoc 1986;188:1178–82.
39. Moss G. Efficient gastroduodenal decompression with simultaneous full enteral nutrition: a new gastrostomy catheter technique. JPEN J Parenter Enteral Nutr 1984;8:203–7.

40. Whiteside OJ, Tytherleigh MG, Thrush S, et al. Intra-operative peritoneal lavage—who does it and why? Ann R Coll Surg Engl 2005;87:255–8.
41. Schein M, Gecelter G, Freinkel W, et al. Peritoneal lavage in abdominal sepsis. A controlled clinical study. Arch Surg 1990;125:1132–5.
42. Nicks BA, Ayello EA, Woo K, et al. Acute wound management: revisiting the approach to assessment, irrigation, and closure considerations. Int J Emerg Med 2010;3:399–407.
43. Schneider RK, Meyer DJ, Embertson RM, et al. Response of pony peritoneum to four peritoneal lavage solutions. Am J Vet Res 1988;49:889–94.
44. Szabo SD, Kieri Jermyn K, Neel J, et al. Evaluation of postceliotomy peritoneal drain fluid volume, cytology, and blood-to-peritoneal fluid lactate and glucose differences in normal dogs. Vet Surg 2011;40:444–9.
45. Rotondo MF, Schwab CW, McGonigal MD, et al. Damage control: an approach for improved survival in exsanguinating penetrating abdominal injury. J Trauma 1993;35:375–82.
46. Brasel KJ, Weigelt JA. Damage control in trauma surgery. Curr Opin Crit Care 2000;6:276–80.
47. Loveland JA, Boffard KD. Damage control in the abdomen and beyond. Br J Surg 2004;91:1095–101.
48. Wagner AE, Dunlop CI. Anesthetic and medical management of acute hemorrhage during surgery. J Am Vet Med Assoc 1993;203:40–5.
49. Giger U. Transfusion medicine. In: Silverstein DC, Hopper K, editors. Small animal critical care medicine. St Louis (MO): Saunders; 2009. p. 281–6.
50. Shock. In: American College of Surgeons Committee on Trauma. Advanced trauma life support for doctors. 8th edition. Chicago (IL): American College of Surgeons; 2008. p. 65–71.
51. Hirshberg A, Sheffer N, Barnea O. Computer simulation of hypothermia during "damage control" laparotomy. World J Surg 1999;23:960–5.
52. Waibel BH, Rotondo MF. Damage control in trauma and abdominal sepsis. Crit Care Med 2010;38:S421–30.
53. Rice TW, Morris S, Tortella BJ. Deviations from evidence-based clinical management guidelines increase mortality in critically injured trauma patients. Crit Care Med 2012;40:778–86.
54. Kirby KA, Wheeler JL, Farese JP, et al. Vacuum-assisted wound closure: application and mechanism of action. Compend Contin Educ Pract 2009;31:568–76.
55. Chisholm CD, Cordell WH, Rogers K, et al. Comparison of a new pressurized saline canister versus syringe irrigation for laceration cleansing in the emergency department. Ann Emerg Med 1992;21:1364–7.
56. Bansal BC, Wiebe RA, Perkins SD, et al. Tap water for irrigation of lacerations. Am J Emerg Med 2002;20:469–72.
57. Hall S. A review of the effect of tap water versus normal saline on infection rates in acute traumatic wounds. J Wound Care 2007;16:38–41.
58. Hranjec T, Swenson BR, Sawyer RG. Surgical site infection prevention: how do we do it. Surg Infect (Larchmt) 2010;11:289–94.
59. Morain WD, Colen LB. Wound healing in diabetes mellitus. Clin Plast Surg 1990; 17:493–501.
60. Greif R, Akça O, Horn EP, et al. Supplemental perioperative oxygen to reduce the incidence of surgical-wound infection. N Engl J Med 2000;342:161–7.
61. Cavanaugh RP, Kovak JR, Fischetti AJ, et al. Evaluation of surgically placed gastrojejunostomy feeding tubes in critically ill dogs. J Am Vet Med Assoc 2008;232:380–8.

62. Moss G, Greeenstein A, Levy S, et al. Maintenance of GI function after bowel surgery and immediate enteral full nutrition. I. Doubling of canine colorectal anastomotic bursting pressure and intestinal wound mature collagen content. JPEN J Parenter Enteral Nutr 1980;4:535–8.
63. Moore FA, Feliciano DV, Andrassy RJ, et al. Early enteral feeding, compared with parenteral, reduces postoperative septic complications. The results of a meta-analysis. Ann Surg 1992;216:172–83.
64. Feliciano DV. Trauma to the peripheral vascular system. In: Schwartz GR, Cayten CG, Mangelsen MA, et al, editors. Principles and practice of emergency medicine. 3rd edition. Philadelphia: Lea & Febiger; 1992. p. 1098.
65. Markowitz J, Archibald J, Downie HG, editors. Surgery of the liver. In experimental surgery including surgical physiology. 2nd edition. Baltimore (MD): Williams & Wilkins; 1964. p. 507–59.

Updates in the Management of the Small Animal Patient with Neurologic Trauma

Jillian DiFazio, DVM[a], Daniel J. Fletcher, PhD, DVM[b],*

KEYWORDS

- Neurotrauma • Traumatic brain injury • Head trauma • Acute spinal cord injury
- Resuscitation • Dog • Cat • Cerebral ischemia

KEY POINTS

- Neurotrauma, including traumatic brain injury (TBI) and acute spinal cord injury (SCI), is a cause of significant morbidity and mortality in veterinary patients.
- Damage to neuronal cells can be divided into primary and secondary injury.
- Pharmacologic and nonpharmacologic therapies are directed at addressing primary injury in SCI as well as minimizing the effects of secondary injury in both TBI and SCI.
- Prognosis for neurotrauma patients depends on the severity of injury, the site of the lesion, and the timing and efficacy of the treatment of primary and secondary injury.

Neurologic trauma, encompassing traumatic brain injury (TBI) and acute spinal cord injury (SCI), is a cause of significant morbidity and mortality in veterinary patients. In one recent retrospective study evaluating blunt trauma in dogs, a diagnosis of TBI was made in 25% of cases and was associated with increased mortality.[1] Acute SCIs occurring secondary to trauma (including vertebral fracture or luxation [VFL], traumatic intervertebral disk herniation, spinal cord parenchymal contusions, and extra-axial hemorrhage) are also common, with an estimated incidence rate of 14% in cats and 9% in dogs based on the information from single-center retrospective studies.[2,3] The causes of neurologic trauma in dogs and cats include motor vehicular trauma, falls, crush injuries, bite wounds, missile injuries (eg, gunshot wounds), and either accidental or purposeful human-inflicted trauma.[4–7] Essential to the management of TBI and SCI is a thorough understanding of the pathophysiology of the primary and secondary injury that occurs following trauma.[8] This article reviews the

a Section of Emergency and Critical Care, Cornell University Hospital for Animals, Upper Tower Road, Ithaca, NY 14853, USA; b Department of Clinical Sciences, Cornell University College of Veterinary Medicine, DCS Box 31, Ithaca, NY 14853, USA
* Corresponding author.
E-mail address: djf42@cornell.edu

Vet Clin Small Anim 43 (2013) 915–940
http://dx.doi.org/10.1016/j.cvsm.2013.03.002
0195-5616/13/$ – see front matter © 2013 Elsevier Inc. All rights reserved.
vetsmall.theclinics.com

pathophysiology of this primary and secondary injury, as well as recommendations regarding clinical assessment, diagnostics, pharmacologic and nonpharmacologic therapy, and prognosis.

MANAGEMENT GOALS

Damage to nervous tissue can be divided into primary and secondary injury. Primary injury occurs immediately after trauma and is the direct result of traumatic impact.[9–12] Secondary injury is often referred to as delayed injury, but usually begins within minutes of injury and can last several days to weeks afterward.[4,6,7,11,13–15] These categories may seem artificial at first, but are important when considering management.

Most TBI therapies are aimed at minimizing the effects of secondary injury. Because instability contributes to exacerbation of primary injury, depending on the type, management of acute SCI may include surgical therapy directed at stabilization to prevent further primary injury in addition to therapies directed at minimizing the effects of secondary injury.[15]

Primary Injury

Primary injury associated with TBI and SCI involves the physical disruption of intracranial structures (eg, TBI) and the spinal cord, vertebrae, and supporting structures (eg, SCI) that occurs at the time of impact. Primary injury is broadly classified as focal or diffuse depending on the extent of injury, and more specifically can be defined based on the location and type of injury.[11] The principal mechanical forces involved in neurologic trauma include concussion (eg, acceleration and deceleration), compression, shear, laceration, distraction, and contusion.[15–17] Primary injuries associated with TBI include epidural hematomas, subdural hematomas, subarachnoid hemorrhage, cortical contusions/hematomas, and traumatic axonal injury.[10] Primary SCI includes VFL, traumatic intervertebral disc herniation, intraparenchymal contusion, and extraaxial hemorrhage.

Secondary Injury

Box 1 summarizes the local factors contributing to secondary injury in neurologic trauma.[4,7,13,15–21] In addition, multiple systemic factors can potentiate secondary injury, most importantly hypoxia and hypotension but also hypercapnia, hypocapnia, hyperglycemia, hypoglycemia, acid-base disturbances, electrolyte abnormalities, hyperthermia, and systemic inflammation.[17,18] Other intracranial factors can also exacerbate secondary injury in TBI, including intracranial hypertension, edema, compromise of the blood-brain barrier (BBB), vasospasm, hemorrhage, infection, mass effects, and seizure activity.[17]

Secondary injury is potentiated by compromise of perfusion. Cerebral perfusion pressure (CPP) is defined as the net pressure facilitating blood flow to the brain, and is the difference between the mean arterial blood pressure (MAP) and intracranial pressure (ICP): $CPP = MAP - ICP$. Similarly, spinal cord perfusion pressure (SCPP) is the difference between MAP and cerebrospinal fluid pressure (CSFP): $SCPP = MAP - CSFP$.[22]

The Monroe-Kellie doctrine states that the cranial vault is a rigid, defined space that has a fixed volume with contributions from the brain parenchyma, cerebrospinal fluid (CSF), blood, and mass lesions (if present). An increase in the volume of any of these will result in a compensatory decrease in 1 or more of the others (defined as intracranial compliance; mainly reliant on changes in CSF or blood volumes), without which a pathologic increase in ICP will occur. With TBI the compensatory capacity of intracranial compliance can be overwhelmed, and intracranial hypertension may occur. Increases in ICP combined with decreases in MAP, a finding that is common in trauma patients, can result in decreases in CPP. In addition, compromise of autoregulatory mechanisms (eg, vasodilation/constriction of cerebral arterioles that maintain constant cerebral and spinal cord blood flow over a wide range of MAP ([0–150 mm Hg]) results in a more linear association between blood flow and MAP, leading to a greater risk of hypoperfusion or hyperemia.[11]

Severe, acute intracranial hypertension may result in the Cushing reflex or central nervous system (CNS) ischemic response. Decreased cerebral blood flow results in elevations in carbon dioxide (CO_2) levels sensed locally at the vasomotor center, causing a dramatic increase in sympathetic tone, ultimately leading to systemic vasoconstriction and increased cardiac output.[23] Increases in MAP stimulate baroreceptors in the aortic and carotid sinuses, resulting in a reflex sinus bradycardia. This response signifies potentially life-threatening intracranial hypertension and should be treated immediately.[4,7,17]

DIAGNOSTIC EVALUATION
Systemic Assessment

Initial triage assessment of the trauma patient should focus on global patient stability with special emphasis on the respiratory and cardiovascular systems. In patients with neurotrauma, this is perhaps even more important because hypotension, hypoxemia, and changes in ventilation contribute to secondary injury and worsen outcome.

Neurologic Assessment

The initial neurologic examination should occur before administration of any analgesic therapy to allow adequate assessment of the neurologic system. Initial neurologic examination should include an evaluation of mentation, cranial nerve reflexes, ambulatory status, presence of voluntary motor function (assessed only in recumbency in the nonambulatory patient with potential VFL), presence of superficial pain perception in the patient who does not demonstrate voluntary motor function, presence of deep pain sensation in the patient who does not demonstrate intact superficial pain perception, spinal reflexes, panniculus reflex, anal tone, and perineal reflex. If the patient is ambulatory and the clinician is not suspicious of a VFL, assessment of gait and proprioceptive function can also occur. Gentle palpation of the spinal column should be done in all patients presenting with possible acute SCI to localize regions of malalignment (eg, "step" fracture), instability, discomfort, or crepitus. When performing a neurologic assessment, it is important that the patient has been adequately resuscitated, as shock can affect neurologic status. In addition, it is important that a thorough recumbent orthopedic examination also be performed to rule out orthopedic injury as a potential cause for apparent neurologic signs.[13,15]

Whenever SCI secondary to VFL is suspected in the nonambulatory patient, minimal movement of the patient should occur. The patient should be immobilized and secured to a backboard until definitive assessment for fractures and luxations can occur.[13,15]

Patients should be neurolocalized and graded based on severity of signs. The Modified Glasgow Coma Scale (MGCS) has been validated in dogs, and is useful in the assessment of TBI patients, as it provides a means of more objectively determining improvement or progression of clinical signs. It also yields prognostic information (**Box 2**).[24,25] One retrospective study showed that the MGCS correlated well with the probability of survival in the first 48 hours after TBI in dogs.[25] Repeated neurologic

Box 1
Mechanisms of secondary injury

Secondary Injury

Glutamate accumulation

- Occurs secondary to:
  - Adenosine triphosphate (ATP) depletion
  - Neuronal cell injury
  - Positive feedback
  - Decreased conversion
  - Potentiated by low interstitial magnesium
- Results in:
  - Loss of ionic gradients
  - Excitotoxicity
  - Generation of free radical oxygen species

Influx of sodium into neuronal cells

- Occurs secondary to:
  - Glutamate accumulation
- Results in:
  - Cytotoxic edema

Influx of calcium into neuronal cells

- Occurs secondary to:
  - Glutamate accumulation
  - Primary injury
- Results in:
  - Cytotoxic edema
  - Neuronal cell destruction through activation of proteases, lipases and endonucleases
  - Reactive oxygen species production through calpain activation
  - Inflammatory mediator release
  - Mitochondrial dysfunction and ATP depletion

Free radical production

- Occurs secondary to:
  - Glutamate accumulation
  - Inflammatory mediator release
  - Increased cytosolic calcium concentrations
  - Ischemia-reperfusion injury
- Results in:
  - Neuronal cell destruction

Inflammatory mediator release

- Occurs secondary to:
  - Primary injury

- ○ Neuronal cell destruction with secondary injury
- Results in:
  - ○ Activation of nitric oxide with alterations in blood flow and vascular permeability
  - ○ Inflammatory cell influx
  - ○ Coagulation cascade activation and thrombosis

Loss of autoregulation

- Occurs secondary to:
  - ○ Primary injury
- Results in:
  - ○ Ischemia

All mechanisms contribute to neuronal cell death

Box 2
Modified Glasgow Coma Scale

Level of Consciousness

6. Occasional periods of alertness and responsive to environment
5. Depression or delirium, capable of responding but response may be inappropriate
4. Semicomatose, responsive to visual stimuli
3. Semicomatose, responsive to auditory stimuli
2. Semicomatose, responsive only to repeated noxious stimuli
1. Comatose, unresponsive to repeated noxious stimuli

Brainstem Reflexes

6. Normal pupillary light reflexes and oculocephalic reflexes
5. Slow pupillary light reflexes and normal to reduced oculocephalic reflexes
4. Bilateral unresponsive miosis with normal to reduced oculocephalic reflexes
3. Pinpoint pupils with reduced to absent oculocephalic reflexes
2. Unilateral, unresponsive mydriasis with reduced to absent oculocephalic reflexes
1. Bilateral, unresponsive mydriasis with reduced to absent oculocephalic reflexes

Motor activity

6. Normal gait, normal spinal reflexes
5. Hemiparesis, tetraparesis, or decerebrate activity
4. Recumbent, intermittent extensor rigidity
3. Recumbent, constant extensor rigidity
2. Recumbent, constant extensor rigidity with opisthotonus
1. Recumbent, hypotonia of muscles, depressed or absent spinal reflexes

assessment is recommended every 30 to 60 minutes after initial presentation to assess clinical response to therapy or progression of clinical signs. There are currently 3 validated scoring systems available for assessing the severity of deficits associated with SCI: the Modified Frankel Score, the 14-Point Motor Score, and the Texas Spinal Cord Injury Score.[26,27]

Brachial plexus injuries should be suspected if a patient has decreased reflexes in only one of the forelimbs, Horner syndrome on the affected side, and decreased panniculus reflex on the affected side.[13] The presence of spinal shock may affect neurolocalization in patients with acute SCI. Spinal shock leads to deficits in segmental spinal reflexes caudal to a lesion, even though the reflex arcs remain physically intact, causing flaccid paralysis, due to a sudden interruption in descending supraspinal input that occurs with acute SCI. Recovery from spinal shock in humans is protracted, but in dogs and cats occurs much more rapidly, typically within 12 to 24 hours.[28]

Imaging

Extra-CNS assessment
As with any trauma patient, imaging should include thoracic radiographs to rule out pulmonary contusions, pneumothorax, and other chest or pulmonary trauma, as well as imaging of the abdomen. Ideally, additional diagnostics such as ultrasonographic imaging via focused assessment with sonography for trauma can also be performed to rule out organ fracture and peritoneal effusion (eg, hemoperitoneum, uroperitoneum, septic peritonitis).[29,30]

Intracranial and spinal assessment
Intracranial imaging for the TBI small animal patient is indicated in patients who fail to respond to aggressive medical management, patients who deteriorate after an initial response to medical therapy, and/or those patients with focal or asymmetric neurologic signs. Computed tomography (CT) is the modality of choice for characterization of TBI in the acute setting, as it is quick, relatively inexpensive, and has excellent ability to identify extra-axial hemorrhage (eg, epidural, subdural, and subarachnoid/intraventricular hemorrhage), intra-axial hemorrhage (eg, cortical contusion, intraparenchymal hematoma, and traumatic axonal injury), cerebral swelling, and cerebral herniation.[9–11] Beyond the acute setting, magnetic resonance imaging (MRI) is recommended when patients continue to be nonresponsive to medical therapy or deteriorate with continued aggressive management despite having normal CT scans.[10,11]

Although plain radiography can yield important information regarding SCI in small animal patients, it has been shown to have relatively low sensitivity for detecting vertebral fractures (72%) and subluxations (77.5%) in dogs.[31] Orthogonal radiographs (ie, both views obtained in lateral recumbency using the horizontal beam technique) should be obtained if more advanced imaging is unavailable. The entire spine should be imaged, as approximately 20% of patients with spinal trauma have multiple VFLs.[32] Absence of VFLs on radiographs should not be used to definitively exclude their presence. Radiographic signs associated with intervertebral disk herniation include narrowing of the disk space, mineralized disk material, narrowing of the articular facets, and narrowing or increased opacity of the intervertebral foramen.[33,34] These signs have relatively low accuracy (51%–61%), sensitivity (64%–69%), and positive predictive value (63%–71%) in diagnosing disk herniation.[33] In addition, other SCIs can occur with trauma that may not be evident with radiography alone.

CT is the imaging modality of choice for bone, and therefore is recommended in the patient whose clinical signs are suggestive of an unstable VFL. CT has been documented to have sensitivity of up to 100% in some human studies for the diagnosis of VFLs.[13] Myelography and CT can be combined, and yields the highest sensitivity for detecting intervertebral disk herniation sites, though CT alone still maintains relatively good sensitivity. Although CT requires sedation or general anesthesia, modern CT scanners are very quick, making this a feasible imaging approach for the polytrauma patient. Whole-body CT scans can often be obtained in less than a minute and allow assessment of the skull, brain, spine, thorax, and abdomen.

Myelography involves injecting contrast into the subarachnoid space and identifying attenuation of the ventral, dorsal, or lateral contrast columns at sites of extradural compression. Myelography provides more information than plain radiography regarding the site of intervertebral disk herniation. Studies have shown agreement between myelographic and surgical findings of approximately 81% to 98%, with accuracy for lateralization of the lesion being approximately 53% to 100%.[34-37] However, myelography provides little additional information regarding presence of VFLs or intraparenchymal injury. Myelography requires general anesthesia and also carries risks associated with contrast administration, including postprocedure seizures.[38,39]

MRI is considered the superior imaging modality for soft tissue including the spinal cord parenchyma, intervertebral disks, and nerve roots. However, it provides relatively poor detail of bony structures and, therefore, is not the modality of choice when pursuing further imaging for VFLs.[40] This modality is more expensive than other techniques and requires longer periods of anesthesia. At the authors' institution it is typically used when other techniques (eg, CT) fail to reveal a cause for neurologic dysfunction in the traumatic SCI patient.

PHARMACOLOGIC STRATEGIES
Systemic Therapy

Oxygen therapy
Oxygen should be supplemented if needed to maintain normoxemia (oxygen partial pressure [Pa_{O_2}] = 80–100 mm Hg and pulse oxygen saturation [Sp_{O_2}] = 94%–98%), but should be titrated to avoid hyperoxemia, which could worsen reperfusion injury.[7] Methods for providing oxygen include flow-by mask, nasal or nasopharyngeal cannulation, oxygen cages or tents, and endotracheal administration.[41] Flow-by mask administration is typically recommended during initial assessment and resuscitation until oxygenation monitoring can be initiated. Nasal or nasopharyngeal cannulation has the benefit of ensuring high concentrations of inspired oxygen, but nasal stimulation can induce sneezing, which can lead to increases in ICP. Because of reduced levels of consciousness, most TBI patients tolerate nasal oxygen quite well. Oxygen cages also can provide relatively high levels of inspired oxygen, but unfortunately minimize access to the critically ill patient.[42] Each patient should be evaluated and the best modality for oxygen administration determined for the individual. If adequate oxygenation cannot be maintained with high fractional oxygen concentrations (Fi_{O_2}) greater than 60%, mechanical ventilation is indicated.[43]

Intravenous fluid therapy
Controversy exists in veterinary medicine regarding the best choice of fluid for resuscitation in the neurotrauma patient. Options for fluid resuscitation include isotonic crystalloids, hypertonic solutions, artificial colloidal solutions, and blood products. Concern exists particularly in TBI management regarding the injured brain's capacity to protect against increases in cerebral edema when faced with fluids containing large amounts of free water caused by disruption of cellular tight junctions and subsequent influxes of ions and larger, colloid-sized molecules with secondary osmotic pull.[4] It is therefore recommended that isotonic fluids containing the least amount of free water (eg, 0.9%

NaCl) be administered, barring significant sodium derangements already present on presentation. Because fluid shifts between the interstitial and intracellular compartments of the brain are predominantly dictated by osmolality as opposed to plasma oncotic pressure, colloidal solutions have not demonstrated any significant benefit over crystalloid therapy.[44] However, owing to rapid redistribution of crystalloids after administration, a combination of colloidal therapy with crystalloid therapy (either isotonic or hypertonic) can be considered to provide longer-lasting volume resuscitation.[7]

Hypertonic saline (HTS) has several potential benefits in the neurologic trauma patient (particularly the TBI patient), including rapidly increasing intravascular volume, increasing cardiac output, improving regional cerebral and spinal cord blood flow by dehydrating cerebrovascular endothelial cells, increasing vessel diameter, decreasing ICP, and enhancing cerebral oxygen delivery.[45–50] It is important that the concentration of HTS being used is noted, as this will affect the dosing of the solution.[4] HTS should be used only in euhydrated patients without significant sodium derangements. In addition, it is imperative that HTS be followed by crystalloid therapy to maintain adequate tissue hydration.

Anemic patients should be treated with packed red blood cells or whole blood to maintain adequate arterial oxygen content and oxygen delivery to damaged nervous tissue. Transfusion goals include normalization of perfusion parameters (including central venous oxygenation saturation >70%). Fresh frozen plasma should be administered to the coagulopathic patient.[7] Those patients that do not respond to fluid resuscitation warrant vasopressor support.[7] After initial fluid resuscitation, fluid therapy should be continued to account for maintenance needs, deficits, and any ongoing losses. Recommended initial bolus dosing of intravenous fluids are listed in **Table 1**.

Pain management

Analgesic therapy is essential in the management of the neurotrauma patient. The degree of analgesia and sedation must be balanced with preservation of blood pressure and ventilatory status, as depression of each of these parameters can contribute to secondary injury, and if possible should not impede reassessment of neurologic status. Adequate analgesia in the TBI patient avoids transient increases in ICP caused by pain and agitation, which can lead to increased cerebral metabolic rate and, consequently, cerebral blood flow and volume.[51]

Opioids are the analgesic drugs of choice in critical care medicine, because of their ease of reversal and relative safety when titrated to effect. Several studies suggest that bolus infusion of opioids should be avoided, and constant-rate infusions (CRIs) are preferred.[51–55] Because of the ease of reversal, it is recommended that full agonist opioids be used.[56,57]

Ketamine noncompetitively inhibits the N-methyl-D-aspartate (NMDA) receptor; therefore, this agent may have neuroprotective properties against ischemic and glutamate-induced injury in addition to its cardiovascular and respiratory-sparing properties. Recent studies have failed to demonstrate that ketamine results in the ICP increases typically reported in the older literature.[51] However, it has been shown to increase cerebral oxygen consumption, possibly through inhibition of the γ-aminobutyric acid (GABA) receptor. Therefore, administration with a GABA agonist (eg, propofol) potentially could decrease these negative effects.

Medetomidine, an α2-agonist, has been documented to have no effect on ICP in anesthetized dogs.[58] Caution must be exercised in using this class of drugs for their analgesic or sedative properties, as they can cause clinically significant reductions in heart rate and cardiac output, thereby affecting CNS perfusion.[23] **Table 2** lists the recommended analgesics and their respective doses.

Table 1
Intravenous fluid therapy and recommended doses

Fluid Type	Recommended Dose
Isotonic crystalloid (0.9% NaCl preferred)	20–30 mL/kg dogs; 10–20 mL/kg cats Administered over 15–20 min Reassess after
Synthetic colloid (eg, 6% hydroxyethylstarch)	5–10 mL/kg Administered over 15–20 min Reassess after
7.5% NaCl	4 mL/kg Administered over 15–20 min Reassess after Always follow with crystalloid therapy
3% NaCl	5.4 mL/kg Administered over 15–20 min Reassess after Always follow with crystalloid therapy
1:2 Ratio of 23.4% NaCl and 6% hydroxyethylstarch or other synthetic colloid	4 mL/kg Administered over 15–20 min Reassess after Always follow with crystalloid therapy
Packed red blood cells	∼10–15 mL/kg Administer over less than 4 h/unit Target normalization of perfusion parameters and packed cell volume (PCV) = 25%–30%
Whole blood	∼20–30 mL/kg Administer within 4 h/unit Target normalization of perfusion parameters and PCV = 25%–30%
Fresh frozen plasma	10–15 mL/kg Administer within 4 h/unit Target normalization of coagulation times

Pharmacologic Strategies Specific for TBI

Hyperosmolar therapy

Intracranial hypertension has consistently been associated with poor outcomes in patients with TBI.[59] Hyperosmolar therapy has been the cornerstone of managing intracranial hypertension since the early twentieth century when HTS and glucose solutions were documented to decrease CSF pressure in cats.[60] The brain is composed

Table 2
Analgesic therapy and recommended doses

Analgesic	Recommended Dose
Fentanyl	Dogs: 2 µg/kg, then constant-rate infusion (CRI) at 2–5 µg/kg/h Cats: 1 µg/kg, then CRI at 1–2 µg/kg/h
Morphine	Dogs: 0.15–0.5 mg/kg slow, then CRI at 0.1–1 mg/kg/h
Ketamine	0.1–1 mg/kg, then CRI at 2–10 µg/kg/min
Lidocaine	Dogs: 1–2 mg/kg, then CRI at 25–80 µg/kg/min
Dexmedetomidine	0.5–1 µg/kg/h

of approximately 80% water, making its volume very responsive to changes in water content. An osmotic agent is only effective if the BBB is impermeable to it. Sodium and mannitol have near perfect exclusion by the BBB, making HTS and mannitol extremely effective for addressing intracranial hypertension. Hyperosmolar therapy in TBI predominantly affects normal, rather than injured, brain tissue.[61] Mannitol is a sugar alcohol that is not significantly metabolized and is excreted unchanged in the urine after intravenous infusion. It is recommended as a first-line treatment for intracranial hypertension.[62] **Table 3** summarizes mannitol's mechanisms of action, recommended dosing, and side effects.[4,63–81] Mannitol is not recommended for prophylactic use in patients with TBI unless there is concern for elevations in ICP, because its effectiveness is related to the degree of intracranial hypertension and its associated response decreases as the cumulative dose increases (ie, it may be less effective when actually necessary).[64,65] Mannitol administration should always be followed by isotonic crystalloid and/or colloid therapy to avoid hypovolemia caused by its diuretic effect, and serum osmolarity should ideally be measured, if possible, when repeated doses are administered.[7]

Table 3 Mannitol versus hypertonic saline		
	Mannitol	**Hypertonic Saline**
Mechanism of action	Increases osmotic gradient across BBB Plasma expansion with decreased blood viscosity Improves brain oxygen delivery and autoregulation Results in cerebral vasoconstriction, decreasing cerebral blood volume and ICP Free radical scavenger	Increases osmotic gradient across BBB Volume expansion Increases cardiac output and blood pressure
Recommended dose	0.5–1.0 g/kg slow over 15–20 min Effects begin within minutes, peak within 15–120 min, duration 1–5 h No benefit of CRIs over boluses	7.5% NaCl: 4 mL/kg 3% NaCl: 5.4 mL/kg 1:2 ratio 23.4% NaCl to 6%, Hetastarch: 4 mL/kg Administered over 15–20 min Reassess after Always follow with crystalloid therapy
Side effects	Volume depletion Electrolyte abnormalities (hyponatremia [pseudo-], hypernatremia, hypokalemia) Acid-base derangements (eg, metabolic acidosis) Congestive heart failure Acute kidney injury (osmolality >320 mOsm/L)	Electrolyte abnormalities (hypernatremia, hyperchloremia) Acid-base derangements (eg, metabolic acidosis) Congestive heart failure Acute kidney injury (less common than with mannitol)
Relative contraindications	Hypovolemia	Significant sodium derangements Dehydration

Abbreviations: BBB, blood-brain barrier; CRI, constant-rate infusion; ICP, intracranial pressure.

Hypertonic saline therapy affords similar osmotic benefits as mannitol therapy, but is a less potent diuretic. **Table 3** summarizes HTS's mechanisms of action, recommended dosing, adverse effects, and relative contraindications.[63,66] It is generally recommended that sodium concentrations be maintained at less than 160 mEq/L, although concentrations of up to 180 mEq/L have been reported in humans treated with hypertonic saline with no complications.[67]

There is no evidence that mannitol is superior to HTS in the treatment of intracranial hypertension or vice versa. The small number of studies available have shown conflicting results.[68–71] It is likely that HTS is preferable in hypovolemic patients, but in euvolemic patients, either is reasonable. When patients do not respond to treatment with one agent, the alternative should be considered.

Administration of furosemide alone or concurrently with mannitol to treat intracranial hypertension has not been shown to have any additional benefit and increases the risk of volume depletion.[72] Therefore, its use is not recommended.

Corticosteroids

Corticosteroids were previously advocated for in the treatment of TBI patients on the basis that corticosteroids decreased cerebral edema. Ground-breaking evidence from the CRASH trials showed that high-dose methylprednisolone was associated with an increase in mortality at 2 weeks and 6 months after injury.[73,74] Corticosteroids are therefore no longer recommended in the treatment of TBI patients.

Anticonvulsant therapy

Posttraumatic seizures are classified as immediate (occurring within 24 hours of injury), early (occurring 24 hours to 7 days after injury), or late (occurring more than 7 days after injury).[62] Seizures increase secondary brain injury by increasing cerebral metabolic demands, increasing ICP, and leading to the release of excessive neurotransmitters. A recent Cochrane meta-analysis concluded that prophylactic antiepileptic drugs are effective in reducing early seizures, but there is no evidence that they are effective in preventing late-onset seizures. Therefore, prophylactic antiepileptic drugs are recommended for 7 days post-TBI in humans.[75] There are few data in veterinary medicine, but if seizures develop, aggressive antiepileptic drug (AED) therapy is indicated to reduce secondary brain injury. The incidence of posttraumatic seizures in small animals is not well documented, but seizures are known to occur. At present, there are no clear recommendations for prophylactic AED therapy in veterinary medicine. If risk factors for seizures are present (eg, penetrating head wounds, depressed skull fractures, and so forth), it is reasonable to consider prophylactic AED therapy for the first 7 days after injury, based on human recommendations. The duration of AED therapy is debatable. Should seizures occur, benzodiazepines should be used as a first-line treatment to stop seizure activity.[76] A variety of AEDs for continued seizure control are available for use in dogs and cats, and these are listed in **Table 4**. At the authors' institution, levetiracetam is frequently used for its rapid onset of action, minimal side effects, and low toxicity potential.

Barbiturate therapy

Barbiturates are considered secondary therapy for the treatment of refractory intracranial hypertension in people, as high-dose therapy can control ICP when other medical and surgical therapies have failed. However, no outcome benefit has been documented.[62] The neuroprotective effects of barbiturates are related to their ability to cause cerebral vasoconstriction, decrease cerebral metabolism, reduce ICP, decrease excitotoxicity, and decrease free radical–mediated injury.[77] Barbiturates also have anticonvulsant properties. Complications associated with the use of barbiturates

Table 4
Antiepileptic drugs and recommended doses

Antiepileptic Drug	Recommended Dose
Diazepam	0.5 mg/kg IV, rectally, intranasally CRI 0.2–1 mg/kg/h
Phenobarbital	Loading 12–20 mg/kg IV, PO divided q 4–6 h over 24 h Dogs: 2.5 mg/kg IV, PO q 12 h initially Targeting trough levels of 20–30 μg/mL Cats: 1–2 mg/kg IV, PO q 24 h initially Targeting trough levels of 10–20 μg/mL
Potassium bromide	Loading 400–600 mg/kg KBr PO/rectally divided q 6–12 h over 24–48 h Loading 600–1200 mg/kg NaBr IV as CRI over 8–24 h 30–50 mg/kg/d as a monotherapy 15–30 mg/kg/d as an add-on drug Targeting trough levels of 0.8–3 mg/mL Not recommended in cats (because of high risk of lower airway signs)
Levetiracetam (Keppra)	20–30 mg/kg IV, PO q 8 h No load necessary
Zonisamide	Loading 10 mg/kg PO q 12 h × 3 d 5–10 mg/kg q 12 h thereafter Targeting therapeutic range described for humans (10–40 μg/mL)
Gabapentin	Dogs: 30–60 mg/kg q 24 h divided q 8–12 h Cats: 5–10 mg/kg q 12–24 h
Propofol	1–4 mg/kg IV bolus CRI 0.05–0.4 mg/kg/min
Pentobarbital Antiepileptic drug used most commonly for induction of barbiturate coma	2–15 mg/kg bolus over 20 min CRI 0.2–1 mg/kg/h

Abbreviations: CRI, constant-rate infusion; IV, intravenously; PO, by mouth; q, every.

include cardiovascular and respiratory depression, with potentially clinically significant hypotension (and associated decreases in CPP) and hypoventilation. The most widely used barbiturate for TBI is pentobarbital.[4] Barbiturate coma (induced with drugs such as phenobarbital or other sedatives) was recently described in association with therapeutic hypothermia (TH) in a dog with TBI and refractory seizure activity.[78] Patients in which barbiturate therapy is instituted must be monitored closely for hypoventilation, and may require mechanical ventilation.

Novel therapies

New therapies targeting excitotoxicity and production of reactive oxygen species are currently being investigated in human medicine, but none have been examined in veterinary practice to date. A recent randomized controlled trial of amantadine in vegetative or minimally conscious humans recovering from TBI showed significantly faster functional recovery over a 4-week period in treated patients.[79] In the near future, more options specifically targeting secondary injury may become available to veterinary practitioners.

Pharmacologic Strategies Specific for Acute SCI

Corticosteroids

The use of corticosteroids in the treatment of acute SCI in humans and animals remains controversial despite extensive clinical research. Proposed mechanisms supporting the use of corticosteroids in SCI include free radical scavenging, anti-inflammatory effects, and improved regional blood flow.[13,15] Much of the clinical and experimental research on corticosteroid therapy in SCI has focused on methylprednisolone sodium succinate (MPSS). The main neuroprotective property of MPSS appears to be its free radical–scavenging ability. Other corticosteroids (eg, prednisone and dexamethasone) lack this property, and are unlikely to have any beneficial effect in the treatment of secondary SCI.[80] Specific evaluation of dexamethasone therapy in dogs has also failed to reveal any benefit in SCI, either experimentally or clinically.[81,82] A series of 3 human clinical trials (National Acute Spinal Cord Injury Studies [NASCIS] I–III) provide the majority of primary evidence relating to the use of MPSS for the treatment of acute SCI.[83–85] None of these studies convincingly demonstrated a benefit of steroids in improving motor function scores, as most of the statistically significant results were based on post hoc subgroup analyses.[86] An experimental study in dogs comparing urgent surgical decompression with MPSS for the treatment of experimentally induced SCI showed that surgical decompression 6 hours after injury (with or without MPSS) resulted in better neurologic outcomes than treatment with MPSS alone.[87] Another experimental dog study showed no improvement in outcome with MPSS administration.[88] There are no published clinical placebo-controlled trials evaluating the efficacy of MPSS in the treatment of SCI in dogs, although there is currently one under way.[16] Given the potential for significant adverse side effects, such as gastrointestinal ulceration, immunosuppression, and compromise of renal perfusion in hypovolemic patients, the routine administration of corticosteroids (including MPSS) is not recommended.[13]

Box 3 summarizes additional pharmacologic therapies directed at minimizing secondary injury in acute SCI that have been investigated.[89–101]

NONPHARMACOLOGIC STRATEGIES
Systemic Therapy

Airway management and ventilation

The upper airway should be directly examined and suctioned if necessary when a neurotrauma patient is initially presented. If the airway is deemed nonpatent or if the patient is unable to control its airway, immediate endotracheal intubation or emergency tracheostomy (if unable to intubate) is indicated.[7] Carbon dioxide has profound effects on cerebral and spinal cord blood flow and blood volume.[102] Both hypoventilation and hyperventilation should be avoided in neurotrauma patients, and close monitoring of CO_2 using end-tidal CO_2 ($ETCO_2$) monitors or blood-gas analysis is warranted. Normal partial pressure of carbon dioxide (Pco_2) (venous, 40–45 mm Hg; arterial, 35–40 mm Hg) should be targeted in all cases.[62] Titration of analgesic medication, positioning in sternal recumbency, and ensuring that the airway is unobstructed can help address ventilation issues, but if these interventions are unsuccessful, endotracheal intubation and mechanical ventilation are indicated. Those patients at risk of cerebral herniation or that have experienced significant neurologic decompensation can be hyperventilated for short periods of time. However, the targets of short-term hyperventilation should be conservative ($ETCO_2 = 30–35$ mm Hg) to prevent excessive cerebral vasoconstriction and ischemic brain injury. Studies evaluating prophylactic hyperventilation during initial resuscitation consistently have shown poor outcomes.[103–105]

Box 3
Pharmacologic agents for the treatment of secondary injury in acute SCI

Agents Directed at Free Radical Injury

- Vitamin E and selenium
  - Pretreatment of cats before SCI resulted in improved neurologic outcome and spinal cord blood flow following injury
- Tirilazad (21-aminosteroid)
  - Reduced spinal cord ischemia in cats
  - Effect not documented in dogs
- *N*-Acetylcysteine
  - No improvement in outcome in dogs with intervertebral disk herniation
- Sulfoxide and ε-aminocaproic acid
  - No improvement in outcome in dogs

Antioxidants require a prolonged period of administration to achieve therapeutic concentrations within the CNS, limiting their use in the acute phase of SCI

Agents Directed at Ionic Disturbances and Excitotoxicity

- Verapamil, diltiazem, nifedipine (calcium-channel antagonists)
  - Improved spinal cord blood flow in cats postinjury with diltiazem and nifedipine; not verapamil
- Sodium-channel blockers
  - Beneficial effects noted in experimental models
- NMDA and non-NMDA glutamate receptor antagonists
  - Delayed administration improved tissue sparing and functional recovery in rodent models
  - Most have adverse side effects and have largely failed clinical trials

Agents Directed at Inflammation

- Minocycline (second-generation tetracycline derivative)
  - Reduces activation of microglia and macrophages experimentally
  - Not yet evaluated in a trial
- Tacrolimus, cyclosporine, mycophenolate mofetil
  - Neuroprotective effects in experimental models of injury

Polyethylene Glycol

- Hydrophilic polymer that seals damaged neuronal membranes
- Evaluated in deep pain perception negative dogs; resulted in restored function in 60% of dogs
- Randomized, controlled trial in dogs currently underway

4-Aminopyridine

- Potassium-channel blocker
  - Improves conduction by blocking the channels that would ordinarily be blocked by intact myelin
- Improves conduction in vitro and vestibulospinal reflexes in cats
- Phase I clinical trial with 39 dogs with SCI

- ○ 64% of dogs had transient improvements in neurologic function
- ○ Side effects rare, but significant

Additional Therapies

- Naloxone (opiate receptor antagonist)
  - ○ Failed to yield a benefit in human clinical trial
- Thyrotropin-receptor antagonist
  - ○ Failed to yield a benefit in canine clinical trial
- Erythropoietin, progesterone and estrogen, magnesium, atorvastatin, melatonin

Supportive care

Supportive care of the patient with neurologic trauma should include the provision of dry, clean bedding; frequent turning; passive range of motion exercises; bladder care; ocular care (eg, frequent lubrication and inspection for corneal ulceration); and nutrition. Hypermetabolic states have been documented in patients with neurotrauma, and early feeding is recommended.[106] The method of feeding should be based on the assessment of a patient's ability to protect the airway. Although hyperglycemia has been associated with worsened mortality rates and neurologic outcome scores in humans with TBI[107] and degree of hyperglycemia has been associated with severity of TBI in animals,[108] intensive insulin therapy is not recommended for the control of hyperglycemia, based on the available human literature.[109–111]

Bladder dysfunction is common in SCI patients, and depends on the location and severity of the lesion. **Table 5** summarizes therapies for upper and lower motor neuron bladder dysfunction.[112] Bladder care should include frequent (minimum every 12 hours) manual bladder expression or urinary catheterization. Compared with indwelling catheterization, intermittent urinary catheterization using a diligent aseptic technique is associated with a decreased risk of urinary tract infection, and there is no increased risk of infection with intermittent catheterization in comparison with manual expression.[113,114]

Nonpharmacologic Strategies Specific for TBI

Decreasing cerebral blood volume

Elevation of the head by 15° to 30° reduces cerebral blood volume, thereby decreasing ICP and increasing CPP without harmful reductions in cerebral oxygenation.[115] A stiff slant board should be used for head elevation to avoid bending of the neck and occlusion of the jugular veins. Elevation should not exceed 30°, as this can contribute to a decrease in CPP with associated effects on cerebral oxygenation.[7]

Table 5
Pharmacologic agents for bladder dysfunction

Upper Motor Neuron Bladder	Lower Motor Neuron Bladder
α-Adrenergic antagonist Prazosin Phenoxybenzamine	Parasympathomimetic Bethanechol
Skeletal muscle relaxant Diazepam	α-Adrenergic agonist Phenylpropanolamine

Therapeutic hypothermia

Many of the processes of neurotraumatic secondary injury are temperature dependent.[116] TH, targeting temperatures of 32° to 34°C (89.6–93.2°F), decreases basal and cerebral metabolism, prevents apoptosis and necrosis and decreases cerebral edema formation and disruption of the BBB by decreasing release of excitotoxic amino acids (EAAs), decreases production of proinflammatory cytokines, and decreases excitatory signaling that can result in seizure activity.[117] Therapeutic hypothermia is indicated as a second-line treatment in humans for intracranial hypertension and status epilepticus[116,117]; however, it has not gained widespread acceptance as a first-line treatment for TBI, likely because it is challenging to implement and has many potential complications.[116,117] Few veterinary practices have the facilities to offer TH, but its successful use in a dog with protracted seizure activity associated with TBI has been described.[78] As technologies for inducing TH and supporting patients being treated become more accessible in veterinary medicine, this therapy may gain more acceptance.

Decompressive craniectomy

Early craniotomy is indicated for evacuation of extra-axial hematomas. The role of decompressive craniectomy is more controversial in the management of TBI patients. It may be performed prophylactically at the time of mass evacuation if early craniotomy is performed, or later as a second-line, rescue therapy when medical management has failed.[118] The results of the ongoing RESCUEicp trial may provide additional insight into the role of early decompressive craniectomy in the management of patients with TBI.[119]

Nonpharmacologic Strategies Specific for Acute SCI

Surgery is usually indicated in patients with moderate to severe deficits, neurologic deterioration, and/or instability of the vertebral column. Controversy exists regarding the best timing for surgical intervention in spinal cord trauma. Many traumatic SCI patients have extraspinal injuries that require initial stabilization. Nevertheless, earlier surgical treatment of human patients with traumatic SCI has been associated with improved outcomes.[120–122]

Management of vertebral fracture and luxation

The stability of spinal fractures in both humans and veterinary patients can be assessed using a 3-compartment model. This model divides the vertebral column into dorsal, middle, and ventral compartments, and a fracture is considered unstable when 2 or more compartments are disrupted. **Table 6** lists the structures included in each of the 3 compartments.[123,124]

General indications for surgical management include moderate to severe neurologic deficits (eg, minimal to no motor function), evidence of vertebral column instability on imaging, and neurologic deterioration despite aggressive conservative management.[13] Spinal cord decompression, reduction, and fixation are the aims of surgical management. There are many surgical techniques for stabilization of VFLs after reduction. The technique chosen depends on the location within the vertebral column, the type of fracture, and surgeon's preference.[123] Stabilization techniques include bone plates, screws, Steinmann pins, Kirschner wires, and polymethylmethacrylate (PMMA) cement.[13] VFLs should be managed by board-certified orthopedic surgeons or neurosurgeons. Although surgical management is often indicated, return to function is generally shorter, and postoperative supportive care is generally less intensive than that required in conservative management, complications can occur, potentially leading to worsening of SCI. Worsening of SCI can occur with surgical manipulation,

Table 6 Three-compartment model for assessing stability of VFLs		
Dorsal Compartment	**Middle Compartment**	**Ventral Compartment**
Vertebral arch (spinous process, articular processes, laminae, pedicles)	Dorsal longitudinal ligament	Ventral portion of the vertebral body
Dorsal ligamentous complex (facet joint capsule, interarcuate ligaments, interspinous ligaments, supraspinous ligaments)	Dorsal aspect of the annulus fibrosus	Nucleus pulposus
Intertransverse ligaments	Dorsal cortex of the vertebral body	Ventral aspect of the annulus fibrosus Ventral longitudinal ligament

loosening of implants, and implant failure or infection (particularly with PMMA). Revisional surgeries are, therefore, sometimes required.[13]

Conservative management of primary injury is most appropriate for patients with minimal deficits, static disease, and good 3-compartment stability. External coaptation has been described, but application of these devices is fraught with complications including inadequate stabilization, increased mobility of VFL sites, and abrasions and ulcerations. Conservative management, therefore, usually consists of strict cage rest for 6 to 8 weeks, analgesia, and nursing care.

Traumatic intervertebral disk herniation

Patients who are nonambulatory, have progressive neurologic deficits, are nonresponsive to conservative management, or have cervical lesions causing severe pain should be considered for surgical management.[34,125,126] With Type III (traumatic) intervertebral disk disease, surgical therapy is often not indicated unless there is an associated compressive extra-axial hematoma. Depending on the site, degree of lateralization, and severity of herniation, dorsal laminectomy, hemilaminectomy or ventral slot procedures may be indicated.[13,34,127–132]

Conservative management can be used in treating patients with hyperpathia (neuropathic pain) alone or with minimal neurologic deficits.[13,34] It is recommended that strict cage rest be instituted for a minimum of 4 to 6 weeks, although a recent retrospective evaluation showed that the duration of rest in the management of thoracolumbar disk disease had no effect on outcome or quality-of-life scores.[133] Conservative management is inappropriate for patients that are surgical candidates based on imaging and/or have lost deep pain perception (DPP).[34]

Spinal cord contusion and extra-axial hemorrhage

A spinal cord contusion is an intraparenchymal hemorrhage that occurs most commonly secondary to other causes of primary injury including VFLs, intervertebral disk extrusion, and penetrating injuries.[13,134] Therapy for parenchymal contusions is aimed at treating concurrent primary injury (see earlier discussion).[13] Extra-axial hemorrhage can occur epidurally or subdurally, and can cause direct compression to the cord. It has also been reported secondary to intervertebral disk extrusion.[135–137] Decompressive surgical techniques are recommended in patients with compressive extra-axial hematomas.[13]

Cellular transplantation therapy

Intraspinal olfactory glial cell transplantation was evaluated in a phase I trial in 9 dogs with thoracolumbar SCI caused by VFLs secondary to vehicular trauma or disk herniation (8 of 9 dogs were DPP negative). Significant functional improvement was noted in this small population of dogs, with 7 of 8 having improved motor function.[138] A recent investigation of the safety of autologous bone marrow stromal cell transplantation in 7 dogs with severe acute SCI caused by VFL found this technique to be feasible and safe, with no complications noted. Two of 7 dogs were able to walk without support during follow-up (29–62 months after SCI).[139] Although these techniques are currently in the early stages of development, they may represent new alternatives for patients with acute SCI.

Prognosis

Prognosis for recovery from neurotrauma depends on the severity of injury, the cause of injury, the site of the lesion, and the timing and efficacy of the treatment of primary and secondary injury.[13] Small animals with neurologic trauma can demonstrate significant neurologic improvement and have a tremendous ability to compensate for neurologic deficits, so serial neurologic reassessments are recommended regardless of the presentation of the patient.

The MGCS can be used to assess prognosis for recovery in dogs with TBI, as it has been documented to be linearly associated with 48-hour survival.[25] The presence of DPP has consistently been associated with improved outcome in acute SCI. A retrospective study evaluating severe thoracolumbar SCI in dogs showed that only 12% of dogs with VFL regained the ability to walk, whereas 69% of dogs with injury attributable to intervertebral disk herniation regained motor function.[140] Surgical management of cases with thoracolumbar disk herniation and intact pain perception is excellent, with expected return of functional motor activity being 80% to 95% (reports range from 72% to 100%).[141] In one study of surgically managed cervical disk herniation, the overall success rate was 99%.[126] A retrospective study of dogs with cervical VFLs found that injuries that could be managed conservatively (ie, nonsurgically) had good functional outcomes in 90% of cases.[142] Those requiring surgical management had a high risk of perioperative mortality (36%), but in those cases that survived the perioperative period the prognosis was excellent (100%). This same study also showed that nonambulatory patients and patients presented at more than 5 days after injury had worse prognoses.[142] Prognostic studies in cats are limited, therefore much of the relevant information is extrapolated from dogs.[143] Finally, neurotrauma rarely occurs independent of other systemic injury. It is therefore crucial to take the entire clinical picture of the patient into account when assessing prognosis and guiding owners in their decision-making process.

REFERENCES

1. Simpson S, Syring R, Otto C. Severe blunt trauma in dogs: 235 cases (1997-2003). J Vet Emerg Crit Care (San Antonio) 2009;19(6):588–602.
2. Marioni-Henry K, Vite CH, Newton AL, et al. Prevalence of diseases of the spinal cord of cats. J Vet Intern Med 2004;18(6):851–8.
3. Fluehmann G, Doherr MG, Jaggy A. Canine neurological diseases in a referral hospital population between 1989 and 2000 in Switzerland. J Small Anim Pract 2006;47(10):582–7.
4. Sande A, West C. Traumatic brain injury: a review of pathophysiology and management. J Vet Emerg Crit Care (San Antonio) 2010;20(2):177–90.
5. Dewey C. Emergency management of the head trauma patient. Vet Clin North Am Small Anim Pract 2000;30:207–25.
6. Hopkins A. Head trauma. Vet Clin North Am Small Anim Pract 1996;26:875–91.

7. Dewey C, Fletcher D. Head trauma management. In: Dewey C, editor. A practical guide to canine and feline neurology. 2nd edition. Ames (IA): Wiley-Blackwell; 2008. p. 221–35.

8. Aries M, Czrosynka M, Budohoski K, et al. Continuous determination of optimal cerebral perfusion pressure in traumatic brain injury. Crit Care Med 2012;40(8): 2456–63.

9. Ling G, Marshall S, Moore D. Diagnosis and management of traumatic brain injury. Continuum 2010;16(6):27–40.

10. Kim J, Gean A. Imaging for the diagnosis and management of traumatic brain injury. Neurotherapeutics 2011;8(1):39–53.

11. Tsang K, Whitfield P. Traumatic brain injury: review of current management strategies. Br J Oral Maxillofac Surg 2012;50:298–308.

12. Proulx J, Dhupa N. Severe brain injury: part I: pathophysiology. Compend Contin Educ Vet 1998;20:897–905.

13. Fletcher DJ, Dewey CW. Spinal trauma management. In: Dewey CW, editor. A practical guide to canine and feline neurology. 2nd edition. Ames (IA): Wiley-Blackwell; 2008. p. 405–17.

14. Johnson K, Vite C. Spinal cord injury. In: Silverstein D, Hopper K, editors. Small animal critical care medicine. 1st edition. St Louis (MO): Elsevier Saunders; 2009. p. 419–23.

15. Park EH, White GA, Tieber LM. Mechanisms of injury and emergency care of acute spinal cord injury in dogs and cats. J Vet Emerg Crit Care (San Antonio) 2012;22(2):160–78.

16. Olby N. The pathogenesis and treatment of acute spinal cord injuries in dogs. Vet Clin North Am Small Anim Pract 2010;40(5):791–807.

17. Fletcher D, Syring R. Traumatic brain injury. In: Silverstein D, Hopper K, editors. Small animal critical care medicine. 1st edition. St Louis (MO): Elsevier Saunders; 2009. p. 658–62.

18. Leonard SE, Kirby R. The role of glutamate, calcium and magnesium in secondary brain injury. J Vet Emerg Crit Care 2002;12(1):17–32.

19. McMichael M, Moore R. Ischemia and reperfusion injury pathophysiology, part I. J Vet Emerg Crit Care (San Antonio) 2004;14(4):231–41.

20. Oyinbo C. Secondary injury mechanisms in traumatic spinal cord injury: a nugget of this multiply cascade. Acta Neurobiol Exp 2011;71(2):281–99.

21. Tator C, Fehlings M. Review of the secondary injury theory of acute spinal cord trauma with emphasis on vascular mechanisms. J Neurosurg 1991;75(1):15–26.

22. Dooney N, Dagal A. Anesthetic considerations in acute spinal cord trauma. Int J Crit Illn Inj Sci 2011;1(1):36–43.

23. Armitage-Chan E, Wetmore L, Chan D. Anesthetic management of the head trauma patient. J Vet Emerg Crit Care (San Antonio) 2007;17(1):5–14.

24. Shores A. Craniocerebral trauma. In: Kirk R, editor. Current veterinary therapy X. X. Philadelphia: WB Saunders; 1983. p. 847–54.

25. Platt S, Radaelli S, McDonnell J. The prognostic value of the Modified Glasgow Coma Scale in head trauma in gods. J Vet Intern Med 2001;15(6):581–4.

26. Levine GJ, Levine JM, Budke CM, et al. Description and repeatability of a newly developed spinal cord injury scale for dogs. Prev Vet Med 2009; 89(1–2):121–7.

27. Olby N, De Risio L, Munana K, et al. Development of a functional scoring system in dogs with acute spinal cord injuries. Am J Vet Res 2001;62(10):1624–8.

28. Smith P, Jeffery N. Spinal shock—comparative aspects and clinical relevance. J Vet Intern Med 2005;19:788–93.

29. Boysen S, Rozanski E, Tidwell A, et al. Evaluation of a focused assessment with sonography for trauma protocol to detect free abdominal fluid in dogs involved in motor vehicle accidents. J Am Vet Med Assoc 2004;225(8):1198–204.

30. Lisciandro GR. Abdominal and thoracic focused assessment with sonography for trauma, triage, and monitoring in small animals. J Vet Emerg Crit Care (San Antonio) 2011;21(2):104–22.

31. Kinns J, Mai W, Seiler G, et al. Radiographic sensitivity and negative predictive value for acute canine spinal trauma. Vet Radiol Ultrasound 2006;47(6):563–70.

32. Vitale C, Coates J. Acute spinal injury. Compendium Standards of Care: Emergency and Critical Care Medicine 2007;9(7):1–11.

33. Lamb CR, Nicholls A, Targett M, et al. Accuracy of survey radiographic diagnosis of intervertebral disc protrusion in dogs. Vet Radiol Ultrasound 2002;43(3):222–8.

34. Brisson BA. Intervertebral disc disease in dogs. Vet Clin North Am Small Anim Pract 2010;40(5):829–58.

35. Israel SK, Levine JM, Kerwin SC, et al. The relative sensitivity of computed tomography and myelography for identification of thoracolumbar intervertebral disk herniations in dogs. Vet Radiol Ultrasound 2009;50(3):247–52.

36. Olby N, Dyce J, Houlton J. Correlation of plain radiographic and lumbar myelographic findings with surgical findings in thoracolumbar disc disease. J Small Anim Pract 1994;35(7):345–50.

37. Griffin J, Levine J, Kerwin S. Canine thoracolumbar intervertebral disk disease: pathophysiology, neurologic examination, and emergency medical therapy. Compend Contin Educ Vet 2009;31(3):E1–13.

38. Lewis D, Hosgood G. Complications associated with the use of iohexol for myelography of the cervical vertebral column in dogs: 66 cases (1988-1990). J Am Vet Med Assoc 1992;200(9):1381–4.

39. Barone G, Ziemer L, Shofer F, et al. Risk factors associated with the development of seizures after use of iohexol for myelography in dogs: 182 cases (1998). J Am Vet Med Assoc 2002;220(10):1499–502.

40. Johnson P, Beltran E, Dennis R, et al. Magnetic resonance imaging characteristics of suspected vertebral instability associated with fracture or subluxation in eleven dogs. Vet Radiol Ultrasound 2012;53(5):552–9.

41. Rozanski EA, Rondeau MP. Respiratory pharmacotherapy in emergency and critical care medicine. Vet Clin North Am Small Anim Pract 2002;32(5):1073–86.

42. Mazzaferro E. Oxygen therapy. In: Silverstein D, Hopper K, editors. Small animal critical care medicine. 1st edition. St Louis (MO): Elsevier Saunders; 2009. p. 78–81.

43. Hopper K. Basic mechanical ventilation. In: Silverstein D, Hopper K, editors. Small animal critical care medicine. 1st edition. St Louis (MO): Elsevier Saunders; 2009. p. 900–4.

44. Zhuang J, Shackford S, Schmoker J, et al. Colloid infusion after brain injury: an effect on intracranial pressure, cerebral blood flow, and oxygen delivery. Crit Care Med 1995;23(1):140–8.

45. Wade C, Grady J, Kramer G, et al. Individual patient cohort analysis of the efficacy of hypertonic saline/dextran in patients with traumatic brain injury and hypotension. J Trauma 1997;42:561–5.

46. Vassar M, Perry C, Gannaway W, et al. Analysis of potential risks associated with 7.5% sodium chloride resuscitation of traumatic shock. Arch Surg 1990;124:1309–15.

47. Vassar M, Perry C, Gannaway W, et al. 7.5% sodium chloride/dextran for resuscitation of trauma patients undergoing helicopter transport. Arch Surg 1991;126:1065–72.

48. Vassar M, Perry C, Holcroft J. Prehospital resuscitation of hypotensive trauma patients with 7.5% NaCl versus 7.5% NaCl with added dextran: a controlled trial. J Trauma 1993;34:622–32.
49. Vassar M, Fisher R, O'Brien P, et al. A multicenter trial for resuscitation of injured patients with 7.5% sodium chloride. Arch Surg 1993;128:1003–11.
50. Cooper J, Myles P, McDermott F, et al. Prehospital hypertonic saline resuscitation of patients with hypotension and severe traumatic brain injury. JAMA 2004;291:1350–7.
51. Roberts D, Hall R, Kramer A. Sedation for critically ill adults with severe traumatic brain injury: a systematic review of randomized controlled trials. Crit Care Med 2012;39(12):2743–51.
52. Sperry R, Bailey P, Reichman M, et al. Fentanyl and sulfentanil increase intracranial pressure in head trauma patients. Anesthesiology 1992;77:416–20.
53. Lauer K, Connolly L, Schmeling W. Opioid sedation does not alter intracranial pressure in head injured patients. Can J Anaesth 1997;44:929–33.
54. Albanese J, Viviand X, Potie F, et al. Sulfentanil, fentanyl, and alfentanil in head trauma patients: a study on cerebral hemodynamics. Crit Care Med 1999;27: 407–11.
55. de Nadal M, Munar F, Poca M, et al. Cerebral hemodynamic effects of morphine and fentanyl in patients with severe head injury: absence of correlation to cerebral autoregulation. Anesthesiology 2000;92:11–9.
56. Hansen B. Acute pain management. Vet Clin North Am Small Anim Pract 2000; 30(4):899–916.
57. Pascoe P. Opioid analgesics. Vet Clin North Am Small Anim Pract 2000;30(4): 757–69.
58. Keegan R, Green S, Bagley R, et al. Effects of medetomidine administration on intracranial pressure and cardiovascular variables of isoflurane-anesthetized dogs. Am J Vet Res 1996;56(2):193–8.
59. Treggiari M, Schultz N, Yanez N, et al. Role of intracranial pressure values and patterns in predicting outcome of traumatic brain injury: a systematic review. Neurocrit Care 2007;6:104–12.
60. Weed L, McKibbon P. Pressure changes in the cerebrospinal fluid following intravenous injection of solutions of various concentrations. Am J Phys 1919; 48:512–30.
61. Ropper A. Hyperosmolar therapy for raised intracranial pressure. N Engl J Med 2012;367(8):746–52.
62. Brain Trauma Foundation, American Association of Neurological Surgeons, Congress of Neurological Surgeons. Guidelines for the management of severe traumatic brain injury. J Neurotrauma 2007;24(1):S1–106.
63. Fink M. Osmotherapy for intracranial hypertension: mannitol versus hypertonic saline. Continuum 2012;18(3):640–54.
64. Kaufmann A, Cardoso E. Aggravation of vasogenic cerebral edema by multiple-dose mannitol. J Neurosurg 1992;77(4):584–9.
65. McManus M, Soriano S. Rebound swelling of astroglial cells exposed to hypertonic mannitol. Anesthesiology 1998;88(6):1586–91.
66. Oddo M, Levine J, Frangos S, et al. Effect of mannitol and hypertonic saline on cerebral oxygenation in patients with severe traumatic brain injury and refractory intracranial hypertension. J Neurol Neurosurg Psychiatr 2009;80(8): 916–20.
67. Aiyagari V, Deibert E, Diringer M. Hypernatremia in the neurologic intensive care unit: how high is too high? J Crit Care 2006;21(2):163–72.

68. Battison C, Andrews P, Graham C, et al. Randomized, controlled trial on the effect of a 20% mannitol solution and a 7.5% saline/6% dextran solution on increased intracranial pressure after brain injury. Crit Care Med 2005;33(1): 196–202.

69. Francony C, Fauvage B, Falcon D, et al. Equimolar doses of mannitol and hypertonic saline in the treatment of intracranial pressure. Crit Care Med 2008;36(3): 795–800.

70. Zeng H, Wang Q, Deng Y, et al. A comparative study on the efficacy of 10% hypertonic saline and equal volume of 20% mannitol in the treatment of experimentally induced cerebral edema in adult rats. BMC Neurosci 2010;11:153.

71. da Silva J, de Lima F, Valenca M, et al. Hypertonic saline more efficacious than mannitol in lethal intracranial hypertension model. Neurol Res 2010;32(2): 139–43.

72. Todd M, Cutkomp J, Brian J. Influence of mannitol and furosemide, alone and in combination, on brain water content after fluid percussion injury. Anesthesiology 2006;105:1176–80.

73. Edwards P, Arango M, Balica L, et al. Final results of MRC CRASH, a randomized placebo-controlled trial of intravenous corticosteroids in adults with head injury- outcomes at 6 months. Lancet 2005;365(9475):1957–9.

74. Roberts I, Yates D, Sandercock P, et al. Effect of intravenous corticosteroids on death within 14 days in 10,008 adults with clinically significant head injury (MRC CRASH trial): randomized placebo-controlled trial. Lancet 2004;364:9442.

75. Schierhout G, Roberts I. Withdrawn: antiepileptic drugs for preventing seizures following acute traumatic brain injury. Cochrane Database Syst Rev 2012;(6):CD000173.

76. Musulin S, Mariani C, Papich M. Diazepam pharmacokinetics after nasal drop and atomized nasal administration in dogs. J Vet Pharmacol Ther 2011;34(1): 17–24.

77. Kassell N, Hitchon P, Gerk M, et al. Alterations in cerebral blood flow, oxygen metabolism, and electrical activity produced by high-dose thiopental. Neurosurgery 1980;7:598–603.

78. Hayes G. Severe seizures associated with traumatic brain injury managed by controlled hypothermia, pharmacologic coma, and mechanical ventilation in a dog. J Vet Emerg Crit Care (San Antonio) 2009;19(6):629–34.

79. Giacino J, Whyte J, Bagiella E, et al. Placebo-controlled trial of amantadine for severe traumatic brain injury. N Engl J Med 2012;366:819–26.

80. Hall E. The neuroprotective pharmacology of methylprednisolone. J Neurosurg 1992;76(1):13–22.

81. Parker A, Smith C. Functional recovery from spinal cord trauma following dexamethasone and chlorpromazine therapy in dogs. Res Vet Sci 1976;21(2):246–7.

82. Levine J, Levine G, Boozer L, et al. Adverse effects and outcome associated with dexamethasone administration in dogs with acute thoracolumbar intervertebral disk herniation: 161 cases (2000-2006). J Am Vet Med Assoc 2008;232(3): 411–7.

83. Bracken M, Shepard M, Collins W. A randomized, controlled trial of methylprednisolone or naloxone in the treatment of acute spinal-cord injury. Results of the second national acute spinal cord injury study. N Engl J Med 1990;322(20): 1405–11.

84. Bracken M, Shepard M, Hellenbrand K. Methylprednisolone and neurological function 1 year after spinal cord injury. Results of the National Acute Spinal Cord Injury Study. J Neurosurg 1985;63(5):704–13.

85. Bracken M, Shepard M, Holford T. Administration of methylprednisolone for 24 or 48 hours or tirilazad mesylate for 48 hours in the treatment of acute spinal cord injury. Results of the Third National Acute Spinal Cord Injury Randomized Controlled Trial. National Acute Spinal Cord Injury. JAMA 1997;277(20):1597–604.
86. Nesathurai S. Steroids and spinal cord injury: revisiting the NASCIS 2 and NASCIS 3 trials. J Trauma Acute Care Surg 1998;45(6):1088–93.
87. Rabinowitz R, Eck J, Harper C. Urgent surgical decompression compared to methylprednisolone for the treatment of acute spinal cord injury. Spine 2008; 33(21):2260–8.
88. Coates J, Sorjonen D, Simpson S, et al. Clinicopathologic effects of a 21-aminosteroid compound (U74389G) and high dose methylprednisolone on spinal cord function after simulated spinal cord trauma. Vet Surg 1995;24: 128–39.
89. Baltzer W, McMichael MA, Hosgood G. Randomized, blinded, placebo-controlled clinical trial of N-acetylcysteine in dogs with spinal cord trauma from acute intervertebral disc disease. Spine 2008;33(13):1397–402.
90. Bains M, Hall E. Antioxidant therapies in traumatic brain injury and spinal cord injury. Biochim Biophys Acta 2012;1822(5):675–84.
91. Hall E, Wolf D. A pharmacological analysis of the pathophysiological mechanisms of posttraumatic spinal cord ischemia. J Neurosurg 1986; 64(6):951–61.
92. Ates O, Cayli S, Gurses I. Comparative neuroprotective effect of sodium channel blockers after experimental spinal cord injury. J Clin Neurosci 2007;14(7): 658–65.
93. Kaptanoglu E, Solaroglu I, Surucu H. Blockade of sodium channels by phenytoin protects ultrastructure and attenuates lipid peroxidation in experimental spinal cord injury. Acta Neurochir 2005;147(4):405–12.
94. Hains B, Saab C, Lo A. Sodium channel blockade with phenytoin protects spinal cord axons, enhances axonal conduction, and improves functional recovery after contusion SCI. Exp Neurol 2004;188(2):365–77.
95. Schwartz G, Fehlings M. Secondary injury mechanisms of spinal cord trauma: novel therapeutic approach for the management of secondary pathophysiology with the sodium channel blocker riluzole. Prog Brain Res 2002;137:177–90.
96. Park E, Velumian A, Fehlings M. The role of excitotoxicity in secondary mechanisms of spinal cord injury: a review with an emphasis on the implications for white matter degeneration. J Neurotrauma 2004;21:754–74.
97. Walters M, Kaste M, Lees K, et al. The AMPA antagonist ZK 200775 in patients with acute ischaemic stroke: a double-blind, multi-centre, placebo-controlled safety and tolerability study. Cerebrovasc Dis 2005;20:304–9.
98. Chan P. White matter injury in spinal cord ischemia: protection by AMPA/kainite glutamate receptor antagonism—Editoral comment. Stroke 2000;31:1952.
99. Chen HS, Lipton S. The chemical biology of clinically tolerated NMDA receptor antagonists. J Neurochem 2006;97:1611–26.
100. Tadie M, D'Arbigny P, Mathe J, et al. Acute spinal cord injury. Early care and treatment in a multicenter study with gacylidine. Soc Neurosci 1999;25:1090.
101. Kwon B, Okon E, Hillyer J. A systematic review of non-invasive pharmacologic neuroprotective treatments for acute spinal cord injury. J Neurotrauma 2011; 28(8):1545–88.
102. Sturges B, LeCouteur R. Intracranial hypertension. In: Silverstein D, Hopper K, editors. Small animal critical care medicine. 1st edition. St Louis (MO): Elsevier Saunders; 2009. p. 423–9.

103. Brain Trauma Foundation T, National Association of State EMS Officials T, National Association of EMTs. Guidelines for prehospital management of traumatic brain injury. Prehosp Emerg Care 2007;12(1):1–52.
104. Davis D, Dunford J, Poste J, et al. The impact of hypoxia and hyperventilation on outcome after paramedic rapid sequence intubation of severely head-injured patients. J Trauma 2004;57(1):1–8.
105. Muizelaar J, Marmarou A, Ward J, et al. Adverse effects of prolonged hyperventilation in patients with severe head injury; a randomized clinical trial. J Neurosurg 1991;75(5):731–9.
106. Deutschman C, Konstantinides F, Raup S. Physiological and metabolic response to isolated closed-head injury. Part i: basal metabolic state: correlations of metabolic and physiological parameters with fasting and stressed controls. J Neurosurg 1986;64:89–98.
107. Jeremitsky E, Omert L, Dunham C, et al. The impact of hyperglycemia on patients with severe brain injury. J Trauma 2005;58(1):47–50.
108. Syring R, Otto C, Drobatz K. Hyperglycemia in dogs and cats with head trauma: 122 cases (1997-1999). J Am Vet Med Assoc 2001;218:1124–9.
109. Vespa P, McArthur D, Stein N, et al. Tight glycemic control increases metabolic distress in traumatic brain injury: a randomized controlled within subjects trial. Crit Care Med 2012;40(6):1923–9.
110. Green D, O'Phelan K, Bassin S, et al. Intensive versus conventional insulin therapy in critically ill neurologic patients. Neurocrit Care 2010;13(3):299–306.
111. Bilotta F, Caramia R, Cernak I, et al. Intensive insulin therapy after severe traumatic brain injury: randomized clinical trial. Neurocrit Care 2008;9(2):159–66.
112. Dewey C. Urinary bladder management. In: Dewey CW, editor. A practical guide to canine and feline neurology. St Louis (MO): Elsevier Saunders; 2003. p. 419–26.
113. Bubenik L, Hosgood G. Urinary tract infection in dogs with thoracolumbar intervertebral disc herniation and urinary bladder dysfunction managed by manual expression, indwelling catheterization or intermittent catheterization. Vet Surg 2008;37:791–800.
114. Smarick S, Haskins S, Aldrich J, et al. Incidence of catheter-associated urinary tract infection among dogs in a small animal intensive care unit. J Am Vet Med Assoc 2004;224(12):1936–40.
115. Ng I, Lim J, Wong H. Effects of head posture on cerebral hemodynamics its influences on intracranial pressure, cerebral perfusion pressure, and cerebral oxygenation. Neurosurgery 2004;54(3):593–7.
116. Sadaka F, Veremakis C. Therapeutic hypothermia for the management of intracranial hypertension in severe traumatic brain injury: a systematic review. Brain Inj 2012;26(7–8):899–908.
117. McCarthy P, Scott L, Ganta C, et al. Hypothermic protection in traumatic brain injury. Pathophysiology 2012;735–57.
118. Wijayatilake D, Shepherd S, Sherren P. Updates in the management of intracranial pressure in traumatic brain injury. Curr Opin Anaesthesiol 2012;25(5):540–7.
119. Hutchinson P, Corteen E, Czosnyka M, et al. Decompressive craniectomy in traumatic brain injury: the randomized multicenter RESCUEicp study. Acta Neurochir 2006;96(S):17–20.
120. La Rosa G, Conti A, Cardali S, et al. Does early decompression improve neurological outcome of spinal cord injured patients? Appraisal of the literature using a meta-analytical approach. Spinal Cord 2004;42(9):503–12.
121. Croce M, Bee T, Pritchard E, et al. Does optimal timing for spine fracture fixation exist? Ann Surg 2001;233(6):851–8.

122. Fehlings M, Perrin R. The timing of surgical intervention in the treatment of spinal cord injury: a systematic review of recent clinical evidence. Spine 2006;31(11): S28–35.

123. Jeffery ND. Vertebral fracture and luxation in small animals. Vet Clin North Am Small Anim Pract 2010;40(5):809–28.

124. Denis F. Spinal instability as defined by the three-column spine concept in acute spinal trauma. Clin Orthop Relat Res 1984;189:65–76.

125. Hillman R, Kengeri S, Waters D. Reevaluation of predictive factors for complete recovery in dogs with nonambulatory tetraparesis secondary to cervical disk herniation. J Am Anim Hosp Assoc 2009;45:155–63.

126. Cherrone K, Dewey C, Coates J, et al. A retrospective comparison of cervical intervertebral disk disease in nonchondrodystrophic large dogs versus small dogs. J Am Anim Hosp Assoc 2004;40:316–20.

127. Gage E, Hoerlein B. Hemilaminectomy and dorsal laminectomy for relieving compressions of the spinal cord in the dog. J Am Vet Med Assoc 1968;152: 351–9.

128. Seim H 3rd, Prata R. Ventral decompression for the treatment of cervical disk disease in the dog: a review of 54 cases. J Am Anim Hosp Assoc 1982;18: 233–40.

129. Gill P, Lippincott C, Anderson S. Dorsal laminectomy in the treatment of cervical intervertebral disk disease in small dogs: a retrospective study of 30 cases. J Am Anim Hosp Assoc 1996;32:77–80.

130. Felts J, Prata R. Cervical disk disease in the dog: intraforaminal and lateral extrusions. J Am Anim Hosp Assoc 1983;19:755–60.

131. Tanaka H, Nakayama M, Takase K. Usefulness of hemilaminectomy for cervical intervertebral disk disease in small dogs. J Vet Med Sci 2005;67:679–83.

132. McCartney W. Comparison of recovery times and complication rates between a modified slanted slot and the standard ventral slot for the treatment of cervical disc disease in 20 dogs. J Small Anim Pract 2007;48:498–501.

133. Levine J, Levine G, Johnson S, et al. Evaluation of the success of medical management for presumptive thoracolumbar intervertebral disk herniation in dogs. Vet Surg 2007;36:482–91.

134. Kent M. Intraaxial spinal cord hemorrhage secondary to atlantoaxial subluxation in a dog. J Am Anim Hosp Assoc 2010;46(2):132–7.

135. Cerda-Gonzalez S, Olby NJ. Fecal incontinence associated with epidural spinal hematoma and intervertebral disk extrusion in a dog. J Am Vet Med Assoc 2006; 228(2):230–5.

136. Caswell JL, Nykamp SG. Intradural vasculitis and hemorrhage in full sibling Welsh springer spaniels. Can Vet J 2003;44(2):137–9.

137. Tidwell AS, Specht A, Blaeser L, et al. Magnetic resonance imaging features of extradural hematomas associated with intervertebral disc herniation in a dog. Vet Radiol Ultrasound 2001;43(4):319–24.

138. Jeffery N, Lakatos A, Franklin R. Autologous olfactory glial cell transplantation is reliable and safe in naturally occurring spinal cord injury. J Neurotrauma 2005; 22(11):1282–93.

139. Nishida H, Nakayama M, Tanaka H. Safety of autologous bone marrow stromal cell transplantation in dogs with acute spinal cord injury. Vet Surg 2012;41: 437–42.

140. Olby N, Levine J, Harris T. Long-term functional outcome of dogs with severe injuries of the thoracolumbar spinal cord: 87 cases (1996-2001). J Am Vet Med Assoc 2003;222(6):762–9.

141. Dewey CW. Myelopathies: disorders of the spinal cord. In: Dewey CW, editor. A practical guide to canine and feline neurology. 2nd edition. Ames (IA): Wiley-Blackwell; 2008. p. 323–88.

142. Hawthorne J, Blevins W, Wallace L, et al. Cervical vertebral fractures in 56 dogs: a retrospective study. J Am Anim Hosp Assoc 1999;35:135–46.

143. Eminaga S, Palus V, Cherubini G. Acute spinal cord injury in the cat: causes, treatment and prognosis. J Feline Med Surg 2011;13(11):850–62.

Analgesia, Anesthesia, and Chemical Restraint in the Emergent Small Animal Patient

Jane Quandt, DACVAA, DVM, MS

KEYWORDS

- Anesthesia • Analgesics • Opioids • Stabilization

KEY POINTS

- Appropriate stabilization of the critically ill animal before sedation or anesthesia is imperative to minimize anesthetic complications.
- Problems should be anticipated and an appropriate and efficient therapeutic plan should be formulated before anesthetic induction.
- Consider the use of a balanced anesthesia technique to minimize potential deleterious effects of single-use drug therapy. Using a combination of different classes of analgesics may be more effective in the treatment of established pain than the use of a single agent.
- The critically ill animal should have drugs titrated to effect to minimize the amount of drug needed and to lessen potential side effects.

INTRODUCTION

The emergent veterinary patient needs a thorough preoperative assessment to define what type of trauma or compromise the patient is undergoing. The critically ill patient has altered physiology and decreased reserves that will affect the pharmacokinetic and pharmacodynamic behavior of analgesic and anesthetic drugs. These patients benefit from minimizing stress levels and optimizing oxygen delivery.

Stabilization of the critically ill patient before anesthetic drug exposure is ideal, because the risk of anesthesia in an unstable patient increases the risk of anesthetic complications. In some of these patients analgesia and chemical restraint may be required to facilitate handling and stabilization. The administration of analgesics may not result in complete pain relief; however, the goal is to achieve a state whereby the pain is bearable and some of the protective aspects of pain, such as inhibiting the use of a fractured leg, remain.[1] It is vital that the underlying disease process be addressed at the same time while pain relief is provided.

Department of Small Animal Medicine & Surgery, College of Veterinary Medicine, University of Georgia, 501 DW Brooks Drive, Athens, GA 30602, USA
E-mail address: quand003@uga.edu

Vet Clin Small Anim 43 (2013) 941–953
http://dx.doi.org/10.1016/j.cvsm.2013.03.008   vetsmall.theclinics.com
0195-5616/13/$ – see front matter © 2013 Elsevier Inc. All rights reserved.

STABILIZATION

Venous access is imperative in the critically ill patient because it will allow administration of intravenous (IV) fluids and analgesics. A dehydrated or hypovolemic state, along with fluid, acid-base, and electrolyte deficits should be corrected, if possible, before anesthesia. Once the patient has been stabilized, thorough diagnostics, such as serial physical examinations, radiographs, blood chemistry, complete blood count, coagulation profile, acid-base status, and blood glucose and lactate levels, should be performed before anesthesia.

The emergent patient often benefits from having more than one IV catheter, either peripherally or centrally, to administer multiple agents and fluids during and after the anesthetic period. If a central venous catheter is to be used for drug administration, the drug should be titrated carefully to avoid a sudden delivery of drug to the brain, causing a profound depressive effect on the animal.

Chemical Restraint

Because of pain, fear, or an ill-natured temperament, some trauma patients cannot be safely examined or handled without some form of chemical restraint, and using chemical restraint may be safest to avoid further injury to the animal or personnel. In animals that can be handled but need analgesia to facilitate radiography or other diagnostics, a physical examination and blood work before drug administration is recommended if possible. In patients that are unable to be handled, choosing the appropriate agents may be difficult, because blood work or a complete physical examination may not be possible. Restraint drugs usually include a combination of a dissociative, alpha-2 agonist, an opioid and possibly a tranquilizer. These agents can be mixed in the same syringe, which will improve ease of administration. If a benzodiazepine is chosen, midazolam may be the preferred drug as it is compatible with other agents and has better intramuscular (IM) absorption than does diazepam. In the extremely painful or vicious animal, a mu-agonist narcotic combined with the alpha-2 agonist (eg, dexmedetomidine) given IM will provide analgesia, sedation, and restraint.

In cats, various combinations of drugs have been used for restraint and sedation, and to ease handling. Midazolam combined with butorphanol IM may not be effective in aggressive or responsive cats, because it has been shown to create anxiousness and difficulty in restraint, and may lead to aggressive behavior.[2] This combination, therefore, should ideally be limited to geriatric cats or cats that are very ill.[2] The addition of ketamine or dexmedetomidine to midazolam and butorphanol improves sedation and restraint.[2] The use of ketamine and dexmedetomidine will also provide excellent sedation, but this combination may induce vomiting.[2] The use of dexmedetomidine can result in bradycardia and increased blood glucose concentrations, which are known side effects of alpha-2 agonists.[2]

Premedication

Premedication may not be necessary unless the animal is fractious or extremely painful. Premedication can calm and quiet the patient, and therefore decrease the amount of induction drugs needed. Analgesic premedication can decrease the amount of inhalant anesthesia that will be required, and provide preemptive, preventive, analgesia before surgery.

Opioids

If it is decided that patients who are critically ill would benefit from premedication, opioids such as morphine, hydromorphone, or oxymorphone in combination with a tranquilizer (eg, midazolam) can be administered IM to provide analgesia and sedation.

Opioids are the preferred agents in the critically ill because of their minimal effect on cardiac output, systemic blood pressure, and oxygen delivery.[3] Opioids provide analgesia and sedative effects and can be reversed with naloxone if necessary. The mu-agonist opioids are used for their significant analgesic effects. The mu-antagonist/kappa-agonist opioid butorphanol does not provide sufficient analgesia for severe pain; however, it does have antiemetic properties, and is the preferred analgesic in the vomiting patient.[3] The partial mu-agonist buprenorphine can be used to treat moderate pain but is difficult to reverse if adverse clinical events occur.[3] Finally, significant histamine release and profound vasodilation can be seen when certain opioids (eg, morphine, meperidine) are given as a rapid IV injection.[3]

Tranquilizers

Benzodiazepines are unreliable anxiolytics when given alone unless the animal has central nervous system (CNS) depression; however, they are can provide improved sedation when given in combination with opioids and dissociatives.[3,4] Likewise, the use of acepromazine should be used cautiously (if at all) in critically ill patients because of its hypotensive effect. One indication for the use of acepromazine would be for the patient with upper airway obstruction (eg, laryngeal paralysis) because of its sedative and antianxiety effects. Acepromazine has minimal respiratory depressant effects, making it an ideal sedative for this population of patients. Sufficient time must be allowed for complete drug effect (even when administered IV), because it can take up to 30 minutes to exhibit its full effect.[4] Oxygen supplementation should also be provided to these patients while sedation is being achieved.[3]

Anticholinergics

Anticholinergics are not routinely administered unless the patient is bradycardic. Anticholinergics may increase myocardial oxygen consumption because of induced tachycardia, and can decrease the threshold for cardiac dysrhythmias.[5]

Dissociative medications

Dissociatives are N-methyl-D-aspartate (NMDA) receptor agonists, and work by providing analgesia peripherally and somatically.[4] The most common dissociative used in veterinary medicine is ketamine, which can be easily included in the premedication protocol as an IM or IV analgesic. As a single agent, ketamine causes muscle rigidity, and is best combined with a benzodiazepine or alpha-2 agonist to provide muscle relaxation. Ketamine causes tachycardia, increases blood pressure, and has some respiratory depression properties.[3,4] Ketamine will have a prolonged effect in cats with renal disease, because excretion is impaired, and should be used cautiously in azotemic patients.[3,4] In addition, ketamine will increase intracranial and intraocular pressure, and is therefore not recommended for use in patients that have sustained traumatic brain injury.[3,4]

Alpha-2 agonist

Alpha-2 agonists can be used to provide sedation and analgesia in extremely painful or fractious animals. Alpha-2 agonists work primarily by decreasing norepinephrine release centrally and peripherally and reducing nociceptive transmission; a decrease in CNS sympathetic outflow and circulating catecholamines also occurs. They can be safely combined with dissociatives, opioids, and tranquilizers for analgesia and anesthesia. Dexmedetomidine, a potent alpha-2 agonist, is commonly used to provide restraint, sedation, analgesia, and muscle relaxation. It can be used IM and IV, and as a constant rate infusion (CRI). Potential side effects of dexmedetomidine include vomiting, peripheral vasoconstriction, and hypertension; a reflex bradycardia may then be seen secondary to hypertension. Adding ketamine to the dexmedetomidine can help to modulate this response.[6] Anticholinergics (eg, atropine) are not recommended to treat the dexmedetomidine-induced bradycardia, because increased heart rate in combination with the peripheral vasoconstriction can worsen cardiac performance and exacerbate hypertension, and induce cardiac arrhythmias.[4] If the bradycardia induced by administration of dexmedetomidine is significant or clinically relevant, IM reversal with atipamezole is the preferred treatment.[4] In cats, dexmedetomidine has been safely used to provide analgesia and sedation, and helps to decrease the amount of anesthetic inhalant that is required.[6,7] Potential side effects of dexmedetomidine include polyuria and interference with insulin production, contributing to hyperglycemia. Because of this, dexmedetomidine is not recommended for use in patients with urinary obstruction or in animals with diabetes mellitus.[4]

Reversal
The reversal of either opioids with naloxone or alpha-2 agonists with atipamezole results in loss of analgesic and sedative effects, which may lead to excitement, pain, and distress for the animal. To minimize these potential side effects, only one reversal agent should be used; for example, if both an opioid and alpha-2 agonist are used in combination, only the alpha-2 agonist should be reversed, leaving the analgesic effects of the opioid active. If a mu-agonist opioid (eg, fentanyl, hydromorphone, or morphine) requires reversal, it is advisable to use a kappa-agonist/mu-antagonist, such a butorphanol or nalbuphine, to reverse the sedative effect of the opioid, because this retains some of the analgesic effects of the kappa-agonist.[4]

The other drug class that can be reversed is the benzodiazepines. If reversal of benzodiazepines is necessary (eg, diazepam, midazolam), the antagonist flumazenil can be administered intravenously.[4]

INDUCTION

Critically ill patients are often depressed and lethargic, and require minimal drug therapy for induction. In the compromised, critically ill patient, anesthetic drug doses can often be reduced to as much as half of the dose used in more stable patients. Induction drugs should be slowly titrated IV to effect, and the minimal amount of drug necessary to intubate the patient should be used. In addition, a balanced anesthetic technique (eg, the use of multiple drug classes) will help minimize the side effects from the use of a single agent or drug class. The use of local anesthesia and epidural analgesia should be used, if appropriate, to decrease the amount of general anesthesia that is required. Intubation should always be performed to control the airway, provide the ability to ventilate the patient, and protect the airway from aspiration of gastric contents into the lungs. The critically ill animal that presents emergently should be considered to have a full stomach, and therefore at risk for aspiration.

Protocols should be implemented to minimize the amount of time the animal is under anesthesia; therefore, techniques such as preclipping the surgical site with the animal awake should be performed if possible. Preoxygenation of the animal before induction will allow for additional time that may be needed to intubate the animal; this is especially helpful in animals in respiratory distress or with an airway that may be difficult to intubate. Finally, electrocardiography and blood pressure monitoring should be in place before induction to detect evidence of arrhythmias, hypotension, or cardiovascular collapse that may occur during induction of the critically ill animal.

Ideally a slow transition to general anesthesia should occur that would allow time for the cardiovascular and nervous system to appropriately respond to and accommodate the medications.[8] However, the critically ill patient may not be able to respond appropriately, and therapeutic intervention must be available to prevent clinical deterioration of the patient. For example, the patient in respiratory distress will require a rapid-sequence intubation to gain control of the airway and provide ventilation with an inspired oxygen concentration of 100%.

Thiopental and Propofol

A rapid-sequence induction can be accomplished with agents that have a short onset time, such as thiopental or propofol. These agents have an onset time of approximately 30 seconds and must be given IV.[9] The duration of action is also short, with thiopental lasting 10 to 15 minutes and propofol lasting 5 to 10 minutes. Propofol may be the preferred agent because of its shorter duration of action.[9] Both of these drugs can be used in combination with a benzodiazepine (eg, diazepam or midazolam) to improve relaxation and decrease the overall dose of thiopental or propofol needed. Both thiopental and propofol are capable of creating cardiac arrhythmias, hypotension, and apnea; hence, intermittent positive pressure ventilation (IPPV) may be necessary.[9] Neither agent will provide analgesia, and therefore additional analgesics must be given before the surgical procedure. Thiopental and propofol decrease intracranial and intraocular pressure and would be indicated for induction of the patient with a traumatic brain injury.[3]

The new formulation of propofol, PropoFol 28, is not labeled for use in cats. The new formulation contains the preservative benzyl alcohol, which can be toxic to cats when administered in large doses. Although PropoFol 28 has been safely used in healthy cats with no indications of toxicity (and normal recoveries have been reported), propofol is less well tolerated in cats compared with dogs because of slower metabolism and excretion.[10] Cats have a low capacity for glucuronic acid conjugation, and therefore have limited ability to metabolize benzoic acid.[10] Repeated doses or infusions can lead to prolonged anesthetic recoveries.[10] Propofol has been reported to increase the presence of Heinz bodies in cats, potentially leading to hemolytic anemia.[10] PropoFol 28 should be avoided in cats that are significantly debilitated or that have or are suspected to have liver impairment.

Alfaxalone

A new induction agent, alfaxalone, may be useful for induction of the critically ill animal. Alfaxalone is a synthetic neuroactive steroid that is rapidly metabolized and eliminated from the body.[11] Alfaxalone, like thiopental and propofol, has dose-dependent changes such as hypoventilation and apnea, but has a wide margin of safety.[11] Alfaxalone has a short duration of action, reported as 14 to 50 minutes.[11] It can also be used as a CRI with good muscle relaxation and rapid recovery.[11] Because excitement on recovery can occur (seen as paddling, muscle twitching, or even violent movements), the administration of sedative drugs in combination with alfaxalone will improve recovery.[11] In dogs that were considered a poor anesthetic risk, alfaxalone administered at a dose of 1 to 2 mg/kg IV over 60 seconds was shown to be an acceptable induction agent with a smooth recovery.[12] It can also be safely combined with a fentanyl CRI.[12] Cats recovering from alfaxalone may be more disoriented and nervous compared with those recovering from propofol.[13]

Opioids

In the critically ill patient that is more cardiovascularly stable, a more gradual induction technique can be performed, such as neuroleptanalgesic techniques, such as hydromorphone, oxymorphone, or fentanyl and diazepam or midazolam, with the addition of either propofol or ketamine to facilitate induction. In dogs and cats with severe liver compromise, remifentanil can also be considered for analgesia. Remifentanil is a synthetic opioid with direct action on the mu-receptors with an ultra-short duration of action.[14] The elimination of remifentanil is independent of hepatic or renal function, which makes it an attractive agent for use in animals with hepatic or renal compromise.[14] It is metabolized by nonspecific esterases in the blood and tissues.[14] Recovery from remifentanil is rapid, even after long-term IV infusions.[14] It has been used in dogs at an initial IV dose of 3 μg/kg IV, followed by a CRI of 0.1 to 0.3 μg/kg/min, with the drug diluted in normal saline.[14,15] Because of the drug's short duration of action, an additional analgesic should be administered on termination of the remifentanil if the painful condition persists. The clinical effects of remifentanil are rapidly dissipated on discontinuation of the infusion, with dogs recovering in 5 to 20 minutes regardless of the duration of the infusion.[14,15] Remifentanil, like other opioids administered as a CRI, is a potent respiratory depressant. IPPV may be required with severe cases; however, this respiratory depression does not persist after discontinuation of the drug.[15] Remifentanil has been used in cats; however, at doses greater than 1 μg/kg/min, dysphoric behavior and frenetic locomotor activity was reported.[16]

Etomidate

The use of etomidate for induction of critically ill patients that are cardiovascularly unstable is appealing because of its minimal cardiovascular effect. Etomidate should not be used as the sole induction agent, because it may lead to retching and myoclonus.[5] Giving a benzodiazepine or opioid IV before administering etomidate minimizes these adverse effects.[5] Repeated use of etomidate in cats may lead to hemolysis secondary to the propylene glycol vehicle.[5] The use of etomidate in the critically ill human patient is controversial because of its ability to lead to adrenal dysfunction, which may lead to an increase in morbidity and mortality.[17] The duration of the adrenal dysfunction can range from 24 to 48 hours in the critically ill patient.[17] The use of hydrocortisone to treat the etomidate-induced adrenal insufficiency had no effect on outcome.[18] The recommendation in human medicine is to use etomidate cautiously in septic shock patients who may have relative adrenal insufficiency secondary to their disease.[17,18] In addition, etomidate should not be used in patients who have or are suspected of having hypoadrenocorticism.

Ketamine

Ketamine can be safely used in the critically ill patient as part of induction (IV). It is commonly used in combination with a benzodiazepine. Ketamine increases heart rate, blood pressure, and cardiac output via a centrally mediated sympathetic response and endogenous catecholamine release.[4] Because of the potential for increased cardiac contractility, it should be used cautiously in animals with hypertrophic cardiomyopathy.[4] Ketamine can have direct myocardial depressant effects, and in debilitated patients with a decreased endogenous catecholamine response, hypotension and cardiovascular instability may result.[4] Ketamine also has the potential to induce seizures when given as a sole agent.[3,4]

Multiple Agents

The use of multiple agents (eg, hydromorphone, diazepam, ketamine, lidocaine, propofol) is an example of balanced anesthesia. Using these drugs in combination results in a slower onset of action, but provides superior analgesia and is more cardiovascularly sparing.[19] Ketamine may be used to enhance analgesia and will increase heart rate and blood pressure.[20] Lidocaine is often beneficial in the critically ill patient because of its free radical scavenging abilities, analgesic effects, and antiarrhythmic properties, which may help minimize the effects of compromised viscera, reperfusion injury, or ventricular arrhythmias.[21] In cats, the use of lidocaine is not recommended because of its cardiovascular depressive effects.[22] Using some of these medications as a combination CRI results in a slower onset of action; therefore, loading doses before starting the CRI is required. The CRI doses of these medications in one study were morphine at 3.3 µg/kg/min, lidocaine at 50 µg/kg/min, and ketamine at 10 µg/kg/min.[19]

Propofol is not recommended for use as a single agent for major surgical procedures because it does not prevent hemodynamic responses to noxious stimulation.[23] It can be used in combination with other agents such as lidocaine and ketamine in the dog for total IV anesthesia.[23] Propofol has negative chronotropic and inotropic effects, and causes venodilation, which can lead to significant hypotension.[23]

In animals with splenic disease, using an induction agent that does not result in splenomegaly is recommended, because splenomegaly/splenic congestion can lead to worsening of splenic hemorrhage. The administration of acepromazine, thiopental, and propofol has been reported to cause splenomegaly.[24] In addition, a reduction in packed cell volume was reported in dogs receiving acepromazine, thiopental, and propofol, which may be of concern in the anemic patient.[24] Therefore, avoiding these agents in animals with splenic disease or if laparoscopy is planned is recommended. Two alternative drugs to consider are hydromorphone and dexmedetomidine, which do not result in splenomegaly.[24]

MAINTENANCE

Once the animal is intubated and stabilized, anesthesia can be maintained via an inhalant agent such as isoflurane or sevoflurane. These agents are the most commonly used, but both create dose-dependent myocardial depression, hypotension, and respiratory depression.[3,25] Both agents have a rapid onset and recovery time, allowing for rapid change in anesthetic concentration.[3,25] Alternatively, maintenance can also be performed with a CRI of anesthetic agents if the patient cannot tolerate the hypotensive effects of inhalant anesthesia. Ketamine/propofol and ketamine/propofol/dexmedetomidine infusions have been used in cats for ovariectomy.[26] Cats were given one of the combinations IV and then maintained on a ketamine/propofol infusion for the surgical procedure.[26] No adverse effects were seen with either group; however, sedation was more profound in the group receiving dexmedetomidine.[26]

Morphine, lidocaine, and ketamine can be used in dogs as a CRI to provide analgesia and to decrease the amount of inhalant required. Additional mu-agonists that can be used as a CRI include fentanyl, oxymorphone, and hydromorphone.[3] Alpha-2 agonists can also be used as a CRI to enhance analgesia and minimize the level of inhalant needed.[27] These CRIs can then be administered postoperatively at lower doses to provide continued analgesia as needed.

Maintenance anesthesia requires careful and constant monitoring to avoid excessive anesthetic depth and preserve cardiovascular function. The electrocardiogram should be monitored closely for changes in heart rate and rhythm, and for the presence of malignant arrhythmias, which may be more prevalent in animals with trauma, splenic disease, septic peritonitis, or hypoxia, or dogs with gastric dilatation volvulus. Additional monitoring during the maintenance phase of anesthesia includes keeping the mean arterial blood pressure (MAP) at greater than 60 mm Hg to maintain renal perfusion. Physical examination findings for perfusion, such as the capillary refill time, mucous membrane color, heart rate, and pulse quality, should also be monitored continuously. Depth of anesthesia should be frequently assessed through monitoring eye position, pupil size, jaw tone, response to stimulus, heart rate, blood pressure, and respiratory rate during the duration of anesthesia. Other monitoring techniques should be implemented, both during and after anesthesia, to enhance the quality of care and decrease morbidity and mortality. The use of pulse oximetry helps to continually assess hemoglobin saturation (Hb) and, therefore, blood oxygenation.[28] Arterial blood gas monitoring may be necessary as the gold standard in some critically ill patients while under anesthesia to assess oxygenation, ventilation, Hb saturation, electrolyte abnormalities, and overall acid-base status. Capnography allows monitoring of the adequacy of ventilatory function and provides an indication of sufficient cardiac output.[28] Capnography will also monitor for signs of esophageal intubation, breathing circuit disconnection, and cardiac arrest; in these situations, carbon dioxide levels become unreadable.[28]

INTRAOPERATIVE HYPOTENSION

Because critically ill patient are often hypotensive during anesthesia, an MAP of less than 60 mm Hg or a systolic blood pressure less than 90 mm Hg requires prompt treatment to maintain appropriate organ perfusion.[29] The initial step should be to decrease the administration of inhalant anesthetic agents because of their depressant and vasodilatory properties. Next, a fluid bolus should be administered. A crystalloid at a rate of 10 to 20 mL/kg IV over 15 to 20 minutes or an artificial colloid bolus of 5 to 10 mL/kg IV over 10 to 20 minutes should be implemented. If no effect occurs, multiple small boluses can be attempted, keeping in mind the total volume of fluids that have been administered. If the hypotension persists during fluid therapy, inotropic support may be needed through administering dopamine or dobutamine. These agents are given as an IV CRI because of their short half-life, at a dose of 2 to 10 µg/kg/min.[29] Dopamine and dobutamine can be used concurrently. Patients on inotropes and vasopressors should be monitored carefully for tachycardia; if this occurs, the rate of the infusion should be decreased or the addition of another inotrope should be considered. Other agents that may be used include ephedrine (0.05–0.5 mg/kg IV as a single bolus), norepinephrine (0.1–1 µg/kg/min IV as a CRI), and vasopressin (0.01–0.04 U/kg/h IV as a CRI).[29,30] If the initial inotrope is not successful in correcting the hypotension, a second agent is added while continuing administration of the first agent. For example, norepinephrine is most often used in combination with dopamine or dobutamine, and vasopressin can also be used in combination with these agents.[30]

If the patient has persistent hypotension after appropriate fluid therapy and inotropic support, discontinuation of the inhalant anesthetic should be considered, and injectable anesthetic drug therapy should be instituted. An example of an injectable anesthetic regimen used in this situation includes a CRI of fentanyl in combination with ketamine and lidocaine. Some very critical patients may only need fentanyl as an intermittent IV bolus or as a CRI. The use of multiple agents to maintain injectable anesthesia can be considered; however, in cats, recent research suggests that the use of a lidocaine CRI should be avoided because of the cardiovascular depressant effects it produces.[22]

RECOVERY

In critically ill patients, continuous cardiovascular support, monitoring, supportive care, and analgesia are imperative during the recovery period. The recovering patient may still require inotropic support, which should be continued in the intensive care unit during recovery, if necessary. Patients should be kept dry and warm, and should recover in a quiet, stress-free environment where they can be continuously and carefully monitored. A shivering animal has greatly increased demands for glucose and oxygen, and oxygen supplementation and heat support should be provided until clinical signs resolve.[31] Acid-base, electrolyte, and blood glucose levels should also be monitored in the recovering and shivering animal. The use of forced warm air heating blankets will help in the treatment of postoperative hypothermia. Finally, the use of analgesics is imperative in these critically ill patients experiencing pain. Although these patients may not exhibit classic pain response symptoms because of their debilitated state, they should be carefully but appropriately treated with analgesics. Pain can lead to catabolism and complications such as delayed wound healing, sepsis, and nosocomial disease.[32]

SUMMARY

Critically ill patients that need to be sedated or anesthetized should be stabilized before drug administration. Appropriate monitoring should be performed at all times to ensure that these patients survive sedation or emergent surgery. Postoperative care includes continued vasopressor and inotropic support, aggressive colloid and/or crystalloid therapy, analgesic support, antibiotic therapy, oxygen therapy, blood pressure monitoring, and nursing care to improve the survivability in this critically ill patient population.

Drugs dosages

Anticholinergics

    Atropine, 0.04 mg/kg IM, 0.02 mg/kg IV

    Glycopyrrolate, 0.01 mg/kg IM, IV

    May make secretions more viscous

    Increase heart rate and can increase myocardial work and oxygen consumption

    Glycopyrrolate does not cross the blood brain barrier or the placenta

Opioids, mu-agonists

    Morphine, 0.2 to 2.0 mg/kg IM, subcutaneous (SC)

        CRI, 0.1 to 0.3 mg/kg loading dose, then 0.1 to 0.3 mg/kg/h

    Oxymorphone, 0.05 to 0.20 mg/kg IM, IV, SC

    Meperidine, 2 to 11 mg/kg IM, SC

    Hydromorphone, 0.1 to 0.2 mg/kg IV, IM, SC

        CRI, 0.025 to 0.050 mg/kg IV loading dose, then 0.01 to 0.04 mg/kg/h

    Fentanyl, 0.005 to 0.08 mg/kg IM, IV, SC

        CRI loading dose for dog, 5 to 10 µg/kg, then 0.7 to 1.0 µg/kg/min

        CRI loading dose for cat, 5 µg/kg, then 0.3 to 0.4 µg/kg/min. May need to give anticholinergic before CRI if bradycardic

    Remifentanil, 3 µg/kg IV, then CRI, 0.1 to 0.3 µg/kg/min

    Complete reversal with naloxone

    Analgesic

    Respiratory depression

    Bradycardia

    Minimal effect on cardiovascular performance

(Continued)

Partial mu-agonist

    Buprenorphine, 0.005 to 0.020 mg/kg IM, IV

        Slow onset, difficult to reverse

        Good for moderate pain

Kappa-agonist/mu-antagonist

    Butorphanol, 0.1 to 0.8 mg/kg intramuscularly, IV, SC

        CRI, 0.1 to 0.2 mg/kg IV loading dose, then 0.1 to 0.2 mg/kg/h

        Minimal cardiovascular effects, not good for severe pain

        Can be used for partial reversal of mu-agonist opioids

Antagonist

    Naloxone, 0.002 to 0.02 mg/kg IM, IV

        Used for reversal of opioids

Dissociatives

    Ketamine, 4 to 11 mg/kg IV, IM

        CRI, 0. 5 mg/kg IV loading dose, then 0.1 to 1.2 mg/kg/h

    Telazol, 2 to 4 mg/kg IM, 2 mg/kg IV (tiletamine and zolazepam)

    Salivation

    Increases heart rate

    Increases intracranial and intraocular pressure

    Analgesic effects

Benzodiazepines

    Diazepam, 0.2 to 0.5 mg/kg IM, IV

    Midazolam, 0.07 to 0.4 mg/kg IM, IV

        CRI, 0.1 to 0.5 mg/kg/h

    Can decrease other drug doses

    Mild sedation and muscle relaxation

    Treat seizures

    Not analgesic

    Diazepam has propylene glycol

Antagonist

    Flumazenil, 0.08 to 0.2 mg/kg IV

Phenothiazines

    Acepromazine, 0.01 to 0.2 mg/kg intramuscularly, intravenously

        No more than 3 mg total dose

        Vasodilation

        Long duration

        Not analgesic

Barbiturates

    Thiopental, 4 to 20 mg/kg IV

        Cardiovascular and respiratory depression

        Rapid induction

Decreases intracranial and intraocular pressure

Effects may be potentiated by concurrent acidosis or hypoproteinemia

Propofol

Propofol, 2 to 8 mg/kg intravenously

CRI, 0.1 to 0.4 mg/kg/min

Rapid-acting with short duration

Respiratory depression

Decreases intracranial and intraocular pressure

Peripheral vasodilation

Myocardial depressant

Etomidate

Etomidate, 0.5 to 4 mg/kg IV

Maintains cardiovascular stability

Not used as a single agent; commonly combined with a benzodiazepine

Suppresses adrenocortical function

Alpha-2 agonists

Dexmedetomidine, 3 to 40 μg/kg IM, IV

CRI, 1 μg/kg intravenous loading dose, then 1 to 3 μg/kg/h

Cardiovascular depression

Vomiting

Good sedation and analgesia

Can combine with opioid or dissociative

Antagonist

Atipamazole, 0.04 to 0.5 mg/kg IM, IV

Lidocaine

Loading dose, 1 to 2 mg/kg IV, then CRI, 1–3 mg/kg/h

CRI not recommended for use in cat

Alfaxalone

Alfaxalone, 2 to 5 mg/kg intravenously.

May need sedation to improve recovery

Neuroleptanalgesics

Combination of an opioid with a tranquilizer or sedative

Analgesic

Noise-sensitive

Maintain cardiovascular stability

Inhalants

Isoflurane, sevoflurane

All inhalants will produce a dose-dependent cardiovascular depression

Cause peripheral vasodilation

Anesthetic depth is rapidly adjusted

Rapid uptake and recovery

REFERENCES

1. Hellebrekers LJ. Pathophysiology of pain in animals and its consequences for analgesic therapy. In: Hellebrekers LJ, editor. Animal pain in a practice-oriented approach to an effective pain control in animals. Utrecht (The Netherlands): Van Derr Wees; 2000. p. 71–83.
2. Biermann K, Hungerbuhler S, Mischke R, et al. Sedative, cardiovascular, haematologic and biochemical effects of four different drug combinations administered intramuscularly in cats. Vet Anaesth Analg 2012;39:137–50.
3. Macintire DK, Drobatz KJ, Haskins SC, et al. Anesthetic protocols for short procedures. In: Macintire DK, Drobatz KJ, Haskins SC, et al, editors. Manual of small animal emergency and critical care. Philadelphia: Lippincott Williams & Wilkins; 2005. p. 38–54.
4. Perkowski S. Sedation of the critically ill patient. In: Silverstein DC, Hopper K, editors. Small animal critical care medicine. St Louis (MO): Saunders Elsevier; 2009. p. 700–4.
5. Carroll G, Martin DD. Trauma and critical patients. In: Tranquilli WJ, Thurmon JC, Grimm KA, editors. Lumb & Jones veterinary anesthesia and analgesia. 4th edition. Ames (IA): Blackwell Publishing; 2007. p. 969–84.
6. McSweeney PM, Martin DD, Ramsey DS, et al. Clinical efficacy and safety of dexmedetomidine used as a preanesthetic prior to general anesthesia in cats. J Am Vet Med Assoc 2012;240:404–12.
7. Pypendop BH, Barter LS, Stanley SD, et al. Hemodynamic effects of dexmedetomidine in isoflurane-anesthetized cats. Vet Anaesth Analg 2011;38:555–67.
8. Trim CM. Anesthetic considerations and complications. In: Paddleford RR, editor. Manual of small animal anesthesia. 1st edition. New York: Churchill Livingstone; 1999. p. 147–98.
9. Chan DL, Rozanski EA, Freeman LM, et al. Colloid osmotic pressure in health and disease. Comp for Cont Edu of the Prac Vet 2001;23:896–904.
10. Taylor PM, Chengelis CP, Miller WR, et al. Evaluation of propofol containing 2% benzyl alcohol preservative in cats. J Feline Med Surg 2012;14(8):516–26.
11. Jimenez CP, Mathis A, Mora SS, et al. Evaluation of the quality of the recovery after administration of propofol or alfaxalone for induction of anaesthesia in dogs anaesthetized for magnetic resonance imaging. Vet Anaesth Analg 2012; 39:151–9.
12. Psastha E, Alibhai HI, Jimenez-Lozano A, et al. Clinical efficacy and cardiorespiratory effects of alfaxalone, or diazepam/fentanyl for induction of anaesthesia in dogs that are a poor anaesthetic risk. Vet Anaesth Analg 2011;38:24–36.
13. Mathis A, Pinelas R, Brodbelt DC, et al. Comparison of quality of recovery from anaesthesia in cats induced with propofol or alfaxalone. Vet Anaesth Analg 2012;39:282–90.
14. Anagnostou TL, Kazakos GM, Savvas I, et al. Remifentanil/isoflurane anesthesia in five dogs with liver disease undergoing liver biopsy. J Am Anim Hosp Assoc 2011;47:e103–9.
15. Allweiler S, Brodbelt DC, Borer K, et al. The isoflurane-sparing and clinical effects of a constant rate infusion of remifentanil in dogs. Vet Anaesth Analg 2007;34: 388–93.
16. Brosnan RJ, Pypendop BH, Siao KT, et al. Effects of remifentanil on measures of anesthetic immobility and analgesia in cats. Am J Vet Res 2009;70:1065–71.
17. de la Granville B, Arroyo D, Walder B. Etomidate in critically ill patients: con-do you really want to weaken the frail? Eur J Anaesthesiol 2012;29:511–4.

18. Cutherbertson BH, Sprung CL, Annane D, et al. The effects of etomidate on adrenal responsiveness and mortality in patients with septic shock. Intensive Care Med 2009;35:1868–76.
19. Muir WW, Wiese AJ, March PA. Effects of morphine, lidocaine, ketamine, and morphine–lidocaine–ketamine drug combination on minimum alveolar concentration in dogs anesthetized with isoflurane. Am J Vet Res 2003;64(9):1155–60.
20. Wagnor AE, Walton JA, Hellyer PW, et al. Use of low doses of ketamine administered by constant rate infusion as an adjunct for postoperative analgesia in dogs. J Am Vet Med Assoc 2002;221(1):72–5.
21. Cassutto BH, Gfeller RW. Use of intravenous lidocaine to prevent reperfusion injury and subsequent multiple organ dysfunction syndrome. J Vet Emerg Crit Care 2003;13:137–48.
22. Pypendop BH, Ilkiw JE. Assessment of the hemodynamic effects of lidocaine administered IV in isoflurane anesthetized cats. Am J Vet Res 2005;66:661–8.
23. Mannarino R, Luna SP, Monteiro ER, et al. Minimum infusion rate and hemodynamic effects of propofol, propofol-lidocaine and propofol-lidocaine-ketamine in dogs. Vet Anaesth Analg 2012;39:160–73.
24. Baldo CF, Garcia-Pereira FL, Nelson NC, et al. Effects of anesthetic drugs on canine splenic volume determined via computed tomography. Am J Vet Res 2012;73:1715–9.
25. Hall LW, Clarke KW, Trim CM. General pharmacology of the inhalation anesthetics. In: Hall LW, Clarke KW, Trim CM, editors. Veterinary anaesthesia. 10th edition. London: WB Saunders; 2001. p. 133–47.
26. Ravasio G, Gallo M, Beccaglia M, et al. Evaluation of a ketamine-propofol drug combination with or without dexmedetomidine for intravenous anesthesia in cats undergoing ovariectomy. J Am Vet Med Assoc 2012;241:1307–13.
27. Quandt JE, Lee JA. Analgesia and constant rate infusions. In: Silverstein DC, Hopper K, editors. Small animal critical care medicine. St Louis (MO): Saunders Elsevier; 2009. p. 710–6.
28. Wright B, Hellyer PW. Respiratory monitoring during anesthesia: pulse oximetry and capnography. Comp for Cont Edu of the Prac Vet 1996;18:1083–97.
29. Hall LW, Clarke KW, Trim CM. Anaesthesia of the dog. In: Hall LW, Clarke KW, Trim CM, editors. Veterinary anaesthesia. 10th edition. London: WB Saunders; 2001. p. 385–435.
30. Pablo LS. The use of vasopressin in critical care patients. In: Proceedings North American Veterinary Conference. Gainesville FL: Eastern State Veterinary Association; 2006. p. 280–2.
31. Hall LW, Clarke KW, Trim CM. General pharmacology of the injectable agents used in aneaesthesia. In: Hall LW, Clarke KW, Trim CM, editors. Veterinary anaesthesia. 10th edition. London: WB Saunders; 2001. p. 113–29.
32. Muir WW. Physiology and pathophysiology of pain. In: Gaynor JS, Muir WW, editors. Handbook of veterinary pain management. 1st edition. St Louis (MO): Mosby; 2002. p. 13–45.

Basics of Mechanical Ventilation for Dogs and Cats

Kate Hopper, BVSc, PhD[a], Lisa L. Powell, DVM[b],*

KEYWORDS

- Mechanical ventilation • Hypoxemia • Hypercapnia • Hypoventilation • Intubation
- Positive pressure ventilation • Respiratory

KEY POINTS

There are 3 main indications for mechanical ventilation:

- Severe hypoxemia (defined as a Pao_2 <60 mm Hg at sea level) that fails to respond to supplemental oxygen.
- Severe hypoventilation (defined as $Paco_2$ >60 mm Hg).
- Excessive work of breathing.

Intermittent positive pressure ventilation (PPV) through the use of mechanical ventilators has been a mainstay of therapy in people with respiratory failure since the poliomyelitis epidemic in the 1940s. Veterinary patients with respiratory failure can also benefit from the use of mechanical ventilation. Two major indications for initiation of PPV include hypoxemia refractory to conventional therapy and ventilatory failure. In addition, patients with severe sepsis and septic shock and those with respiratory muscle fatigue can benefit from mechanical ventilation. An intensive care unit (ICU) ventilator differs from an anesthesia ventilator through its ability to vary the inspired oxygen concentration and to humidify the inspired air. Thus, patients can be maintained on an ICU ventilator for as many days as is necessary. With the advent of positive pressure ventilators, intensivists emerged as the primary physicians caring for these patients in the ICU. In veterinary medicine, the role of long-term mechanical ventilation has been primarily assumed by specialists in emergency and critical care. However, patients that present with imminent respiratory failure must be managed quickly and assuredly by the primary attending veterinarian. First and foremost, an adequate and patent airway must be established. Following rapid sedation, hand ventilation with an Ambu bag connected to an oxygen source can be administered. An anesthesia ventilator

[a] Department of Veterinary Surgical and Radiological Sciences, University of California, Davis, CA, USA; [b] University of Minnesota Veterinary Medical Center, St Paul, MN, USA
* Corresponding author.
E-mail address: powel029@umn.edu

Vet Clin Small Anim 43 (2013) 955–969
http://dx.doi.org/10.1016/j.cvsm.2013.03.009
0195-5616/13/$ – see front matter © 2013 Elsevier Inc. All rights reserved.
vetsmall.theclinics.com

can be temporarily used (eg, for up to 8 hours); however, because of the potential for oxygen toxicity from delivery of 100% fraction of inspired oxygen (FiO_2) by the anesthesia ventilator, the use of an ICU ventilator is more suitable if longer ventilation is necessary. With support, veterinary patients with severe respiratory failure have the potential to survive.

INDICATIONS FOR VENTILATION

Mechanical ventilation is indicated when adequate gas exchange can no longer be maintained and there is a significant risk of patient death as a consequence. There are 4 main indications for mechanical ventilation. These are[1–3]

1. Severe hypoxemia despite oxygen therapy (PaO_2 <60 mm Hg)
2. Severe hypoventilation (defined as PcO_2 >60 mm Hg)
3. Excessive work of breathing
4. Severe circulatory shock

Severe Hypoxemia Despite Oxygen Therapy

The oxygenation status of a patient is ideally assessed by measurement of the partial pressure of oxygen in an arterial blood sample (PaO_2). Hypoxemia is commonly defined as a PaO_2 of less than 80 mm Hg at sea level, while a PaO_2 of less than 60 mm Hg is considered severe hypoxemia. Severe hypoxemia is also known as hypoxemic respiratory failure.[1] The need for mechanical ventilation in the hypoxemic patient will depend on the underlying mechanism of hypoxemia and the patient's response to oxygen therapy. Also, if the arterial sample is taken at significant altitude, the cut-off for hypoxemia will be lower. In the emergency room setting, collection of an arterial blood gas (ABG) may not be feasible and unfortunately venous blood gas (VBG) samples cannot be used to evaluate oxygenation. In the absence of ABG samples, pulse oximetry can provide a measure of oxygenation. Pulse oximetry is appealing, as it is noninvasive; however, it is prone to inaccuracies. A pulse oximeter reading of 95% is equivalent to a PaO_2 of ~80 mm Hg, while 90% is approximately 60 mm Hg (indicating severe hypoxemia).[1,4] Mechanical ventilation is a consideration for patients with severe hypoxemia despite oxygen therapy, in other words, patients with a PaO_2 of less than 60 mm Hg or an SpO_2 of less than 90% despite oxygen therapy.

General mechanisms of hypoxemia include

1. Inadequate inspired oxygen
2. Hypoventilation
3. Venous admixture

Inadequate inspired oxygen is not likely to be relevant to the emergency room patient. It can occur in patients on a breathing circuit when the oxygen supply is disconnected or the oxygen tank is empty. It is also the cause of hypoxemia when at high altitude. This problem is readily resolved with oxygen administration.

Hypoventilation is defined by an elevation in the partial pressure of carbon dioxide (PcO_2). Elevations in PcO_2 will reduce the partial pressure of alveolar oxygen as defined by the alveolar air equation.[4] When patients are breathing room air, moderate-to-severe hypercapnia will be associated with hypoxemia. This cause of hypoxemia is readily resolved with oxygen administration and is not an indication for PPV.[4] It is important to note that hypercapnia itself may be an indication for PPV.

Venous admixture describes any mechanism by which blood can pass from the right side of the heart to the left side of the heart without being fully oxygenated.

This includes ventilation–perfusion (V/Q) mismatch, right-to-left anatomic shunts, and diffusion defects. Right-to-left anatomic shunts are associated with congenital cardiovascular defects (eg, right-to-left patent ductus arteriosus) and generally become clinically relevant in young animals. These cases are not usually considered candidates for PPV. Lung diseases associated with a true diffusion defect are associated with changes to the gas exchange surface of the alveoli. In small animal patients, such diseases include smoke inhalation, oxygen toxicity, and acute respiratory distress syndrome (ARDS). The alveolar changes typified by these diseases are the loss of the type 1 pneumocytes and their replacement with the large, cuboidal type 2 pneumocytes. This process is slow, taking several days after the initial pulmonary insult to occur.[5] Hypoxemia subsequent to a diffusion defect improves with oxygen therapy and should not require PPV. As the diseases that can cause a diffusion defect can also cause severe V/Q mismatch, PPV maybe indicated in those patients failing to respond to therapy. V/Q mismatch refers to pulmonary parenchymal disease that leads to alveoli receiving decreased ventilation for the degree of perfusion (low V/Q) or no ventilation but ongoing perfusion (no V/Q or shunt). In small animal medicine, V/Q mismatch is associated with all forms of pulmonary parenchymal disease including pulmonary edema, hemorrhage, and pneumonia. When pulmonary parenchymal disease is associated with severe hypoxemia despite high levels of oxygen therapy, PPV is indicated. As a general guideline, a Pao_2 of less than 60 mm Hg despite greater than 60% Fio_2 is an indication for PPV unless the underlying cause for the hypoxemia can be readily resolved.[1]

Severe Hypoventilation

Hypoventilation is marked by hypercapnia (Pco_2 >50 mm Hg). As arterial and venous carbon dioxide levels correlate well in hemodynamically stable patients, with $Pvco_2$ running approximately 4 mm Hg higher than $Paco_2$, venous blood gases can be used to evaluate ventilation (but not oxygenation) status in most patients.[4] In hemodynamically unstable animals, measurement of $Paco_2$ is ideal, as carbon dioxide can accumulate in venous blood in association with low flow states and is no longer representative of ventilation. Hypoventilation is defined as a Pco_2 greater than 50 mm Hg, while severe hypoventilation is a Pco_2 greater than 60 mm Hg (eg, hypercapnic respiratory failure).[1] Severe hypoventilation that cannot be readily resolved by treatment for the primary disease (eg, reversal agent for a sedative) may be an indication for PPV. The extreme of hypoventilation is apnea, a clear indication for manual or PPV. As elevations of Pco_2 may be associated with increases in intracranial pressure, animals considered at risk of intracranial hypertension (eg, head trauma) may require PPV to maintain a $Paco_2$ less than 45 mm Hg and greater than 35 mm Hg.

The Pco_2 is controlled primarily by alveolar minute ventilation, which is equal to the product of the respiratory rate and effective (alveolar) tidal volume (TV). Consequently, causes of severe hypoventilation are diseases that impair the ability of patients to maintain an adequate respiratory rate and/or TV. Such diseases include brain disease, cervical spinal cord disease, peripheral neuropathies, diseases of the neuromuscular junction, and myopathies. Hypoventilation will cause hypoxemia when the patient is breathing room air, as it reduces (dilutes out) the partial pressure of oxygen in the alveolus.[4] The higher the Pco_2, the lower the alveolar oxygen partial pressure and hence the greater the severity of hypoxemia. Oxygen therapy will increase the partial pressure of oxygen in the alveolus, and hypoxemia should rapidly resolve (although the Pco_2 will be unchanged). For this reason, oxygen therapy should be provided as soon as hypoventilation is identified. Hypoventilation is life-threatening, because it is associated with inadequate respiratory rate and/or TV, which can easily result in apnea and death. When hypoventilation is severe or the underlying disease thought to be progressive in nature, PPV is indicated.[1]

Excessive Work of Breathing

Animals that are breathing so hard that they are becoming exhausted or appear to be at risk of developing exhaustion (eg, orthopnea or eyes closed during breathing) may require PPV to prevent imminent death. While some of these patients may be maintaining adequate blood gases, they are at risk for respiratory fatigue and arrest. Also, in these fragile patients, there may be no time for blood gas evaluation to be performed. This decision is based on clinical judgment and is particularly important in the emergency room setting where patients can present in a near-death state, and rapid intervention is the only chance to stabilize them.

Animals in severe respiratory distress due to lung disease are expected to have increased respiratory rate and effort with hypoxemia and hypocapnia (Pco_2 <35 mm Hg). The presence of normal or elevated Pco_2 in the respiratory distress patient can be a sinister sign suggestive of respiratory muscle fatigue and may support the decision to initiate PPV even if hypoxemia can be adequately resolved with oxygen therapy. Again, this should be determined based on clinical evaluation of work of breathing and signs consistent with respiratory fatigue.

Severe Circulatory Shock

Clinical signs of circulatory shock include obtundation, mucous membrane pallor, tachycardia or bradycardia, tachypnea, weak pulse quality, and cold extremities. Circulatory shock can be due to hypovolemia, cardiac disease, and loss of vasomotor tone. In patients with severe circulatory shock that is persistent despite initial resuscitation efforts, PPV may be indicated. The main goal of PPV in these patients is to reduce oxygen consumption by relieving the work of the respiratory muscles.[1] Both experimental animal studies and human clinical studies have found that PPV can improve outcome from shock, and PPV is part of the early goal-directed therapy algorithm for the treatment of septic shock.[6–8] A secondary goal is to allow airway protection by supporting the animal appropriately during anesthesia.

Prognosis

Mechanical ventilation in emergency room patients plays several important roles. In many situations, PPV may need to be initiated before any specific diagnosis can be obtained as part of life-saving stabilization efforts. In this setting, stabilization of the ABCDs (ie, airway, breathing, circulation, dysfunction) is imperative, and further prognostication of the patient can be made once the patient is successfully stabilized, allowing further diagnostic tests to be performed. Some animals may not need PPV for more than a few hours, and the owners of patients that need longer term PPV will have the benefit of a more informed prognosis once further diagnostic tests have been performed in a more controlled manner. That said, it is important to keep in mind that some patients may be difficult to wean off PPV once initiated, and the costs associated with short-term (or long-term) PPV is high. Another important role for PPV in the emergency room patient is to relieve suffering and prevent further clinical deterioration while owners spend some time to consider all their options or say good bye to their pet.

The prognosis of weaning from PPV is largely dependent on the underlying disease for which the animal requires ventilation. In general, patients that require PPV for hypoventilation (eg, cervical disc disease) have a greater likelihood of weaning than those with pulmonary parenchymal disease (eg, ARDS, pulmonary contusions, fungal pneumonia).[9–11] For example, in a study evaluating 128 dogs and cats that received PPV for more than 24 hours, 50% of animals with hypoventilation were weaned, while only 36% of animals with pulmonary parenchymal disease were weaned.[10] It is more helpful to consider prognosis of weaning from PPV in terms of the primary disease process present. For example, in the pulmonary parenchymal group in this study, 50% of animals with aspiration pneumonia were successfully weaned, while only 8% of animals with ARDS were weaned. This study largely reflects ICU patients, not emergency room patients, and only enrolled patients ventilated for 24 hours or longer. Other factors that have been reported to be associated with a poorer outcome from PPV include age, weight, and species. The weaning rates reported for feline patients are consistently lower than that of canine patients, reported to be 10% to 25%, overall.[10,12]

Disease processes that may have a fair prognosis for weaning from PPV include

- Congestive heart failure
- Pulmonary contusions
- Aspiration pneumonia
- Cervical spinal cord compression
- Polyradiculoneuritis
- Intoxications

Disease processes that may have a poor prognosis to be weaned from PPV include

- Cardiopulmonary arrest
- Intracranial disease
- ARDS

OVERVIEW OF VENTILATION MODES

To understand how to appropriately manage a patient undergoing PPV, an understanding of the ventilation modes and ventilator settings is imperative.[1,13]

Pressure Versus Volume Control

Modern ICU ventilators have the capability to generate several different breath types to the patient. The more basic machines tend to be either volume control ventilators or pressure control ventilators. These ventilators can generate a breath in 1 of 2 basic ways. It can deliver a preset TV over a given inspiratory time (volume control, or VC), or the machine can maintain a preset airway pressure for a given inspiratory time (pressure control, or PC). In a volume-controlled breath, the peak inspired airway pressure (PIP) generated will be dependent on the preset TV chosen by the operator and the compliance of the respiratory system. In a pressure-controlled breath, the TV will depend on the preset airway pressure chosen by the operator and the compliance of the respiratory system.

Assist-Control Ventilation

In this mode of ventilation, a minimum respiratory rate is set by the operator. If the trigger sensitivity is set appropriately, the patient can increase the respiratory rate, but all breaths delivered will be full ventilator breaths, either pressure- or volume-controlled. Breaths triggered by the ventilator are controlled breaths, while breaths triggered by the patient are considered assisted breaths (eg, patient initiates the breath, but the ventilator generates the full breath). This mode of ventilation provides maximum support of the respiratory system and is used in patients with severe disease or patients with no respiratory drive.

Synchronized Intermittent Mandatory Ventilation

In this mode of ventilation, a set number of mandatory breaths is delivered. Between these breaths, the patient can breathe spontaneously. In modern ventilators, the machine tries to synchronize the mandatory breaths with the patient's inspiratory efforts, thus the term synchronized intermittent mandatory ventilation (SIMV). Between these mandatory breaths, the patient can breathe spontaneously, as often or as few times as desired. The operator can only control the minimum respiratory rate and minute ventilation; there is no control over the maximum rate or maximum minute ventilation. As this mode combines full ventilator breaths with spontaneous patient breaths, it is generally used for animals that do not require 100% assistance from the ventilator, such as neurologically inappropriate animals with an unreliable respiratory drive (eg, brain injury), or patients with lung disease that are improving and do not need as much support as assist–control provides.

Continuous Positive Airway Pressure

Continuous positive airway pressure (CPAP) is a completely spontaneous mode of ventilation; in other words, the patient determines both the respiratory rate and TV. The ventilator delivers no breaths; the operator can only control the baseline airway pressure, a form of positive end-expiratory pressure (PEEP). This mode of ventilation provides support for the patient's spontaneous breaths and is only suited for patients with a strong respiratory drive and minimal pulmonary dysfunction. The ventilator will alarm if the animal does not generate adequate breaths or develops apnea, so it is a useful monitoring mode for weaning patients or for monitoring intubated patients.

Pressure Support Ventilation

Pressure support ventilation (PSV) allows the operator to augment the TV of spontaneous breaths. For example, a patient has a PSV of 6 cm H_2O. This patient will begin and end inspiration, and the ventilator will maintain a pressure of 6 cm H_2O in the airway during this inspiration; this effectively provides the patient with a greater tidal volume for less patient effort. Pressure support ventilation is generally used in conjunction with CPAP or to support the spontaneous breaths in SIMV.

OVERVIEW OF VENTILATOR SETTINGS

The parameters the operator is able to adjust on a ventilator will vary between machines. On advanced ICU ventilators, there tend to be more options for adjusting breath parameters compared with simpler, anesthesia-type machines. It is important to note that there is no consistency in the terminology for ventilator settings between companies; therefore, it may be necessary to read the manufacturer's instructions to fully understand how the settings on an individual machine operate.

Trigger Variable

This is the parameter that initiates a ventilator breath. In patients that are not making any respiratory effort, the trigger variable will be time (which is determined from the set respiratory rate). The patient trigger setting is usually a change in airway pressure or a change in flow of the circuit. Appropriate trigger sensitivity is an essential safety measure to ensure ventilator breaths are synchronized with genuine respiratory efforts made by the patient.[14,15] This increases patient comfort and allows the patient to increase its RR as required. The trigger variable can be too sensitive, such that nonrespiratory efforts such as patient handling may initiate breaths; this should also be avoided.

Respiratory Rate and Inspiration: Expiration Ratio

The respiratory rate can be set on all ventilators either directly or by manipulation of variables such as minute ventilation, inspiratory time, or exhalation time. The ideal respiratory rate for an individual patient generally needs to be titrated according to patient comfort and Pco_2. Respiratory rates are commonly set in the range of 10 to 20 breaths per minute initially. The ratio of the duration of inspiration to expiration (called the I:E ratio) may be preset by the operator or may be a default setting within the machine. Commonly, an I:E ratio of 1:2 is used to ensure the patient has fully exhaled before the onset of the next breath.[2] This is similar to a physiologic normal breath, where expiration lasts approximately twice as long as inspiration. As respiratory rates are increased, the expiratory time will have to be reduced accordingly. It is advised to prevent the I:E ratio from increasing more than 1:1 to avoid a situation known as breath stacking or intrinsic PEEP.[15,16]

Inspiratory Time and Flow Rate

Inspiratory time is commonly set at 1 second, but shorter inspiratory times are suitable for patients with high respiratory rates.[2] Many smaller patients seem to tolerate shorter inspiratory times well. Many volume control ventilators have the option to set the flow rate instead of the inspiratory time. The faster the inspiratory flow rate, the more quickly the breath is delivered. Flow rates of 60 L/min are suggested as a good starting point.[2] The flow rate may be adjusted between 40 and 80 L/min as needed to provide an inspiratory time that suits the patient's needs.[16]

Tidal Volume

The normal TV reported for dogs and cats is in the range of 10 to 15 mL/kg. Lower TV (6–8 mL/kg) may be targeted in animals with severe lung disease.[15,16] When using volume control ventilation, the operator presets the desired TV. Overdistension of the lung is extremely dangerous, as it is a major mechanism of ventilator-induced lung injury and can have severe, even fatal consequences. It is recommended to start with no more than 10 mL/kg as a preset TV. The TV can always be increased if it is determined to be insufficient once the patient is connected to the machine. If pressure control ventilation is used, then the operator presets the pressure used to generate inspiration; once the animal is connected to the machine, the TV achieved with the preset pressure is assessed. A TV of around 10 mL/kg would be a very acceptable result. A simple evaluation of TV is to observe the patient's chest movements to see if normal chest excursions are occurring, although direct measurement of TV should be performed when ever possible.

Positive End-Expiratory Pressure

Pulmonary parenchymal disease can lead to areas of poorly ventilated alveoli (eg, alveoli smaller than normal) and alveolar collapse; this is the primary cause of inefficient oxygenating ability of the diseased lung. PEEP will maintain pressure in the airway during exhalation. This prevents full exhalation occurring, holding the lung in a semiinflated state, which can help open up previously collapsed alveoli to improve lung-oxygenating ability and potentially protect against some forms of ventilator-associated lung injury.[2,17] As lung disease tends to be heterogeneous, there is a risk that while increases in PEEP may recruit areas of diseased lung, it may also cause overdistension or volutrauma of healthier lung regions. In general, PEEP is likely to be beneficial in patients with cardiogenic and noncardiogenic pulmonary edema and acute lung injury (ALI) or ARDS.[13]

There are some potential dangers from the use of PEEP that must be considered. The use of PEEP in diseases such as pneumonia, where the diseased lung may not be recruited, should be done with caution. Also, as PEEP increases peak airway pressure, it can contribute to barotrauma (eg, pressure trauma to the lung). Also, as PEEP maintains elevated intrathoracic pressure during exhalation, it may compromise venous return (eg, hypotension). Cardiovascular monitoring is recommended for all ventilator patients and is essential when high levels of PEEP and/or more aggressive ventilator settings are used. Ultimately, optimizing PEEP requires balancing the potential gain with the concern for adverse effects.[2,17]

Peak Inspired Airway Pressure

Patients with normal lungs (such as anesthetic patients or patients with ventilatory failure) typically only require low PIPs in the range of 8 to 15 cm H_2O, ideally not exceeding 20 cm H_2O. Patients with lung disease often have stiff, noncompliant lungs and consequently will require higher airway pressures to achieve the same TV. Peak airway pressures as high as 30 cm H_2O may be required in animals with very severe lung disease.[18] High airway pressure can cause lung injury (barotrauma) and should be avoided where possible. When using pressure control ventilation, the desired airway pressure is preset by the operator. Once the animal is connected to the ventilator, the TV achieved with that airway pressure can be assessed. Alternatively in volume control, the TV is preset, and the associated airway pressure must be assessed once PPV commences. Initially, airway pressures of 10 to 15 cm H_2O should be targeted; higher airway pressures can be used if indicated by inadequate pulmonary function.

SELECTION OF INITIAL SETTINGS

There is no way to accurately predict the ideal ventilator settings for a specific patient. The choice of initial settings is based on an understanding of the underlying disease process present.[2,15,16] Once the patient is attached to the ventilator, the settings are then titrated to target adequate blood gases with an acceptable F_{IO_2}.

Animals that do not have pulmonary disease are expected to have compliant, easy-to-ventilate lungs. As a result, low airway pressures, higher TV, and less PEEP are likely to be well tolerated (**Table 1**). When initially placing a patient on the ventilator, the use of 100% oxygen should be utilized as a safety measure (and weaned down once ventilator settings are determined and the patient stabilized).

Table 1 Suggested initial ventilator settings for patients with normal pulmonary function	
Ventilator Parameter	**Initial Setting**
Fraction of inspired oxygen	100%
Tidal volume	8–15 mL/kg
Respiratory rate	10–20 breaths per minute
Inspiratory pressure (above PEEP)	8–12 cm H_2O
PEEP	0–4 cm H_2O
Inspiratory time	~1 s
Inspiratory: Expiratory (I:E) ratio	1:2
Inspiratory trigger	−1 to −2 cm H_2O or 0.5 to 2.0 L/min

Animals that require PPV for pulmonary disease are expected to have poor lung compliance and will require higher airway pressures than animals with healthy lungs (**Table 2**). PEEP may improve the oxygenating efficiency of the diseased lung and can be a very important aspect of management of some ventilator patients. Studies have shown that limiting TV to approximately 6 mL/kg in human patients with ALI and ARDS improves survival.[18] The role of small TV ventilation in other lung diseases is unknown, but limiting TV when possible may be beneficial.

Once the patient is attached to the ventilator, the patient's chest should be observed for appropriate movement (eg, if there is insufficient or overaggressive chest inflation, the ventilator settings should be adjusted appropriately). The thorax should then be auscultated bilaterally to ensure there is ventilation of bilateral lung fields. All monitoring parameters need to be rapidly and continuously evaluated including blood pressure, electrocardiography (ECG), pulse oximeter and end-tidal carbon dioxide ($ETCO_2$) monitoring. Any concerning changes should be addressed immediately.

Once the patient is adequately stabilized on the ventilator, assessment of ABGs is ideally performed. The target of PPV is to maintain adequate gas exchange while minimizing the likelihood of ventilator-associated lung injury. Target values are commonly a PaO_2 between 80 and 120 mm Hg and a $PaCO_2$ of 35 to 50 mm Hg.[19]

PaO_2

The first aim in titration of ventilator settings is to lower the FIO_2 to no more than 60% while maintaining an acceptable PaO_2. In the absence of ABGs, reductions in the FIO_2 will have to be based on the saturation of oxygen (SpO_2) based off the pulse oximeter. The implantation of PEEP may help increase the oxygenating efficiency of the sick lung. If the PaO_2 is not high enough to allow adequate reductions in FIO_2, increases in PEEP may be of benefit.

$PaCO_2$

The $PaCO_2$ will be inversely proportional to alveolar minute ventilation (eg, TV × respiratory rate). When titrating the initial ventilator settings, if $PaCO_2$ is higher than desired, increases in TV and/or respiratory rate are made and vice versa if the $PaCO_2$ is too low. If ABGs are not available, venous PCO_2 can be used to guide ventilator settings. Initially, PCO_2 should be measured on a blood gas machine to evaluate the correlation with $ETCO_2$. Once this relationship has been established, $ETCO_2$ can be used as a noninvasive measure to titrate ventilator settings further. If a significant change in the patient

Table 2	
Suggested initial ventilator settings for patients with pulmonary disease	
Ventilator Parameter	**Initial Setting**
Fraction of inspired oxygen	100%
Tidal volume	6–8 mL/kg
Respiratory rate	20–30 breaths per minute
Inspiratory pressure (above PEEP)	10–15 cm H_2O
PEEP	4–8 cm H_2O
Inspiratory time	~1 s
I:E ratio	1:2
Inspiratory trigger	−1 to −2 cm H_2O or 0.5 to 2.0 L/min

status occurs, the Pco_2 should be measured directly, as the relationship and accuracy with $ETCO_2$ can rapidly change.

Initial Patient Stabilization on the Ventilator

Placing a veterinary patient on an ICU ventilator requires knowledge about how the specific ventilator is connected with inflow and outflow tubing, a humidifier, and airway suction. Because of the time it takes to assemble the ventilatory equipment, the unstable patient should be anesthetized, intubated, and manually ventilated in the emergency room until the ventilator is ready to use. An anesthesia circuit breathing bag or purpose-made practice lung can be placed on the Y-piece of the ventilator circuit, allowing for input of initial ventilator settings before placing the patient directly on the breathing circuit. The initial settings used are based on general guidelines such as those described previously. When the ventilator settings are verified and the patient is anesthetized, transfer to the ventilator breathing circuit can occur. Intensive monitoring should be initiated before or soon after anesthetic induction. As the patient is being placed on the ventilator, an inspired oxygen concentration of 100% should be provided. Once the patient has stabilized on the ventilator, the aim is to decrease the FIo_2 in an effort to decrease the likelihood of oxygen toxicity. A sustained FIo_2 of less than 60% oxygen within the first 12 hours is desired, especially in patients with severe hypoxemic respiratory failure.[20] Sustaining a minimally adequate oxygenation (Pao_2 of 60 mm Hg, SpO_2 of ~90% or above) is essential, and this may limit the degree to which FIo_2 can be reduced.

Mechanically ventilated patients require intense monitoring and supportive care. Intravenous catheters (ideally, a multilumen catheter), an arterial catheter, a body temperature probe, and urinary catheterization should be used. Monitoring should include continuous ECG, continuous pulse oximetry, continuous direct arterial blood pressure, intermittent blood gas analysis (via an arterial catheter), and $ETCO_2$ measurements. Nursing care should include catheter asepsis, oral antibacterial rinse, tracheal tube suction, passive range of motion of all limbs, ocular care, and intermittent change of body position.[21] The ventilator itself requires management, including emptying water traps that collect condensation from the tubing and filling of the humidifier with sterile water as needed. Most ventilator patients need a dedicated veterinary nurse constantly, and an attentive veterinarian who can troubleshoot ventilator problems and make adjustments to ventilator settings as needed. As such, placing and maintaining a patient on a mechanical ventilator is a significant financial and time obligation.

Induction and Maintenance of Anesthesia

To successfully ventilate neurologically intact dogs and cats, appropriate anesthesia must be maintained. This is to allow maintenance of the endotracheal tube (ETT), to prevent patient movement, to provide patient comfort, and to stop animals from bucking or fighting the ventilator, as the sensation of receiving a positive pressure breath is unpleasant. In neurologically inappropriate animals, anesthesia may not be necessary. Paralyzed animals may only need anesthesia to allow ETT intubation or placement of a tracheostomy tube (which allows PPV with minimal to no anesthetic or sedative drugs). Comatose patients may also tolerate ETT intubation without drug administration and are another group of patients that often can be ventilated without anesthesia.

There are several options for induction and maintenance of anesthesia in the ventilated patient. Induction of anesthesia should be performed using at least 1 fast-acting intravenous drug allowing rapid ETT placement (eg, fentanyl or midazolam). All animals should be preoxygenated before induction. Consideration of the patient's cardiovascular status when selecting induction drugs is important. Propofol, administered slowly and to effect, is an ideal induction drug for hemodynamically stable patients. In the emergency room, where animals are often hemodynamically unstable or there is insufficient time to assess the cardiovascular system adequately, the use of induction drugs such as ketamine or etomidate may be preferable.

Maintenance anesthesia of the PPV patient is generally achieved by combinations of injectable drugs, as inhalant anesthesia is not an option when ventilating patients on an ICU ventilator. However, if an anesthesia ventilator is temporarily used, low concentrations of inhalant anesthesia can also be employed. Care must be taken, however, as inhalants can exacerbate hypotension and worsen pulmonary gas exchange. The choice of anesthesia protocol for individual PPV patients will be influenced by their cardiovascular stability, the duration of PPV anticipated, and in some situations, cost. A further consideration is recovery time. It is ideal to be able to recover animals as soon as they are ready to be weaned from PPV. This may require reducing drug doses ahead of time or changing the anesthetic protocol when weaning is thought to be imminent. Injectable anesthetics such as propofol and pentobarbital will provide an adequate plane of anesthesia when used as constant rate infusions (CRI) and generally are the basis for most ventilator patient anesthetic protocols. It is ideal to provide balanced anesthesia by the addition of drugs such as benzodiazepines and/or opioids. This allows minimal dosing of any 1 drug to reduce the likelihood of adverse effects. Sample protocols include fentanyl-lidocaine-ketamine and fentanyl-dexmedetomidine in addition to propofol or pentobarbital. See **Table 3** for suggested dosing regimens. Long-term administration of propofol in dogs can lead to lipemia, which can have adverse effects and should be avoided. By minimizing the dose of propofol with the addition of other drugs, lipemia can often be avoided. Cats cannot tolerate long-term (>48 hours) propofol administration, as it leads to Heinz body formation; therefore, other anesthetic regimes need to be considered for long-term PPV in this species.[22] Another concern for PPV in cats is the delayed recovery time they have after prolonged injectable anesthesia. After 24 hours of anesthesia, recovery time has been reported to be 18 to 35 hours in one study.[23] In the authors' experience, it can take many days for cats to recover from long-term anesthesia. As they often require ventilator support during the

Table 3	
Anesthetic/analgesic agents commonly used in ventilated patients	
Anesthetic/Analgesic Agent	**Suggested Dose**
Fentanyl	1–7 μg/kg/h CRI Loading dose: 2–5 μg/kg
Midazolam	0.1–0.5 mg/kg/h CRI Loading dose: 0.2–0.4 mg/kg
Diazepam	0.1–1.0 mg/kg/h CRI Loading dose: 0.5 mg/kg
Morphine-lidocaine-ketamine CRI	Morphine: 0.2 mg/kg/h; loading dose: 0.1–0.2 mg/kg slow intravenously Lidocaine: 3 mg/kg/h; loading dose 1–2 mg/kg Ketamine: 0.6 mg/kg/h; loading dose 0.5 mg/kg
Propofol	0.05–0.4 mg/kg/min CRI
Dexmedetomidine	0.5 to 1.0 μg/kg/h

All doses indicate intravenous route.

prolonged recovery period, it adds significantly to the cost and challenge of management of cats needing PPV.

Monitoring

Continuous monitoring of cardiovascular parameters, respiratory parameters, body temperature, and fluids both administered and lost (eg, evaporative, urinary, gastrointestinal losses, etc.) is of utmost importance when managing a patient on a mechanical ventilator. Continuous pulse oximetry, ECG, ETCO$_2$, blood pressure, and body temperature should be measured. In addition, charting of results on an hourly basis will help to identify trends, diagnosing both clinical improvement and areas of concern that must be addressed. Ideally, an arterial catheter should be placed to measure both blood pressure and intermittent blood gas analysis. In smaller dogs and cats, placement of an arterial catheter may not be possible; in these cases, one must rely on results of pulse oximetry readings and VBG analysis to assess presence of significant hypoxemia and effective ventilation.[21]

Po$_2$ and Pco$_2$ Targets

Traditionally, patients should be ventilated to endpoints of normal blood levels of Po$_2$ and Pco$_2$: Pao$_2$ of 80 to 120 mm Hg (SpO$_2$ of 95%–99%) and a Paco$_2$ of 35 to 45 mm Hg. In most patients, these goals can be reached with an Fio$_2$ of no more than 60% and mild-to-moderate ventilator settings. In patients with severe lung disease, far more aggressive ventilator settings (eg, higher PEEP, Fio$_2$, and PIP) may be necessary to achieve the normal blood gas goals. Ventilating with high TV and pressures can cause lung trauma, including pulmonary biotrauma and barotrauma and worsening patient outcome. A study by the ARDSnet group in 2000 showed a decrease in mortality when using a low TV strategy when ventilating patients with ARDS.[18] Current recommendations for ARDS patients include ventilating to an oxygen saturation of 85% to 90% (eg, Pao$_2$ 55–80 mm Hg) and allowing Paco$_2$ to rise above normal, as long as blood pH is maintained above 7.2 (eg, permissive hypercapnia).[18,24] Although this strategy may not be as relevant to patients with other forms of lung disease, lowering the target Pao$_2$ to 60 mm Hg (SpO$_2$ of 90%) and increasing the tolerance for hypercapnia (eg, Pco$_2$ >50 mm Hg) may reduce the magnitude of the ventilator settings needed in animals with severe hypoxemic respiratory failure. This may reduce the likelihood of ventilator-induced lung injury.

Troubleshooting

Problems involving PPV include hypoxemia/oxygen desaturation, hypercapnia, hypotension, patient–ventilator dyssynchrony, air leak, resistance to air flow, and barotrauma.

Hypoxemia is a common problem faced by patients undergoing PPV. The approach to management of hypoxemia differs when it is an acute development versus a more gradual onset. If acute desaturation is detected on the pulse oximeter, repositioning of the pulse oximeter or confirmation with an ABG is ideal. Acute desaturation of a ventilator patient that was previously oxygenating adequately indicates a dramatic decrease in pulmonary function. Potential causes include pneumothorax, machine malfunction, circuit disconnection, and loss of oxygen supply. The Fio$_2$ should be immediately increased to 100%, the thorax auscultated, and the ventilator function reviewed. If a pneumothorax is suspected, thoracocentesis should be performed immediately. A gradual decline in oxygenating efficiency of the lung is not uncommon in the ventilator patient and is more suggestive of progressive pulmonary disease such as pneumonia, ARDS, or ventilator-induced lung injury rather than a pneumothorax or machine issue. This can be addressed in several ways. The F_{IO_2} can be increased; however, high levels of inspired oxygen over a long period of time can induce ALI and secondary oxygen toxicity. Other methods include increasing the PEEP level, increasing the TV, and increasing the peak pressure at which the tidal breath is delivered.

Hypercapnia in the ventilator patient may be due to one or more of the following causes:

- Pneumothorax
- ETT or tracheostomy tube kink or obstruction
- Increased apparatus dead space—excess tubing/connectors between the patient and the ventilator circuit Y-piece
- Incorrect assembly of the ventilator circuit, including large airway leaks, obstruction of the exhalation circuit, or any problem that would prevent effective generation or delivery of a TV
- Increased pulmonary dead space, which may occur with overdistension of alveoli or large pulmonary embolism
- Inadequate ventilator settings, in particular inadequate TV, inadequate respiratory rate, or both; settings that can impair exhalation such as insufficient expiratory time can also cause hypercapnia

A sudden increase in $Paco_2$ (eg, hypoventilation or hypercapnia) in a previously stable patient is suggestive of an acute abnormality such as an ETT or tracheostomy tube obstruction or dislodgement, ventilator circuit leak, or pneumothorax. If evaluation of the machine and patient rules out major complications, then it is to be assumed that there is insufficient alveolar minute ventilation, and appropriate changes in the ventilator settings should be made.

Hemodynamic compromise can be an adverse effect of PPV. Subatmospheric pressure generated within the thoracic cavity during normal, spontaneous inspiration promotes venous return to the right side of the heart (eg, preload). When a patient is placed on PPV, it causes positive intrathoracic pressure during inspiration, which opposes venous return. As a result, venous return occurs primarily during exhalation during PPV and may be reduced. With the addition of PEEP, which generates positive intrathoracic pressure during exhalation, venous return may be further compromised. Perfusion parameters and blood pressure should be closely monitored in the PPV patient, especially when high PEEP levels and high peak pressures are used. If hemodynamic compromise occurs, volume support to improve preload may be beneficial. In patients that are hypotensive despite fluid therapy, vasopressor therapy may be indicated.

Patient–ventilator dyssynchrony occurs when the patient's breath and the mechanical breath conflict with one another. When a patient fights or bucks the ventilator, it can prevent effective ventilation of the animal and may lead to desaturation and hypercapnia. In addition, it increases the work of breathing and can increase both patient discomfort and patient morbidity. Bucking the ventilator is 1 of the most common challenges for PPV patient management. It is ideal to have a thorough, systematic approach to this problem to avoid missing potential causes. Potential causes of patient–ventilator dyssynchrony include

- Hypoxemia— loss of oxygen supply, worsening of underlying disease, or development of new pulmonary disease such as pneumothorax, pneumonia, or ARDS
- Hypercapnia— circuit disconnect/leak, tube obstruction or kink, pneumothorax

- Pneumothorax— Typified by a rapidly climbing Pco_2 and a plummeting Pao_2; auscultation and diagnostic thoracocentesis is warranted
- Hyperthermia
  - Anesthetized animals like to have relatively low temperatures, and even a rectal temperature of 102°F/38.9°C may cause dogs to pant on the ventilator; active cooling is required to control panting in hyperthermic ventilator patients
  - A common cause of hyperthermia is increased breathing efforts when patients fight the ventilator; airway humidification makes it difficult for patients to lose heat, and humidification may have to be discontinued for short periods to allow hyperthermia to be resolved.
- Inappropriate ventilator settings— observe when the patient is trying to inhale and exhale and evaluate if the patient's breathing pattern is appropriate or consistent with the ventilator settings
- Inadequate depth of anesthesia— monitor routine clinical signs of anesthetic depth; this may be the most common cause of bucking, but care should be taken not to blindly increase the anesthetic drug dose when patients begin bucking the machine without fully assessing the patient or the ventilator settings

It is very important to appropriately set the high- and low-pressure alarms on the ventilator. Low pressure in the ventilator circuit indicates air leak, which is usually due to inadvertent disconnection of the ventilator tubing. The high-pressure alarm is activated due to increased resistance to airflow. This may be caused by ETT obstruction from a mucous plug or a large amount of secretions or due to the development of a pneumothorax. Resistance to airflow can also be due to worsening of pulmonary disease, requiring higher pressures to adequately ventilate the patient. Plateau airway pressures of greater than 30 cm H_2O should be avoided.[18]

SUMMARY

Mechanical ventilation can be a life saving tool for dogs and cats experiencing hypoxemic respiratory failure and those that develop ventilatory failure. Ventilation of patients with ventilatory failure has been shown to have a better prognosis than ventilation of those ventilated for hypoxemic respiratory failure.[9,10] An anesthesia machine can be used to provide PPV to patients for a short period of time; this may be suitable for initial stabilization of animals in the emergency room. If longer-term ventilation is required, referral to a veterinary hospital with an ICU ventilator should be considered. Recognizing and treating dogs and cats with imminent respiratory failure with anesthesia, intubation, and PPV can be practical and life saving.

REFERENCES

1. Laghi F, Tobin MJ. Indications. In: Tobin MJ, editor. Indications for mechanical ventilation. 2nd edition. New York: McGraw-Hill; 2006. p. 129–62.
2. Hess DR, Kacmarek RM. Essentials of mechanical ventilation. 2nd edition. New York: McGraw-Hill; 2002.
3. Pilbeam SP. Establishing the need for mechanical ventilation. In: Pilbeam SP, Cairo JM, editors. Mechanical ventilation physiological and clinical applications. St Louis (MO): Mosby; 2006. p. 63–80.
4. West JB. Respiratory physiology: the essentials. 8th edition. Baltimore (MD): Lippincott Williams & Wilkins; 2008.
5. Lumb AB. Nunn's applied respiratory physiology. 7th edition. Toronto: Elsevier; 2010.

6. Aubier M, Trippenbach T, Roussos C, et al. Respiratory muscle fatigue during cardiogenic shock. J Appl Physiol 1981;51:499–508.
7. Kontoyannis DA, Nanas JN, Kontoyannis SA, et al. Mechanical ventilation in conjunction with the intra-aortic balloon pump improves the outcome of patients in profound cardiogenic shock. Intensive Care Med 1999;25:835–8.
8. Rivers E, Nguyen B, Havstad S, et al. Goal directed therapy in the treatment of severe sepsis and septic shock. N Engl J Med 2001;345:1368–77.
9. King LG, Hendricks JC. Use of positive-pressure ventilation in dogs and cats: 41 cases (1990-1992). J Am Vet Med Assoc 1994;204:1045–52.
10. Hopper K, Haskins SC, Kass PH, et al. Indications, management and outcome of long-term positive-pressure ventilation in dogs and cats: 148 cases (1990–2001). J Am Vet Med Assoc 2007;230:64–75.
11. Campbell VL, King LG. Pulmonary function, ventilator management, and outcome of dogs with thoracic trauma and pulmonary contusions: 10 cases (1994–1998). J Am Vet Med Assoc 2000;217:1505–9.
12. Lee JA, Drobatz KJ, Koch MW, et al. Indications for and outcome of positive-pressure ventilation in cats: 53 cases (1993–2002). J Am Vet Med Assoc 2005; 226:924–31.
13. Archambault PM, St-Onge M. Invasive and noninvasive ventilation in the emergency department. Emerg Med Clin North Am 2012;30:421–49.
14. Pilbeam SP. Final considerations in ventilator set up. In: Pilbeam SP, Cairo JM, editors. Mechanical ventilation physiological and clinical applications. St Louis (MO): Mosby; 2006. p. 127–49.
15. MacIntyre NR. Mechanical ventilation. In: Vincent JL, Abraham E, Moore FA, et al, editors. Textbook of Critical Care. 6th edition. Philadelphia: Elsevier-Saunders; 2011. p. 328–34.
16. Pilbeam SP. Initial ventilator settings. In: Pilbeam SP, Cairo JM, editors. Mechanical ventilation physiological and clinical applications. St Louis (MO): Mosby; 2006. p. 105–26.
17. MacIntyre NR. Alveolar-capillary gas transport. In: MacIntyre NR, Branson RD, editors. Mechanical ventilation. 2th edition. St Louis (MO): Saunders; 2009. p. 171–81.
18. The Acute Respiratory Distress Syndrome Network. Ventilation with lower tidal volumes as compared with traditional tidal volumes for acute lung injury and the acute respiratory distress syndrome. N Engl J Med 2000;342:1301–8.
19. Haskins SC, King LG. Positive pressure ventilation. In: King LG, editor. Textbook of respiratory disease in dogs and cats. Philadelphia: WB Saunders; 2004. p. 217–29.
20. Marini JJ, Wheeler AP. Indications and options for mechanical ventilation. In: Marini JJ, Wheeler AP, editors. Critical care medicine. 4th edition. Philadelphia: Lippincott Williams & Wilkins; 2010. p. 129–47.
21. Clare M, Hopper K. Mechanical ventilation: ventilator settings, patient management, and nursing care. Compend Contin Educ Pract Vet 2005.
22. Andress JL, Day TK, Day D. The effects of consecutive day propofol anesthesia on feline red blood cells. Vet Surg 1995;24(3):277–82.
23. Boudreau AE, Bersensas AM, Kerr CL, et al. A comparison of 3 anesthetic protocols for 24 hours of mechincal ventilation in cats. J Vet Emerg Crit Care 2012;22:239–52.
24. Hickling KF, Walsh J, Henderson S, et al. Low mortality rate in adult respiratory distress syndrome using low-volume, pressure-limited ventilation with permissive hypercapnia: a prospective study. Crit Care Med 1994;22(10):1568–78.

Updates in Small Animal Cardiopulmonary Resuscitation

Daniel J. Fletcher, PhD, DVM[a],*, Manuel Boller, Dr med vet, MTR[b]

KEYWORDS

- Cardiopulmonary resuscitation • Cardiopulmonary arrest • Basic life support
- Advanced life support • Post-cardiac arrest care

KEY POINTS

- For dogs and cats that experience cardiopulmonary arrest (CPA), rates of survival to discharge are 6% to 7%, as compared with 20% for people who experience CPA.
- To improve outcomes after CPA, a comprehensive strategy that includes preventive and preparedness measures, basic life support, advanced life support, and postcardiac arrest critical care titrated to the patient's needs is necessary.
- Optimization of each of these elements may help improve overall survival and offers an opportunity to work toward that goal.
- The Reassessment Campaign on Veterinary Resuscitation initiative recently completed an exhaustive literature review and generated a set of evidence-based, consensus cardiopulmonary resuscitation guidelines in 5 domains: preparedness and prevention, basic life support, advanced life support, monitoring, and postcardiac arrest care.

CPR AS A CONTINUUM OF CARE

Cardiopulmonary arrest (CPA) is a highly lethal condition in veterinary medicine with only 6% to 7% of small animals surviving to hospital discharge.[1] A comprehensive strategy is necessary to reduce mortality caused by CPA and several opportunities exist to influence outcomes positively.[2] Preventive measures and recognition of animals at imminent risk can lead to a reduction of the numbers that experience CPA, and preparedness of the resuscitation team and tools will optimize early and effective response to CPA. Well-executed basic and advanced life support will then increase the likelihood of a return of spontaneous circulation (ROSC). Last but not least, postcardiac arrest care is the imperative final step to increasing rate of survival-to-hospital discharge. It addresses treatment of neurologic, myocardial, and systemic ischemia

[a] Department of Clinical Sciences, Cornell University College of Veterinary Medicine, DCS Box 31, Ithaca, NY 14853, USA; [b] Faculty of Veterinary Science, The University of Melbourne, 250 Princes Highway, Werribee, Victoria 3030, Australia
* Corresponding author.
E-mail address: djf42@cornell.edu

Vet Clin Small Anim 43 (2013) 971–987
http://dx.doi.org/10.1016/j.cvsm.2013.03.006
0195-5616/13/$ – see front matter © 2013 Elsevier Inc. All rights reserved.

vetsmall.theclinics.com

and reperfusion injury as well as precipitating conditions. The Reassessment Campaign on Veterinary Resuscitation (RECOVER) recently completed an exhaustive literature review and generated a set of evidence-based, consensus guidelines to provide a clear basis for training and practice for the above outlined cardiopulmonary resuscitation (CPR) continuum of care.[3,4] Accordingly, RECOVER provides clinical instructions in 5 domains: preparedness and prevention,[5] basic life support,[6] advanced life support,[7] monitoring,[8] and postcardiac arrest care.[9] This article reviews some of the most important aspects of these new guidelines.

PREPAREDNESS AND PREVENTION

Early initiation of CPR for patients with CPA is of key importance. Thus veterinary practices must be well prepared for early recognition of and response to CPA. **Box 1** summarizes the key recommendations for preparedness and prevention. CPR training for veterinary personnel possibly involved in resuscitation should include both a structured, didactic component and a psychomotor component with opportunities to practice technical skills.[10,11] Integrated individual and team performance should be trained in mock codes with structured feedback conducted at least once every 6 months.[12,13] In addition to well-trained personnel, resuscitation tools must be prepared and ready at all times, specifically a stocked crash cart and cognitive aids. A crash cart containing all necessary drugs and equipment should be maintained in the practice and should be routinely audited to ensure drugs are in date and equipment is functional. Cognitive aids, such as algorithm and dosing charts, were shown to improve adherence to guidelines and individual performance during CPR.[14–16] They should be readily accessible in a standard, central location, and staff should be trained on the use of these aids regularly. After every CPR event, a debriefing session should be held, during which team performance is discussed and critically evaluated. This

---

Box 1
Preparedness and prevention

Preparedness and prevention key guidelines

CPR training

    Both didactic and hands-on training are essential

    Refresher training should be done at least every 6 months

Crash cart

    Available in a central location

    Regularly stocked and audited

Cognitive aids

    Algorithm, drug, and dosing charts

    Personnel should be trained in their use

Diagnosis of CPA

    Standardized ABC assessment in any acutely presenting or decompensating patient

    ABC assessment should take no longer than 15 seconds

    If there is any doubt the patient is in CPA, CPR should be started without delay

debriefing session can improve future performance and, at the same time, serve as refresher training.[17,18]

Early recognition of CPA is the precondition for timely initiation of resuscitation measures and is of paramount importance. In principle, CPA should be ruled out rapidly in any acutely unresponsive patient. In nonanesthetized patients, the diagnosis can be made by physical examination alone and is defined by unconsciousness and apnea. Thus, a rapid assessment lasting no more than 10 to 15 seconds and focused on ruling out CPA should be undertaken immediately in any unresponsive patient. To that end, a standardized diagnostic approach based on evaluation of airway, breathing, and circulation (ABC) will identify CPA efficiently. If CPA cannot be definitively ruled out, CPR should be initiated immediately rather than pursuing further diagnostic assessment. Immediate CPR is important because (1) several studies in human medicine have shown that pulse palpation is an insensitive test for diagnosis of CPA, and this may also be the case in dogs and cats; (2) a large body of literature supports the notion that even short delays in initiating CPR in pulseless patients reduce the likelihood of successful resuscitation; and (3) the risks of performing CPR on an unresponsive patient not in CPA are small.[19,20] Thus the clinician should not delay starting CPR in any patient in which there is a suspicion of CPA.

BASIC LIFE SUPPORT

Once CPA is recognized, basic life support (BLS) should be initiated as quickly as possible by following the treatment mnemonic CAB (circulation, airway, breathing). High-quality BLS is arguably the most important intervention in CPR. **Box 2** summarizes the key BLS guidelines. Circulation should be addressed first by starting chest compressions immediately, because ventilation will be ineffective in the absence of blood flow, and evidence suggests that outcome worsens as delay to the initiation of chest compressions increases.[19]

Circulation: Chest Compressions

Patients with untreated CPA lack forward blood flow out of the heart and oxygen delivery to the tissues ceases. An immediate consequence is the exhaustion of cellular energy stores, followed by cell depolarization and compromise of organ function, which results in increasing severity of ischemic organ injury with time and sets the stage for escalating reperfusion injury on reinstitution of tissue blood flow. Thus early institution of high-quality chest compressions is the most important aspect of effective CPR. The goals of chest compressions include the following: (1) restoration of blood flow to the lungs allowing carbon dioxide (CO_2) elimination and oxygen uptake, and (2) delivery of oxygen to tissues to restore organ function and metabolism. Experimental evidence suggests that even well-executed chest compressions produce approximately 30% of normal cardiac output. Therefore, proper chest compression technique is crucial. Delay in the start of high-quality chest compressions reduces the likelihood of ROSC.

Although not well studied in dogs and cats, some experimental data and anatomic principles suggest that chest compressions should be performed with the dog or cat positioned in either left or right lateral recumbency,[21] with a compression depth of 1/3 to 1/2 the width of the chest and at a rate of 100 to 120 compressions per minute, regardless of animal size or species. Use of visual or acoustic prompts to ensure correct rate of compression, such as a flashing light, a metronome, or a song with the correct tempo (eg, the BeeGee's "Staying Alive"), is recommended. To allow full elastic recoil of the thorax, leaning on the chest between compressions must be avoided.

Box 2
Basic life support

Basic life support key guidelines

Chest compression technique

    Most patients in lateral recumbency

    Rate of 100–120 compressions per minute regardless of species or size

    Compress 1/3–1/2 the width of the chest

    Allow full recoil of the chest between compressions

    Minimize interruptions and delays in starting compressions

    Rotate compressor after every 2-minute cycle of CPR

Chest compression posture

    Lock elbows and interlock hands

    Shoulders directly above hands

    Bend at waist and use core muscles

    Avoid leaning

    If table is too tall, use a stool, climb onto table, or put patient on floor

Chest compression hand position

    Medium and large round-chested dogs: over highest portion of the lateral thoracic wall

    Keel-chested dogs: directly over the heart

    Small dogs and cats: directly over the heart; consider one-handed technique

    Flat-chested dogs (eg, bulldogs): dorsal recumbency; hands on sternum

Ventilation

    Intubated patient (preferred technique)

        10 breaths/minute simultaneously with compressions

        1 second inspiratory time

        Approximately 10 mL/kg tidal volume

    Mouth to snout

        Close patient's mouth tightly

        Make seal over both nares with mouth

        Deliver 2 quick breaths with 1-second inspiratory time

        30:2 technique: 30 chest compressions, 2 quick breaths, immediately resume compressions

---

Excessive leaning will lead to increased intrathoracic pressure, reduced venous return to the chest and heart, and a reduction in cerebral and myocardial blood flow. Pauses in chest compressions are harmful and thus compressions should be delivered without interruption in cycles of 2 minutes. Any interruption in compressions should be as short as possible, as it takes approximately 60 seconds of continuous chest compressions before coronary perfusion pressure reaches its maximum.[22] Coronary perfusion pressure in turn is a critical determinant of myocardial blood flow and increases the likelihood of ROSC. To minimize pauses, all processes requiring interruption of chest compressions, such as electrocardiogram (ECG) analysis or pulse palpation, should be executed in a coordinated fashion at the end of each 2-minute cycle. During this planned pause of a few seconds' duration, a new compressor should take over to reduce the negative effect of rescuer fatigue on chest compression depth, rate, and leaning.

The mechanism of blood flow generation is fundamentally different during CPR compared with spontaneous circulation and 2 distinct models exist to describe how chest compressions generate systemic blood flow. According to the cardiac pump theory, the left and right ventricles are directly compressed, increasing the pressure in the ventricles, opening the pulmonic and aortic valves, and providing blood flow to the lungs and the tissues, respectively.[23] Recoil of the chest between compressions caused by the elastic properties of the rib cage creates negative intrathoracic pressure, leading to filling of the ventricles before the subsequent compression. The thoracic pump theory proposes that external chest compressions increase overall intrathoracic pressure, forcing blood from intrathoracic vessels into the systemic circulation, with the heart acting as a passive conduit.[24] Recommendations for rescuer hand position during chest compressions in dogs and cats are based on these concepts and vary in accordance with the animal's size and chest conformation.

In medium to large-breed dogs with standard round-chested conformations (eg, Labrador retrievers, Rottweilers, etc), blood flow generated by the thoracic pump mechanism likely predominates. Therefore, to maximize the intrathoracic pressure generated, it is recommended that the chest be compressed over the highest point on the lateral thoracic wall with the patient in the lateral recumbency position. To the contrary, in very keel-chested dogs (eg, sight hounds, etc), chest compressions with the hands positioned directly over the heart are reasonable, as the cardiac pump mechanism likely predominates. In markedly flat-chested dogs with dorsoventrally compressed chests like humans (eg, English bulldogs, French bulldogs, etc), compressions with the hands positioned over the sternum and the patient in the dorsal recumbency position may be considered. In these and other large dogs with low chest compliance, considerable compression force is necessary for CPR to be effective. Compression posture is essential for maximal effectiveness, and the compressor should lock the elbows with one hand on top of the other and position the shoulders directly above the hands. Using this posture engages the core muscles rather than the biceps and triceps, maintaining optimal compression force by reducing fatigue. If the patient is on a table and the elbows cannot be locked, a stool should be used or the patient should be placed on the floor.

Most cats and small dogs tend to have chest wall characteristics that favor the cardiac pump mechanism; therefore, chest compressions should be performed directly over the heart. Compressions may be performed using the same 2-handed technique as described above for large dogs, or alternatively by using a single-handed technique whereby the compressing hand is wrapped around the sternum and compressions are achieved from both sides of the chest by squeezing. Circumferential compressions of the chest using both hands may also be considered.

Airway and Breathing: Ventilation

Although immediate initiation of chest compressions on recognition of CPA is essential, ventilation is also important and should commence as soon as possible. If an endotracheal tube (ETT) and laryngoscope are available, the patient should be intubated. To avoid interruption in chest compressions, dogs and cats should be intubated in the lateral recumbency position. Once intubated, chest compressions and ventilations should be performed simultaneously because the inflated cuff of the ETT allows effective alveolar ventilation during a chest compression, prevents gastric insufflation with air, and minimizes interruptions in chest compressions. Intubated patients should be ventilated at a rate of 10 breaths per minute with a short inspiratory time of approximately 1 second. If a spirometer is available, a tidal volume of approximately 10 mL/kg should be targeted. This low minute ventilation is adequate during CPR because pulmonary blood flow is reduced. Care should be taken not to hyperventilate the patient, as low arterial CO_2 tension leads to cerebral vasoconstriction, decreasing oxygen delivery to the brain.

If an ETT is not readily available, mouth-to-snout ventilation will provide sufficient oxygenation and CO_2 removal. The patient's mouth should be held closed firmly with one hand. The neck is extended to align the snout with the spine, opening the airway as completely as possible. The rescuer makes a seal over the patient's nares with his/her mouth and blows firmly into the nares to inflate the chest. The chest should be visually inspected during the procedure and the breath continued until a normal chest excursion is accomplished. An inspiratory time of approximately 1 second should be targeted.

In nonintubated patients ventilated using the mouth-to-snout technique, ventilation cannot be performed simultaneously with chest compressions. Therefore, 30 chest compressions should be delivered, immediately followed by 2 short breaths. Alternating compressions and ventilations at a ratio of 30:2 should be continued for 2-minute cycles, and the rescuers rotated every cycle to prevent fatigue. Because the mouth-to-snout technique requires pauses in chest compressions, it should only be used when endotracheal intubation is impossible because of a lack of equipment or trained personnel.

ADVANCED LIFE SUPPORT

Once BLS procedures have been implemented, the CPR team should initiate advanced life support (ALS), which includes monitoring, drug therapy, and electrical defibrillation. **Box 3** summarizes the key ALS guidelines for veterinary CPR.

Monitoring

Many commonly used monitoring devices are of limited use during CPR because of their susceptibility to motion artifact and the likelihood that decreased perfusion and altered pulse quality will compromise accurate readings. Pulse oximeter and indirect blood pressure monitors, including Doppler and oscillometric devices, are not useful during CPR unless ROSC is restored. The 2 most useful monitoring modalities during CPR are ECG and capnography.

ECG

Although the ECG is highly susceptible to motion artifact and cannot be interpreted during ongoing chest compressions, an accurate rhythm diagnosis is essential to guide drug and defibrillation therapy. The goal of ECG monitoring during CPR is to diagnose which of the 3 most common arrest rhythms are present: (1) asystole, (2) pulseless electrical activity (PEA), or (3) ventricular fibrillation (VF).[1,25,26] As interpretation of the ECG requires interruption of chest compressions, the only time the ECG should be evaluated is between 2-minute cycles of CPR while compressors are being rotated. A clear announcement of the rhythm diagnosis to the group by the team leader with an invitation to express differing opinions on the diagnosis will minimize the risk of an incorrect rhythm diagnosis. However, chest compressions should be

Box 3
Advanced life support

Advanced life support (ALS) key guidelines

Monitoring

   Electrocardiogram

      Apply as soon as possible during CPR

      Determine rhythm diagnosis during intercycle pauses in compressions

   End-tidal carbon dioxide

      Target minimum of 15 mm Hg as an indicator of chest compression efficacy

      Sudden increase indicates possible ROSC

Drug therapy

   Vasopressors (eg, epinephrine, vasopressin)

      Indicated for asystole, PEA, or refractory ventricular fibrillation

      Divert blood from the periphery to core organs

      Repeat every other cycle of CPR (every 4 minutes)

      Use high-dose epinephrine only for prolonged CPR

   Vagolytics (eg, atropine)

      Indicated for asystole or PEA, especially if due to high vagal tone

      Decrease parasympathetic tone

      Repeat every other cycle of CPR (every 4 min)

   Reversal agents (eg, naloxone, flumazenil, atipamezole)

      Administer in any patients treated with reversible drugs before CPA

   Intravenous fluids

      Use cautiously in euvolemic patients

      Administer in patients with known or suspected hypovolemia

   Corticosteroids

      Not recommended for routine use during CPR or after ROSC

      Consider low-dose hydrocortisone in patients after ROSC with refractory hypotension

Defibrillation

   Electrical defibrillation

      Treatment of choice for all patients with ventricular fibrillation

      Continue chest compressions while charging

      Administer ONE shock

      Immediately resume chest compressions for 2 min after defibrillation

   Precordial thump

      Deliver a strong blow using the heel of the hand directly over the heart

      Minimal efficacy—use only if electrical defibrillation is not available

resumed immediately and discussion about the rhythm diagnosis should proceed into the next cycle.

Capnography (end-tidal CO_2 monitoring)

End-tidal CO_2 ($ETCO_2$) can be determined noninvasively and continuously during CPR and is generally feasible to use.[27,28] The presence of measurable CO_2 by $ETCO_2$ monitoring is supportive of (but not definitive for) correct placement of the ETT tube.[29] Because $ETCO_2$ is proportional to pulmonary blood flow, it can also be used as a measure of chest compression efficacy under conditions of constant quality of ventilation. Similarly, a very low $ETCO_2$ value during CPR (eg, <10–15 mm Hg) was found to be associated with a reduced likelihood of ROSC.[1,30] $ETCO_2$ substantially increases on ROSC, and therefore, is a valuable early indicator of ROSC during CPR.

Drug Therapy

Drug therapy is preferably administered by the intravenous (IV) or intraosseus (IO) route. Therefore, placement of a peripheral or central IV or IO catheter is recommended, but should not interfere with continuation of BLS. Depending on the arrest rhythm, the use of vasopressors, parasympatholytics, and/or anti-arrhythmics may be indicated in dogs and cats with CPA. In addition, in some cases the use of reversal agents (eg, naloxone, flumazenil, atipamezole), IV fluids, and alkalinizing drugs (eg, sodium bicarbonate) may be indicated. **Table 1** summarizes the drugs and doses that may be of use during CPR.

Vasopressors

Vasopressors are recommended regardless of the arrest rhythm to increase peripheral vascular resistance, thereby increasing central arterial pressure and thus coronary and cerebral perfusion pressures. During CPR, cardiac output is low even during optimal external chest compressions. Therefore, redirecting blood flow away from the peripheral tissues and toward the core (eg, the heart, lungs, and brain) is essential to maintain perfusion to these vital organs. Epinephrine is a catecholamine that causes peripheral vasoconstriction via stimulation of α_1-receptors, but also acts on β_1-receptors and β_2-receptors. The α_1 effects have been shown to be the most beneficial during CPR.[31] Initially, low doses (0.01 mg/kg IV/IO every other cycle of CPR) are recommended because studies have shown that lower doses are associated with a higher survival to discharge in people.[32] However, after prolonged CPR, a higher dose (0.1 mg/kg IV/IO every other cycle of CPR) may be considered. Epinephrine may also be administered via the ETT (0.02 mg/kg low dose; 0.2 mg/kg high dose) by feeding a long catheter through the ETT and diluting the epinephrine 1:1 with isotonic saline or sterile water.[33]

Vasopressin is an alternative vasopressor that exerts its vasoconstrictive effects via activation of peripheral V1 receptors. It may be used interchangeably with epinephrine during CPR at a dose of 0.8 U/kg IV/IO every other cycle of CPR. Potential benefits of vasopressin include continued efficacy in acidemic environments in which α_1-receptors may become unresponsive to epinephrine, and lack of β_1 effects that may cause increased myocardial oxygen consumption and worsen myocardial ischemia on ROSC.[34] Vasopressin may be administered via ETT using the technique described above.

Atropine

The use of atropine in CPR has been studied extensively.[35–37] It is an anticholinergic, parasympatholytic drug. Only a few studies have shown a beneficial effect, but there is minimal evidence of harm during CPR; atropine at a dose of 0.04 mg/kg IV/IO may be

Table 1
CPR drugs and doses

	Drug	Common Concentration	Dose/Route	Comments
Arrest	Epinephrine (low dose)	1 mg/mL (1:1000)	0.01 mg/kg IV/IO 0.02–0.1 mg/kg IT	Every other BLS cycle for asystole/PEA Increase dose ×2–10 and dilute for IT administration
	Epinephrine (high dose)	1 mg/mL (1:1000)	0.1 mg/kg IV/IO 0.2 mg/kg IT	Consider for prolonged (>10 min) CPR
	Vasopressin	20 U/mL	0.8 U/kg IV/IO 1.2 U/kg IT	Every other BLS cycle Increase dose for IT use
	Atropine	0.54 mg/mL	0.04 mg/kg IV/IO 0.08 mg/kg IT	Every other BLS cycle during CPR Recommended for bradycardic arrests/known or suspected high vagal tone Increase dose for IT use
	Bicarbonate	1 mEq/mL	1 mEq/kg IV/IO	For prolonged CPR/ PCA phase when pH <7.0 Do not use if hypoventilating
Antiarrhythmic	Amiodarone	50 mg/mL	2.5–5 mg/kg IV/IO	For refractory VF/pulseless VT Associated with anaphylaxis in dogs
	Lidocaine	20 mg/mL	2 mg/kg slow IV/IO push (1–2 min)	For refractory VF/pulseless VT *only* if amiodarone is not available
Reversal agents	Naloxone	0.4 mg/mL	0.04 mg/kg IV/IO	To reverse opioids
	Flumazenil	0.1 mg/mL	0.01 mg/kg IV/IO	To reverse benzodiazepines
	Atipamezole	5 mg/mL	0.1 mg/kg IV/IO	To reverse α_2-agonists
Defibrillation (may increase dose once by 50%–100% for refractory VF/pulseless VT)	Monophasic External		4–6 J/kg	
	Monophasic internal		0.5–1 J/kg	
	Biphasic external		2–4 J/kg	
	Biphasic internal		0.2–0.4 J/kg	

Abbreviations: IT, intratracheal; VT, ventricular tachycardia.

considered during CPR in dogs and cats and is reasonable in all dogs and cats with asystole or PEA associated with increased vagal tone. Atropine may also be administered via ETT (0.08 mg/kg).[38]

Anti-arrhythmic drugs

The treatment of choice for nonperfusing VF/ventricular tachycardia is electrical defibrillation, which is discussed later. However, patients with VF refractory to defibrillation may benefit from treatment with amiodarone at a dose of 2.5 to 5 mg/kg IV/IO.[39] It has been reported to cause anaphylactic reactions and hypotension in some dogs, so patients should be closely monitored for signs of allergic reactions once ROSC is achieved. Treatment with diphenhydramine (2 mg/kg intramuscularly) and/or anti-inflammatory corticosteroids (0.1 mg/kg dexamethasone sodium phosphate IV) is warranted should these signs be noted.

If amiodarone is not available, lidocaine (2 mg/kg slow IV/IO push) may be of benefit for patients with VF refractory to electrical defibrillation. Although lidocaine has been shown to increase the defibrillation threshold in dogs in one study, benefit was evident in other studies.[40,41]

Reversal agents

Although specific evidence of efficacy is not available, the use of reversal agents in dogs and cats in which reversible anesthetic/analgesic drugs were recently administered may be considered. Naloxone (0.04 mg/kg IV/IO) can be used to reverse opioids, flumazenil (0.01 mg/kg IV/IO) for benzodiazepines, and atipamezole (0.1 mg/kg IV/IO) or yohimbine (0.1 mg/kg IV/IO) for α_2-agonists.

Intravenous fluids

Euvolemic or hypervolemic patients are unlikely to benefit from IV fluid administration during CPR, because fluids administered IV serve solely to increase right atrial pressure, which may compromise perfusion of the brain and heart. However, in patients with documented or suspected hypovolemia, IV fluids will help to restore adequate circulating volume and may increase the efficacy of chest compressions and improve perfusion.

Corticosteroids

Although one prospective observational study showed an association between administration of corticosteroids and increased rate of ROSC in dogs and cats, the type and dose of steroids administered were highly variable and the study design did not allow determination of a cause-and-effect relationship.[1] Other studies have shown no benefit or harm from the use of steroids during CPR.[42,43] It is well known that even a single high dose of corticosteroids can lead to gastrointestinal ulceration and bleeding in dogs, which could then lead to other ill effects, such as bacterial translocation.[44–46] Immunosuppression and reduced renal prostaglandin production, a primary mechanism used by the kidney to maintain perfusion in the face of hypotension, are also known side effects. Because the documented risks of high-dose steroids far outweigh the potential benefit shown in one study, the use of steroids is not recommended in patients with CPA.

Sodium bicarbonate

Administration of sodium bicarbonate (1 mEq/kg, once, diluted IV) may be considered in patients with prolonged CPA (greater than 10–15 minutes) because of the likelihood of severe acidemia resulting from metabolic acidosis (eg, lactate and uremic acids) and venous respiratory acidosis due to inadequate peripheral perfusion and accumulation of CO_2. Inhibition of normal enzymatic and metabolic activity and severe vasodilation can result from the acidemia. Because these issues may be rapidly resolved once ROSC is achieved, bicarbonate therapy should be reserved for patients with prolonged CPA and with documented severe acidemia (pH <7.0) of metabolic origin.

Electrical Defibrillation

Early electrical defibrillation in patients with VF has been associated with increased ROSC and survival to discharge in numerous studies.[47] If the duration of VF is known or suspected to be 4 minutes or less, chest compressions should be continued until the defibrillator is charged, and the patient should then be defibrillated immediately. If the duration of VF is known or suspected to be more than 4 minutes, one full cycle of CPR should be performed before defibrillating to allow the myocardial cells to generate enough energy substrate to restore a normal membrane potential, thereby increasing the likelihood of success.[48]

Defibrillators may be either monophasic (delivering a current in one direction across the paddles) or biphasic (delivering a current in one direction, then reversing and delivering a current in the opposite direction). The use of biphasic defibrillators is recommended over monophasic defibrillators because of the higher efficacy in terminating ventricular fibrillation and because a lower current (and hence less myocardial injury) is required to defibrillate the patient successfully.[7] For monophasic defibrillators, an initial dose of 4–6 J/kg should be used, while biphasic defibrillation should start at 2–4 J/kg. The second dose may be increased by 50%, but subsequent doses should not be further increased.

After defibrillation, chest compressions should be resumed immediately, without a pause for rhythm analysis, and a full 2-minute cycle of CPR should be administered before reassessing the ECG and determining if the patient is still in VF, requiring additional defibrillation.[49,50] Brief assessment of the ECG immediately after defibrillation to determine if a perfusing rhythm has resulted is reasonable, but should minimally delay resumption of chest compressions.

POSTCARDIAC ARREST CARE

Two-thirds of human in-hospital cardiac arrest victims that initially achieve ROSC die during the postresuscitation phase.[51] In one veterinary study, only 16% of dogs and cats that reached ROSC after CPA were found to survive to hospital discharge.[1] Consequently, postcardiac arrest (PCA) care plays a significant role in the management of CPA and has the potential to save many lives.

In general, patient outcome is determined by (1) patient condition, (2) events that led to CPA, (3) the ischemic injury sustained during the cardiac arrest itself, and (4) the processes unfolding during and after reperfusion. Abnormalities in the PCA phase are the consequence of the 4 following processes: (1) anoxic brain injury, (2) postischemic myocardial dysfunction, (3) the systemic response to ischemia and reperfusion, and (4) the persistent precipitating pathologic abnormality (eg, underlying disease processes).[52] Because these elements vary between patients, the clinical phenotype of the PCA patient is highly variable and can range from virtually no detectable clinical abnormalities to devastating neurologic and multiorgan dysfunction. Consequently, a "one-size-fits-all" therapy cannot be recommended and rather should be titrated to alleviate the resulting clinical signs using critical care principles. The principles listed below have particular relevance to PCA care. Early hemodynamic optimization, similar to algorithms described for severe sepsis and septic shock, has been shown to be effective in human CPA survivors and should be considered in hemodynamically unstable small animals after cardiac arrest.[52–54] Suitable resuscitation endpoints are a central venous oxygen saturation of at least 70% and/or normalization of lactate levels. Central venous pressure monitoring can be useful to limit the risk of fluid overload, given that left ventricular dysfunction predisposes the patient to hydrostatic pulmonary edema and ischemia-reperfusion injury can lead to increased endothelial permeability.[55] In PCA patients, cerebral autoregulation of blood flow may be impaired after cerebral anoxia such that cerebral blood flow depends more directly on cerebral perfusion pressure, requiring a mean arterial pressure of 80 mm Hg or greater.[56]

Neuroprotective measures are of particular importance after cardiac arrest, given the selective vulnerability of the brain to anoxia.[57,58] Mild therapeutic hypothermia (eg, core temperature of 32–34°C [89.6–93.2°F]) for 12 to 24 hours after ROSC improves neurologic outcome after CPA in humans and other species, including dogs, that remain comatose 1 to 2 hours after resuscitation.[59–62] Although therapeutic hypothermia may not be applicable broadly in veterinary patients, individual reports support that it is feasible in principle.[63,64] Current experimental evidence indicates harm associated with rapid active rewarming and hyperthermia in animal models of cerebral ischemia and cardiac arrest. It is therefore important to monitor and control body temperature after CPA. Although optimal rates of rewarming are yet to be established, aggressive, active rewarming should be avoided and passive rewarming should not surpass 1.0°C (1.8°F) per hour, but rather target a slower rate of rewarming of 0.25°C to 0.5°C (0.45–0.9°F) per hour. Seizures should be treated with diazepam (0.5 mg/kg IV/IO) and/or phenobarbital (4 mg/kg IV).

Respiratory optimization is a third important element of PCA care. To assure optimal arterial oxygen tension (eg, partial pressure of arterial oxygen [Pao_2] 80 to 100 mm Hg) and CO_2 levels (eg, partial pressure of arterial carbon dioxide [$Paco_2$] 35–40 mm Hg) and to prevent respiratory arrest in the comatose PCA patient, the routine use of mechanical ventilation immediately after cardiac arrest and then as needed is optimal, if available. However, this is not required for patients in whom spontaneous ventilation is adequate to maintain the above listed target blood gas values. In all cases, adequacy of ventilation should be monitored using $ETCO_2$ or arterial blood gas analysis. Experimental and human clinical evidence substantiates the harm that may be associated with hyperoxic reperfusion.[65–67] As hypoxemia is also harmful, titration of supplemental oxygen to maintain normoxemia (eg, targeting an oxygen saturation [SpO_2] level of 94%–96% or Pao_2 of 80–100 mm Hg) is therefore a reasonable strategy to reduce oxidative injury while reducing the risk of hypoxemia.

Additional supportive patient care is directed toward the patient's precipitating disease process and concomitant organ dysfunctions (eg, ileus, acute kidney injury, etc). A summary of the key concepts for PCA care can be found in **Box 4**.

PROGNOSIS

Prognostic indicators in animals that have achieved ROSC have been poorly studied. Although low overall rates of survival have been reported, the inciting cause of cardiac arrest may be one of the most important prognostic factors. In a retrospective study examining characteristics of 15 dogs and 3 cats that survived to hospital discharge, only 3 animals had significant underlying chronic disease, whereas all other patients were considered systemically healthy before the incident.[25] It is likely that patients experiencing CPA as a consequence of severe, untreatable, or progressive chronic diseases are less likely to survive to hospital discharge, even though these outcomes are confounded by euthanasia. Peri-anesthetic CPA carries a better prognosis for

---

Box 4
Postcardiac arrest care

Postcardiac arrest care key guidelines

Respiratory optimization

  Ventilation

    Maintain normal $Paco_2$ (eg, 35–45 mm Hg)

    Mechanical ventilation required for persistent hypoventilation

  Oxygenation

    Titrate oxygen supplementation to maintain normoxemia (eg, Pao_2 80–100 mm Hg, SpO_2 94%–98%)

    Mechanical ventilation required for persistent hypoxemia nonresponsive to oxygen therapy

Hemodynamic optimization

  Target normotension or mild hypertension (mean arterial pressure 80–120 mm Hg, systolic 100–200 mm Hg)

    Treat hypovolemia with IV fluids

    Treat vasodilation with vasopressors

    Treat poor cardiac contractility with positive inotropes

Neuroprotective therapy

  Treat seizures aggressively

  Prevent hyperthermia/fever

  Therapeutic hypothermia and slow rewarming if comatose

  Mannitol (eg, 0.5–1 g/kg slow IV over 20 min) or hypertonic saline for signs of increased intracranial pressure

---

survival to discharge (as high as 47% in one recent prospective observational veterinary study), and continued CPR efforts in this population are most rewarding.[1]

SUMMARY

CPA is a highly lethal condition. To improve outcomes after CPA, a comprehensive strategy that includes preventive and preparedness measures, BLS, ALS, and PCA critical care titrated to the patient's needs is necessary. Optimization of each of these elements may help improve overall survival and offers an opportunity to work toward that goal.

REFERENCES

1. Hofmeister EH, Brainard BM, Egger CM, et al. Prognostic indicators for dogs and cats with cardiopulmonary arrest treated by cardiopulmonary cerebral resuscitation at a university teaching hospital. J Am Vet Med Assoc 2009; 235(1):50–7.
2. Boller M, Boller EM, Oodegard S, et al. Small animal cardiopulmonary resuscitation requires a continuum of care: proposal for a chain of survival for veterinary patients. J Am Vet Med Assoc 2012;240(5):540–54.

3. Boller M, Fletcher DJ. RECOVER evidence and knowledge gap analysis on veterinary CPR. Part 1: evidence analysis and consensus process: collaborative path toward small animal CPR guidelines. J Vet Emerg Crit Care (San Antonio) 2012;22(Suppl 1):S4–12.

4. Fletcher DJ, Boller M, Brainard BM, et al. RECOVER evidence and knowledge gap analysis on veterinary CPR. Part 7: clinical guidelines. J Vet Emerg Crit Care (San Antonio) 2012;22(Suppl 1):S102–31.

5. McMichael M, Herring J, Fletcher DJ, et al. RECOVER evidence and knowledge gap analysis on veterinary CPR. Part 2: preparedness and prevention. J Vet Emerg Crit Care (San Antonio) 2012;22(Suppl 1):S13–25.

6. Hopper K, Epstein SE, Fletcher DJ, et al. RECOVER evidence and knowledge gap analysis on veterinary CPR. Part 3: basic life support. J Vet Emerg Crit Care (San Antonio) 2012;22(Suppl 1):S26–43.

7. Rozanski EA, Rush JE, Buckley GJ, et al. RECOVER evidence and knowledge gap analysis on veterinary CPR. Part 4: advanced life support. J Vet Emerg Crit Care (San Antonio) 2012;22(Suppl 1):S44–64.

8. Brainard BM, Boller M, Fletcher DJ. RECOVER evidence and knowledge gap analysis on veterinary CPR. Part 5: monitoring. J Vet Emerg Crit Care (San Antonio) 2012;22(Suppl 1):S65–84.

9. Smarick SD, Haskins SC, Boller M, et al. RECOVER evidence and knowledge gap analysis on veterinary CPR. Part 6: post-cardiac arrest care. J Vet Emerg Crit Care (San Antonio) 2012;22(Suppl 1):S85–101.

10. Noordergraaf GJ, Van Gelder JM, Van Kesteren RG, et al. Learning cardiopulmonary resuscitation skills: does the type of mannequin make a difference? Eur J Emerg Med 1997;4(4):204–9.

11. Cimrin AH, Topacoglu H, Karcioglu O, et al. A model of standardized training in basic life support skills of emergency medicine residents. Adv Ther 2005;22(1): 10–8.

12. Isbye DL, Meyhoff CS, Lippert FK, et al. Skill retention in adults and in children 3 months after basic life support training using a simple personal resuscitation manikin. Resuscitation 2007;74(2):296–302.

13. Mpotos N, Lemoyne S, Wyler B, et al. Training to deeper compression depth reduces shallow compressions after six months in a manikin model. Resuscitation 2011;82(10):1323–7.

14. Royse AG. New resuscitation trolley: stages in development. Aust Clin Rev 1989;9(3–4):107–14.

15. Schade J. An evaluation framework for code 99. QRB Qual Rev Bull 1983;9(10): 306–9.

16. Dyson E, Smith GB. Common faults in resuscitation equipment–guidelines for checking equipment and drugs used in adult cardiopulmonary resuscitation. Resuscitation 2002;55(2):137–49.

17. Edelson DP, Litzinger B, Arora V, et al. Improving in-hospital cardiac arrest process and outcomes with performance debriefing. Arch Intern Med 2008; 168(10):1063–9.

18. Dine CJ, Gersh RE, Leary M, et al. Improving cardiopulmonary resuscitation quality and resuscitation training by combining audiovisual feedback and debriefing. Crit Care Med 2008;36(10):2817–22.

19. Rittenberger JC, Menegazzi JJ, Callaway CW. Association of delay to first intervention with return of spontaneous circulation in a swine model of cardiac arrest. Resuscitation 2007;73(1):154–60.

20. Dick WF, Eberle B, Wisser G, et al. The carotid pulse check revisited: what if there is no pulse? Crit Care Med 2000;28(Suppl 11):N183–5.
21. Maier GW, Tyson GS, Olsen CO, et al. The physiology of external cardiac massage: high-impulse cardiopulmonary resuscitation. Circulation 1984;70(1): 86–101.
22. Kern K, Hilwig R, Berg R, et al. Importance of continuous chest compressions during cardiopulmonary resuscitation. Circulation 2002;105(5):645–9.
23. Kouwenhoven WB, Jude JR, Knickerbocker GG. Closed-chest cardiac massage. JAMA 1960;173:1064–7.
24. Niemann JT, Rosborough J, Hausknecht M, et al. Blood flow without cardiac compression during closed chest CPR. Crit Care Med 1981;9(5):380–1.
25. Waldrop JE, Rozanski EA, Swanke ED, et al. Causes of cardiopulmonary arrest, resuscitation management, and functional outcome in dogs and cats surviving cardiopulmonary arrest. J Vet Emerg Crit Care 2004;14(1):22–9.
26. Plunkett SJ, McMichael M. Cardiopulmonary resuscitation in small animal medicine: an update. J Vet Intern Med 2008;22(1):9–25.
27. Grmec S, Klemen P. Does the end-tidal carbon dioxide (EtCO2) concentration have prognostic value during out-of-hospital cardiac arrest? Eur J Emerg Med 2001;8(4):263–9.
28. Pokorná M, Necas E, Kratochvíl J, et al. A sudden increase in partial pressure end-tidal carbon dioxide (P(ET)CO(2)) at the moment of return of spontaneous circulation. J Emerg Med 2010;38(5):614–21.
29. Li J. Capnography alone is imperfect for endotracheal tube placement confirmation during emergency intubation. J Emerg Med 2001;20(3):223–9.
30. Kolar M, Krizmaric M, Klemen P, et al. Partial pressure of end-tidal carbon dioxide successful predicts cardiopulmonary resuscitation in the field: a prospective observational study. Crit Care 2008;12(5):R115.
31. Bassiakou E, Xanthos T, Papadimitriou L. The potential beneficial effects of beta adrenergic blockade in the treatment of ventricular fibrillation. Eur J Pharmacol 2009;616(1–3):1–6.
32. Vandycke C, Martens P. High dose versus standard dose epinephrine in cardiac arrest—a meta-analysis. Resuscitation 2000;45(3):161–6.
33. Manisterski Y, Vaknin Z, Ben-Abraham R, et al. Endotracheal epinephrine: a call for larger doses. Anesth Analg 2002;95(4):1037–41 table of contents.
34. Biondi-Zoccai GG, Abbate A, Parisi Q, et al. Is vasopressin superior to adrenaline or placebo in the management of cardiac arrest? A meta-analysis. Resuscitation 2003;59(2):221–4.
35. Blecic S, Chaskis C, Vincent JL. Atropine administration in experimental electromechanical dissociation. Am J Emerg Med 1992;10(6):515–8.
36. DeBehnke DJ, Swart GL, Spreng D, et al. Standard and higher doses of atropine in a canine model of pulseless electrical activity. Acad Emerg Med 1995;2(12): 1034–41.
37. Coon GA, Clinton JE, Ruiz E. Use of atropine for brady-asystolic prehospital cardiac arrest. Ann Emerg Med 1981;10(9):462–7.
38. Paret G, Mazkereth R, Sella R, et al. Atropine pharmacokinetics and pharmacodynamics following endotracheal versus endobronchial administration in dogs. Resuscitation 1999;41(1):57–62.
39. Anastasiou-Nana MI, Nanas JN, Nanas SN, et al. Effects of amiodarone on refractory ventricular fibrillation in acute myocardial infarction: experimental study. J Am Coll Cardiol 1994;23(1):253–8.

40. Dorian P, Cass D, Schwartz B, et al. Amiodarone as compared with lidocaine for shock-resistant ventricular fibrillation. N Engl J Med 2002;346(12):884–90.
41. Dorian P, Fain ES, Davy JM, et al. Lidocaine causes a reversible, concentration-dependent increase in defibrillation energy requirements. J Am Coll Cardiol 1986;8(2):327–32.
42. Mentzelopoulos SD, Zakynthinos SG, Tzoufi M, et al. Vasopressin, epinephrine, and corticosteroids for in-hospital cardiac arrest. Arch Intern Med 2009;169(1): 15–24.
43. Smithline H, Rivers E, Appleton T, et al. Corticosteroid supplementation during cardiac arrest in rats. Resuscitation 1993;25(3):257–64.
44. Levine JM, Levine GJ, Boozer L, et al. Adverse effects and outcome associated with dexamethasone administration in dogs with acute thoracolumbar interverte-bral disk herniation: 161 cases (2000-2006). J Am Vet Med Assoc 2008;232(3): 411–7.
45. Dillon AR, Sorjonen DC, Powers RD, et al. Effects of dexamethasone and surgical hypotension on hepatic morphologic features and enzymes of dogs. Am J Vet Res 1983;44(11):1996–9.
46. Rohrer CR, Hill RC, Fischer A, et al. Gastric hemorrhage in dogs given high doses of methylprednisolone sodium succinate. Am J Vet Res 1999;60(8): 977–81.
47. Link MS, Atkins DL, Passman RS, et al. Part 6: electrical therapies: automated external defibrillators, defibrillation, cardioversion, and pacing: 2010 American Heart Association Guidelines for Cardiopulmonary Resuscitation and Emergency Cardiovascular Care. Circulation 2010;122(18 Suppl 3):S706–19.
48. Weisfeldt ML, Becker LB. Resuscitation after cardiac arrest a 3-phase time-sensitive model. J Am Med Assoc 2002;288(23):3035–8.
49. Cammarata G, Weil MH, Csapoczi P, et al. Challenging the rationale of three sequential shocks for defibrillation. Resuscitation 2006;69(1):23–7.
50. Tang W, Snyder D, Wang J, et al. One-shock versus three-shock defibrillation protocol significantly improves outcome in a porcine model of prolonged ventricular fibrillation cardiac arrest. Circulation 2006;113(23):2683–9.
51. Peberdy MA, Kaye W, Ornato JP, et al. Cardiopulmonary resuscitation of adults in the hospital: a report of 14720 cardiac arrests from the National Registry of Cardiopulmonary Resuscitation. Resuscitation 2003;58(3):297–308.
52. Neumar RW, Nolan JP, Adrie C, et al. Post-cardiac arrest syndrome: epidemiology, pathophysiology, treatment, and prognostication. A consensus statement from the International Liaison Committee on Resuscitation. Circulation 2008; 118(23):2452–83.
53. Rivers E, Nguyen B, Havstad S, et al. Early goal directed therapy in the treatment of the severe sepsis and septic shock. N Engl J Med 2001;345(19): 1368–77.
54. Gaieski DF, Band RA, Abella BS, et al. Early goal-directed hemodynamic optimization combined with therapeutic hypothermia in comatose survivors of out-of-hospital cardiac arrest. Resuscitation 2009;80(4):418–24.
55. Adams J. Endothelium and cardiopulmonary resuscitation. Crit Care Med 2006; 34(12):S458–65.
56. Sundgreen C, Larsen FS, Herzog TM, et al. Autoregulation of cerebral blood flow in patients resuscitated from cardiac arrest. Stroke 2001;32(1):128–32.
57. Madl C, Holzer M. Brain function after resuscitation from cardiac arrest. Curr Opin Crit Care 2004;10(3):213–7.

58. Ginsberg M, Belayey L. Biological and molecular mechanism of hypothermic neuroprotection. In: Mayer S, Sessler D, editors. Therapeutic hypothermia. New York: Marcel Dekker; 2005. p. 85.

59. Arrich J, Holzer M, Herkner H, et al. Cochrane corner: hypothermia for neuroprotection in adults after cardiopulmonary resuscitation. Anesth Analg 2010;110(4): 1239.

60. The Hypothermia after Cardiac Arrest Study Group. Mild therapeutic hypothermia to improve the neurologic outcome after cardiac arrest. N Engl J Med 2002; 346(8):549–56.

61. Bernard SA, Gray TW, Buist MD, et al. Treatment of comatose survivors of out-of-hospital cardiac arrest with induced hypothermia. N Engl J Med 2002;346(8): 557–63.

62. Nozari A, Safar P, Stezoski SW, et al. Mild hypothermia during prolonged cardiopulmonary cerebral resuscitation increases conscious survival in dogs. Crit Care Med 2004;32(10):2110–6.

63. Kanemoto I, Taguchi D, Yokoyama S, et al. Open heart surgery with deep hypothermia and cardiopulmonary bypass in small and toy dogs. Vet Surg 2010; 39(6):674–9.

64. Hayes GM. Severe seizures associated with traumatic brain injury managed by controlled hypothermia, pharmacologic coma, and mechanical ventilation in a dog. J Vet Emerg Crit Care (San Antonio) 2009;19(6):629–34.

65. Neumar RW. Optimal oxygenation during and after cardiopulmonary resuscitation. Curr Opin Crit Care 2011;17(3):236–40.

66. Kilgannon JH, Jones AE, Parrillo JE, et al. Relationship between supranormal oxygen tension and outcome after resuscitation from cardiac arrest. Circulation 2011;123(23):2717–22.

67. Balan IS, Fiskum G, Hazelton J, et al. Oximetry-guided reoxygenation improves neurological outcome after experimental cardiac arrest. Stroke 2006;37(12): 3008–13.

Index

Note: Page numbers of article titles are in **boldface** type.

Vet Clin Small Anim 43 (2013) 989–1003
http://dx.doi.org/10.1016/S0195-5616(13)00124-1
0195-5616/13/$ – see front matter © 2013 Elsevier Inc. All rights reserved.

vetsmall.theclinics.com

Moving?

Make sure your subscription moves with you!

To notify us of your new address, find your **Clinics Account Number** (located on your mailing label above your name), and contact customer service at:

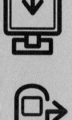

Email: journalscustomerservice-usa@elsevier.com

800-654-2452 (subscribers in the U.S. & Canada)
314-447-8871 (subscribers outside of the U.S. & Canada)

Fax number: 314-447-8029

Elsevier Health Sciences Division
Subscription Customer Service
3251 Riverport Lane
Maryland Heights, MO 63043

*To ensure uninterrupted delivery of your subscription, please notify us at least 4 weeks in advance of move.

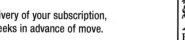

Printed and bound by CPI Group (UK) Ltd, Croydon, CR0 4YY

03/10/2024

01040409-0012